Cuckoldry, Impotence and Adultery in Europe (15th–17th century)

In Renaissance and early modern Europe, various constellations of phenomena—ranging from sex scandals to legal debates to flurries of satirical prints—collectively demonstrate, at different times and places, an increased concern with cuckoldry, impotence and adultery. This concern emerges in unusual events (such as scatological rituals of house-scorning), appears in neglected sources (such as drawings by Swiss mercenary soldier-artists), and engages innovative areas of inquiry (such as the intersection between medical theory and Renaissance comedy). Interdisciplinary analytical tools are here deployed to scrutinize court scandals and decipher archival documents. Household recipes, popular literary works and a variety of visual media are examined in the light of contemporary sexual culture and contextualized with reference to current social and political issues. The essays in this volume reveal the central importance of sexuality and sexual metaphor for our understanding of European history, politics and culture, and emphasize the extent to which erotic presuppositions underpinned the early modern world.

Sara F. Matthews-Grieco is Professor of History and Coordinator of Women's & Gender Studies at Syracuse University in Florence, Italy.
She is also the editor of *Erotic Cultures of Renaissance Italy*.

Cuckoldry, Impotence and Adultery in Europe (15th–17th century)

Edited by Sara F. Matthews-Grieco

Routledge
Taylor & Francis Group
LONDON AND NEW YORK

First published 2014 by Ashgate Publishing

2 Park Square, Milton Park, Abingdon, Oxfordshire OX14 4RN
711 Third Avenue, New York, NY 10017

Routledge is an imprint of the Taylor & Francis Group, an informa business

First issued in paperback 2018

British Library Cataloguing in Publication Data
A catalogue record for this book is available from the British Library

The Library of Congress has cataloged the print edition as follows:
Cuckoldry, impotence and adultery in Europe, 15th–17th century / edited by Sara F. Matthews-Grieco.
pages cm. -- (Visual culture in early modernity)
Includes bibliographical references and index.
ISBN 978-1-4724-1439-7 (hardcover: alk. paper) 1. Cuckolds—Europe—History. 2. Impotence—Europe—History. 3. Adultery—Europe—History. I. Matthews Grieco, Sara F.

HQ806.C83 2014
306.73094—dc23

2014017416

ISBN 978-1-4724-1439-7 (hbk)
ISBN 978-1-138-54816-9 (pbk)

Contents

PART III: HORNS AND VISUAL INNUENDO

List of Illustrations

Black and White Figures

10 Picart's Browbeaten Husbands in 17th-Century France: Cuckoldry in Context

List of Contributors

Francesca Alberti. PhD, Université Paris 1 Panthéon-Sorbonne, currently teaching assistant at the l'Université catholique de l'Ouest-Angers. **Publications**: author/co-editor of *Rire en images à la Renaissance* (Brepols, Turnhout, 2014); author/co-editor of *Penser l'étrangeté. L'histoire de l'art de la Renaissance italienne entre bizarrerie, extravagance et singularité* (Rennes, P.U.R., 2012); "*Bizzarri componimenti e straordinarie invenzioni.* La *Danaé* de Tintoret, une peinture comique," *Studiolo* 7 (2009); "Iconographie, fonction et contexte de la *Descente de croix* de Daniele da Volterra," *Artibus et Historiae*, no. 66 (2012); "*Giove uccellato*: quand les métamorphoses se font extravagantes," in *Extravagances amoureuses: l'amour au-delà de la norme à la Renaissance*, ed. E. Boillet and C. Lastraioli (Paris: Honoré Champion éditeur, 2010); "Le comique dans la peinture mythologique de Tintoret," *Bulletin de l'Association des Historiens de l'Art Italien*, XIV, 2008. **Fellowships/honors**: Académie de France à Rome-Villa Médicis, Deutsches Forum für Kunstgeschichte (Paris); Nederlands Interuniversitair Kunsthistorisch Instituut (Florence); Villa Finaly (Florence); member of the CHAR and of Cinquecento Plurale. **Current research interests**: laughter in 16th century; sacred and profane images; the practice of doodling during the Renaissance period.

Christiane D. Andersson. Professor of Art History, Bucknell University of Pennsylvania. **Publications**: "Urs Graf's Erotic Drawings," *The Sienese Shredder* (New York, vol. 5, 2010). "Dürer's Drawings," L. Silver and J. Chipps (ed.), *The Essential Dürer* (Philadelphia: University of Pennsylvania Press, 2010); *The Language of the Nude: Four Centuries of Drawing the Human Body* (London, Lund Humphreys, 2008); "A rare early woodcut by the Master DS: Christ crucified between Mary and St. John," *Stanford University Museum of Art Journal* 26–7 (1996–1997); "Die Spalatin-Chronik und ihre Illustrationen aus der Cranach-Werkstatt," C. Grimm, J. Erichsen and E. Brockhoff (eds.) *Lucas Cranach. Ein Maler-Unternehmer aus Franken* (Augsburg, 1994); with Charles Talbot, *From A Mighty Fortress: Prints, Drawings and Books in the Age of Luther* (Detroit MUI: Detroit Institute of the Arts, 1983). **Fellowships/honors**: CASVA, National Gallery of Art, Washington, DC, Institute for Advanced

Study, Princeton; Metropolitan Museum of Art, NY; Getty Museum, LA; National Endowment for the Humanities; Humboldt Foundation; Herzog-August-Bibliothek Wolfenbüttel. **Current research interests**: polemical prints of the Reformation; censorship of art in the Renaissance; drawings and prints in the German-speaking countries (especially Dürer and Urs Graf); images of women in Renaissance art.

Molly Bourne. Coordinator, Graduate Program in Renaissance Art and Professor of Art History, Syracuse University in Florence. **Publications**: "Mail Humor and Male Sociability: Sexual Innuendo in the Epistolary Domain of Francesco II Gongaga," S. F. Matthews-Grieco (ed.), *Erotic Cultures of Renaissance Italy* (Farnham, UK/Burlington, VT: Ashgate, 2010); *Francesco II Gonzaga: the Soldier-Prince as Patron* (Rome: Bulzoni, 2008); "Renaissance Husbands and Wives as Patrons of Art: the 'Camerini' of Isabella d'Este and Francesco II Gonzaga," Sheryl E. Reiss and David G. Wilkins (eds.), *Beyond Isabella: Secular Women Patrons of Art in Renaissance Italy* (Kirksville, MO: Truman State University, 2001); "Francesco II Gonzaga and maps as palace decoration in Renaissance Mantua," *Imago Mundi: The International Journal for the History of Cartography* 51:1 (1999); **Fellowships/honors**: member of the Accademia Nazionale Virgiliana; fellowship at Villa I Tatti, the Harvard Center for Italian Renaissance Studies. **Current research interests**: a biographical study of Camilla Faà, lover of Ferdinando Gonzaga, sixth Duke of Mantua; co-editor of a *festschrift* in honor of Gary M. Radke, Syracuse University.

Matteo Duni. Professor of History and Coordinator, Department of Humanities and Social Sciences, Syracuse University in Florence; European Studies Center, Maxwell School (Syracuse University, NY). **Publications**: "Un manuale inedito per cacciatori di streghe. il Formularium pro exequendo Inquisitionis officio di Modesto Scrofeo (c. 1523)," *Archivio Storico Italiano*, 103 (2013); "I dubbi sulle streghe," G. Ernst and G. Giglioni (eds.), *I vincoli della natura. Magia naturale e stregoneria nel Rinascimento* (Roma, Carocci, 2012); *Under the Devil's Spell. Witches, Sorcerers, and the Inquisition in Renaissance Italy* (Florence/Villa Rossa: Syracuse University, 2007); *Tra religione e magia. Storia del prete Guglielmo Campana (1460?–1541)* (Florence: Olschki, 1999); co-editor of *Fratelli d'Italia. Riformatori italiani nel Cinquecento* (Torino: Claudiana, 2011); *Non lasciar vivere la malefica. Le streghe nei trattati e nei processi (secc. XIV-XVII)* (Florence: Firenze University Press, 2008). **Fellowships/honors**: fellowship at Villa i Tatti, Harvard University Center for Italian Renaissance Studies; research associate, Dipartimento di Studi storici e geografici, Università di Firenze; researchassistant, Department of History and Civilization European University Institute; fellowship at the École française de Rome. **Current research interests**: the European witch hunt and its opponents; the Witches' Sabbath and its formation; the Roman Inquisition and magic.

Laura Giannetti. Associate Professor of Italian, University of Miami. **Publications**: "Of Eels and Pears: A Sixteenth-Century Debate on Taste, Temperance, and the Pleasures of the Senses," Wietse de Boer and Christine Gottler (eds.), *Religion and the Senses in Early Modern Europe* (Leiden/Boston, Brill, 2013); "Italian Renaissance Food-Fashioning or the Triumph of Greens," *California Italian Studies* (1.2, 2010), www.escholarship.org/uc/item/1n97s00d; "Ma che potrà succedermi se io donna amo una donna? Female-Female Desire in Italian Renaissance Comedy," *Renaissance Drama* 36/37 (2010); *Lelia's Kiss: Imagining Gender, Sex and Marriage in Italian Renaissance Comedy* (Toronto: University of Toronto Press, 2009); "The Forbidden Fruit or the Taste for Sodomy in Renaissance Italy, *Quaderni d'italianistica* XXVII (2006); "When Male Characters Pass as Women: Theatrical Play and Social Practice in the Italian Renaissance," *Sixteenth Century Journal* XXXVI:3 (2005); ed. and transl.with Guido Ruggiero, *Five Comedies from the Italian Renaissance* (Baltimore: Johns Hopkins University Press, 2003). **Fellowships/honors**: Center for the Humanities, University of Miami, faculty fellow, 2014–2015; Modern Language Association Executive Committee of the Division on Medieval and Renaissance Italian Literature; Provost Award at the University of Miami; fellowship at Villa I Tatti, the Harvard University Center for Italian Renaissance Studies. **Current research interests**: Italian Renaissance comedy, gender and sexuality; food culture and the literary imagination in early modern Italy.

M. A. Katritzky. Barbara Wilkes Research Fellow in Theatre Studies, Department of English, The Open University, Milton Keynes, United Kingdom. **Publications**: series editor with Professor Jim Davis, University of Warwick, *The Ashgate Performance Practice Reprint Series* (four vols., 2014); author, *Healing, performance and ceremony in the writings of three early modern physicians: Hippolytus Guarinonius and the brothers Felix and Thomas Platter* (Farnham, UK/Burlington, VT: Ashgate 2012); *Women, medicine and theatre 1500–1750: literary mountebanks and performing quacks* (Aldershot, UK/ Burlington, VT: Ashgate, 2007); *The Art of commedia: a study in the commedia dell'arte 1560–1620 with special reference to the visual records* (Amsterdam: Rodopi, 2006); co-author, *The Handbook to Literary Research* (Oxford: Routledge, 2010). **Fellowships/honors**: research awards, Arts & Humanities Research Council and British Academy; Kathleen Barker Award, Society for Theatre Research; fellowships from the Herzog August Bibliothek, Wolfenbüttel, the Alexander von Humboldt Foundation and the Netherlands Institute for Advanced Study, Wassenaar. **Current research interests**: early modern English and comparative drama; English actors in Shakespearean Europe; issues of gender and physicality in early modern medical and theatrical practice.

Sara F. Matthews-Grieco. Professor of History and Coordinator of Women's & Gender Studies, Syracuse University in Florence; European Studies Center, Maxwell School (Syracuse University, NY). **Publications**: various essays appear in the collective volumes: *Erotic Cultures of Renaissance Italy* (Aldershot, UK: Ashgate, 2010); *At Home in Renaissance Italy* (London: V&A, 2006), *Histoire du Corps*, vol. I (Paris: Seuil, 2005); *Le désir et le goût, une autre histoire* (Paris: Université de Vincennes, 2005); *Women in Italian Renaissance Culture and Society* (Oxford: European Humanities Research Centre, 2000). Co-editor of *Représentation et identité en Italie et en Europe XVe–XIXe siècle* (Rome: MEFR, 2003); *The Art Market in Italy, 15th–17th centuries* (Modena: Panini, 2003); *Monaca, moglie, serva, cortigiana. Vita e immagine della donna tra rinascimento e controriforma* (Florence: Morgana, 2001). **Fellowships/honors**: Herzog August Bibliothek, American Philosophical Society, John Simon Guggenheim Foundation, Harvard Center for Italian Renaissance Studies (Villa I Tatti), European University Institute. **Current research interests**: women, the family and sexuality in Renaissance and early modern Italy and France; visual literacy and the codification of the iconographic idiom in Europe (1450–1650).

Jacqueline Marie Musacchio. Professor of Art, Wellesley College. **Publications**: "Infesting the Galleries of Europe: The Copyist Emma Conant Church in Paris and Rome," *Nineteenth-Century Art Worldwide* 10:2 (Autumn 2011); *Art, Marriage, and Family in the Florentine Renaissance Palace* (New Haven/London: Yale University Press, 2008); catalog author, *Art and Love in Renaissance Italy* (New York: Metropolitan Museum of Art and Kimbell Art Museum, 2008); "Objects and Identity: Antonio de'Medici and the Casino at San Marco in Florence," J. J. Martin (ed.), *The Renaissance World* (New York: Routledge, 2007); *Marvels of Maiolica* (Boston: Bunker Hill Press, 2004); *Art and Ritual of Childbirth in Renaissance Italy* (New Haven/London: Yale University Press, 1999). **Fellowships/honors**: fellowships at CASVA, Lewis-Walpole Library; Association of Research Institutes in Art History Online Publishing Prize. **Current research interests**: the biography and historiography of Bianca Cappello; late 19th-century American women abroad.

Meredith K. Ray. Associate Professor of Italian, University of Delaware. **Publications**: *In the Shadow of Galileo: Women, Scientific Culture and Literary Discourse in Early Modern Italy* (Cambridge, MA: Harvard University Press, [2015]); ed. and trans. with Lynn Westwater, *Arcangela Tarabotti, Letters Familiar and Formal* (Toronto: Centre for Reformation and Renaissance Studies, 2012); *Writing Gender in Women's Letter Collections of the Italian Renaissance* (Toronto: University of Toronto Press, 2009); ed. with Lynn Westwater, *Arcangela Tarabotti, Lettere familiari e di compliment* (Turin: Rosenberg & Sellier, 2005). Articles include "Prescriptions for Women: Alchemy, Medicine, and the Renaissance Debate over Women," *Women Writing Back/Writing Women Back: Transnational Perspectives From the Middle Ages to the Dawn of the Modern Era*, ed. A. Montoya et al. (Brill: Leiden, 2010), 135–62; "Experiments with

Alchemy: Caterina Sforza in Early Modern Scientific Culture," *Gender and Scientific Discourse in Early Modern Europe*, ed. Kathleen Perry Long (Farnham, UK/Burlington, VT: Ashgate, 2010), 139–64; "Textual Collaboration and Spiritual Partnership in Sixteenth-Century Italy: The Case of Ortensio Lando and Lucrezia Gonzaga," *Renaissance Quarterly* 62:3 (Fall 2009). **Fellowships/honors**: National Endowment for the Humanities, American Association for Italian Studies Book Prize, Society for the Study of Early Modern Women Translation Prize, Renaissance Society of America Research Grant, Penn Humanities Forum, American Association of University Women, Fulbright-Hays Dissertation Fellowship. **Current research interests**: women and early modern scientific culture; 16th-century *libri di segreti*; Renaissance women writers; epistolary writing.

Louise Rice. Associate Professor of Art History, New York University. **Publications**: "The Pre-Mochi Projects for the Veronica Pier in St Peter's," *The Eternal Baroque: Studies in Honour of Jennifer Montagu*, Turin, in press; "Cardinal Rapaccioli and the Turnip-sellers of Rome: A Satire on the War of Castro by Baccio del Bianco," *Master Drawings* XLVII (2009); "Simon Vouet's *Hesperus* and the Mythopoetics of Praise," in E. Cropper (ed.), *Dialogues in Art History, from Mesopotamian to Modern* (New Haven/London, 2009); "Bernini and the Pantheon Bronze," G. Satzinger & S. Schütze (eds.), *Sankt Peter in Rom 1506–2006* (Munich, 2008); "POMIS SVA NOMINA SERVANT: The Emblematic Thesis Prints of the Roman Seminary," *Journal of the Warburg and Courtauld Institutes* (LXX, 2007); "*Apes philosophicae*: Bees and the Divine Design in Barberini Thesis Prints," L. Mochi Onori *et al.* (eds.), *I Barberini e la cultura europea del Seicento* (Rome, 2007); "The Pentecostal Meaning of Borromini's Sant'Ivo alla Sapienza," *Francesco Borromini 1599–1667* (Rome/Milan, 2000). **Fellowships/Honors**: National Humanities Center; Metropolitan Museum of Art; Center for Advanced Study in the Visual Arts; American Academy in Rome; Premio Salimbeni; Premio Salvatore Rebecchini. **Current research interests**: Roman baroque art and architecture; prints and print culture in 16th- and 17th-century Europe; history of education.

Acknowledgments

For this volume, as for others, the hospitality of the Renaissance Society of America has played a key role, not only by hosting sessions where these essays were first aired (Montreal 2011 and Washington, DC, 2012), but also by providing a thought-provoking audience. In this context Elissa Weaver merits special recognition for having sponsored these sessions under the disciplinary umbrella of "Women and Gender Studies." As always, Syracuse University (NY) and Syracuse University in Florence deserve fulsome thanks for support of this project from start to finish, both moral and material. In this context, special recognition is due to (in alphabetical order): Carol Faulkner, Margaret Himley, Sasha Perugini, Gary Radke and Dennis Romano.

In its final stages, this volume particularly benefitted from the generous hospitality of the *Herzog August Bibliothek* in Wolfenbüttel, where Gillian Bepler and the library staff ensure an unrivaled environment for research, reflection and exchange. *Ein herzliches Dankeschön.*

Endeavors such as these permit scattered research on a particular topic to come together despite the artificial boundaries of disciplinary areas, and all of the contributions in this volume have benefitted immeasurably from the synergy of group reflection. Gratitude is furthermore due to Erika Gaffney at Ashgate Publishing (Vermont) for her enthusiastic reaction to this volume and her patience throughout the process of bringing it together. At the same time, the home stretch is the part of such journeys when an editor can no longer see the forest for the trees, which is why sincere thanks are also due to Alexandra Korey, for her patient work and thoughtful observations on the manuscript.

Dulcis in fundo, this volume—which features three essays by Syracuse University in Florence faculty—commemorates the 50th anniversary of the Syracuse University Graduate Program in Renaissance Art.

Sara F. Matthews-Grieco
Florence, March, 2014

Introduction: Sexual Transgression as Social Metaphor

Sara F. Matthews-Grieco

In truth, cuckolds are not those who have a ribald [unfaithful] wife, but rather those who sleep with the wife of another man. The word derives from the nature of the bird, which lays its eggs in the nests of others.

Andrea Alciato, "Les Coquuz," Emblemes, Lyons, 1549[1]

Adultery, cuckoldry and the community control of sexual mores constitute particularly problematic aspects of the history of marriage in the Western World.[2] The structural principle of the double standard, whereby men's marital infidelity is considered a minor peccadillo and women's a serious transgression, has been extremely well documented.[3] Yet, with the exception of studies on humorous *topoi* in literary satire and comic theatre,[4] scholarly attention has focused more on the issue of female adultery than on the notion of cuckoldry, almost as if scholarship unwittingly echoes the early modern mindset according to which both agency and fault lie, above all, in the female body and its appetites. Popularizing biographies of famous courtesans and royal mistresses perpetuate a fascination with the double standard, while accounts of the sexual license of early modern courts provide prurient examples of amorous affairs.[5] Scandalous trials for the annulment of a marriage due to male impotence are sometimes deemed worthy of popular interest,[6] but on the whole the topics of cuckoldry and impotence have rarely been the subject of concerted scholarly attention.

The seriousness with which female adultery was viewed in Renaissance and early modern Europe was, however, but the more visible face of a coin on which male honor and the social stigma of cuckoldry (including a presumed lack of virility) constituted the dark and complex reverse. Social historians attentive to gender studies have accurately diagnosed wifely infidelity as being an issue that implied more than just male personal and sexual honor. A man whose wife was known to have committed adultery was perceived as lacking in two ways: he was deemed neither able to physically satisfy his wife (otherwise why should she stray?), nor was he considered capable of keeping any kind of order in his household. The consequences in terms of personal reputation would spill over into business networks and other areas of a man's "public" persona and threaten, through such a bad example, the stability of the rest of the community. This is not the place to further explore the many studies of collective community action taken against men who tolerated such behavior on the part of their wives, nor the court cases in which church and state were called upon to intervene in disorderly conjugal relations.[7] The premise of this volume is to cast more light on the dark side of the coin, on cuckoldry as opposed to adultery, on impotence as opposed to infidelity.

In Renaissance and early modern Europe, the emergence of constellations of events—ranging from sex scandals to legal debates to flurries of satirical prints—demonstrate, at different times and places, an increased concern with cuckoldry, impotence and adultery. As the essays in this volume repeatedly point out, there are specific moments and contexts in which this topic gains critical mass, be it in the political or diplomatic arena, in religious or medical literature, or in literary and artistic expression. By isolating specific incidences of acute concern with cuckoldry and impotence in the historical past, it is possible to determine how these sexual phenomena were both perceived and instrumentalized according to the specifics of each context. Finally, by focusing on clusters of different but synchronic sources, it is possible to identify the wider scenario: the current social, cultural or political climate that gave rise to a focus on cuckoldry and its consequences.

This volume brings together a series of interdisciplinary essays that examine specific cases or clusters of documents in which issues related to cuckoldry, impotence and adultery emerge as being particularly resonant. From publicly shamed palaces in Medici Florence to satirical prints proposing a *Confraternity of Cuckolds*, each author analyzes the circumstances that made accusations of sexual disorder into an appropriate social strategy or rhetorical tool. Not only does this volume furnish an unprecedented panorama of the various scenarios in which accusations of cuckoldry and impotence could play a central role, but it also places sexual reputation and sexual metaphor into the forecourt of our historical understanding of the presuppositions that underpinned the early modern world.

Genesis

This collective investigation began at a Renaissance Society of America annual meeting in Venice in Spring 2010, during a dinner on the Giudecca. Despite a number of fascinating sessions on the sexual cultures of the European past, a curious lacuna had become evident: there was relative silence, even disinterest, with regard to cuckoldry in the early modern period. Yet a multitude of cultural phenomena, including visual culture, literature and drama, legal tracts and canon law, medical and botanical treatises, dietary advice manuals and popular shaming rituals, all devote a great deal of attention to cuckoldry. Cuckoldry, impotence and adultery constitute a *longue durée* equation that appears in all social and cultural contexts.[8] Female adultery and/or domination over a husband imply both lack of virility (impotence) and a loss of male honor (cuckoldry). This basic equation can be applied in all directions (for example, male impotence = female adultery = cuckoldry) and gives rise to cultural expressions that can range from doubt regarding the ability of a ruling political figure to reassurance about the immaculate virginity of Mary, the mother of God.[9]

Court scandals and shaming rituals can overlap, comic theatre and satirical prints entertain as well as blame, humorous drawings and elite paintings will elicit laughter, and legal treatises can echo medical skepticism with regard to magic being the primary cause of erectile dysfunction. The omnipresence of cuckoldry, impotence and female adultery is a cultural phenomenon whose pervasiveness has long been discounted as being entirely self-evident, which is exactly why it is worthy of closer examination. In order to address this particular issue, a task force of historians, art historians and scholars of drama and literature was brought together to examine these three, often conflated, aspects of early modern sexual culture. The resulting essays in this volume cast light on a variety of arenas in Renaissance and early modern Europe where sexual culture emerges as being embedded with social, medical, political and religious implications.

The tripartite sequence of the essays that appear in this volume responds to three different trends in Renaissance and early modern studies. The first is an ongoing interest in the history of marriage and sexual culture at all levels of the social ladder: cuckoldry and impotence were of acute concern from village to court, and accusations relative to such transgressions provide a privileged window onto marital relations, notions of honor and current perceptions of the body. The second historical trend is the interdisciplinary cross-referencing of sources in an effort to reconstruct the erotic cultures of the past. Sources such as demonological treatises and innovative legislation, contemporary medical theory and household *libri di secreti* as well as literary works such as plays and the *novella,* all evoke a widespread fear of cuckoldry and impotence, portrayed in either a serious or comic vein. The third trend is the use of visual media as a privileged source for social and cultural history. Four out of the ten essays in this volume focus on iconographic documents in which specific attention is paid to cuckoldry and impotence, to henpecked husbands and insubordinate wives. Ranging from comic references to artistic rivalry in Renaissance Venice to the military impotence of German mercenary soldiers, visual discourse reveals a variety of situations in which cuckoldry and impotence were used as a rhetorical tool, a coded means to comment on wider issues.

Contents

The first of the three parts of this volume, Part I: Defamed Buildings and Shamed Bodies, inaugurates the discussion with three examples of public scandals featuring female adultery, complacent cuckolds and community shaming rituals such as the noisy and theatrical skimmington. Set in Renaissance Italy and Restoration England, these essays constitute a concrete reminder of the widespread resonance of such issues. An accusation of cuckoldry was one of the more pervasive forms of social invective in early modern Europe, the metaphorical extensions of this insult were particularly complex, and conjugal (mis)behavior could have repercussions on diplomatic relations and political alliances as well as on local communities. Jacqueline Musacchio's "Adultery, Cuckoldry and House-Scorning in Florence: The Case of Bianca Cappello" subtly examines a celebrated scandal where court and city were at odds with respect to sexual *mores*. She reveals, amongst other neglected aspects of the case, the fact that the urban neighborhood materially expressed its disapproval of sexual disorder amongst the local elite in a time-honored fashion: horns, other animal parts and excrement were deployed to effect on the façades of buildings already "defamed" by the scandalous behavior of their inhabitants. Next, Molly Bourne looks at accusations of impotence rather than cuckoldry by revisiting a celebrated trial that enthralled the entire peninsula. In "Vincenzo Gonzaga and the Body Politic: Impotence and Virility at Court," Bourne provides an analysis of the legal, medical and metaphorical meanings of the body in elevated political circles in 16th-century Italy. In such circumstances, accusations of impotence could become a diplomatic ploy and the bodies of the participants—be they that of a Gonzaga crown prince or a Florentine orphan girl—assume a dual identity, both performative and political. The third essay, M. A. Katritzky's "Historical and Literary Contexts for the Skimmington: Impotence and Samuel Butler's *Hudibras*," looks at theatre, travelogues and historical accounts to cast light on the skimmington ride (an English variant of the European *charivari*), and documents the fact that England and the continent had differing attitudes to "magically" induced impotence. Using contemporary accounts, the author demonstrates how Butler merges features typical of popular skimmingtons, insisting on the sensory and performative dimension of such events: bad smells, rough music, neighbors as proxies for the offending couple and symbolic props (such as horns). Butler, however, uses the skimmington for more than theatrical effect: he also uses this popular ritual to subvert and mock Puritans, Catholics, English royalty and political elites. The three essays in this section bring home the fact that marital fidelity and virile performance were of acute concern to contemporary society as a whole, both literally and metaphorically. Local communities felt impelled to shame transgressing neighbors (even if they had powerful connections), court scandals were international in scope and subject to widespread speculation, and explicit references to popular street theatre could be strategically deployed to critique religious and political authority.

Part II: Impotence, Magic and Medicine shifts the focus from adultery, cuckoldry and impotence in the social and political arena to the legal, literary and medical constructions of these same sexual phenomena. Contextualized by comparisons with other contemporary sources, these essays examine speculation regarding "magical" impotence in Renaissance Italy, Italian comic theater as opposed to humanist writings on the ages of man, and the phenomenon of the household recipe book. What were the legal loopholes regarding conjugal sexual dysfunction, and what were the medical remedies proposed for problems of erotic performance? Matteo Duni's "Impotence, Witchcraft and Politics: a Renaissance Case" looks at contemporary theories with regard to the causes of male impotence. He draws particularly on legal treatises and demonological tracts that deal with the notion that the inability to consummate a marriage might be attributed to magical spells rather than to other causes such as immaturity, physical repulsion or debility. Skepticism with respect to magical impotence and speculation on the failure of certain dynastic unions, such as that of Gian Galeazzo Maria Sforza with Isabella of Aragon (1489), are here explored in terms of witchcraft beliefs, marriage legislation, court politics and international gossip networks. The next essay in this volume, "The Satyr in the Kitchen Pantry" by Laura Giannetti, shifts the focus to early modern drama and remedies for impotence as opposed to the causes thereof. The author looks specifically at Italian Renaissance comedy and its treatment of impotent old men who are presented as being comic in their attempts to regain sexual prowess. Giannetti reveals that plays refer systematically to current medical theory and popular remedies to revive or enhance virile performance, elements that a contemporary audience would have understood as referring to an elderly protagonist's amorous aspirations. This study concludes by pointing out the social and cultural tensions between the comic view of the foibles of elderly men and the normative decorum of humanist discourse, which defined old age as a stage of life when earthly passions were both unseemly and unhealthy. Medical solutions to problems related to sexuality and sexual performance are also the subject of Meredith Ray's essay, "Impotence and Corruption: Sexual Function and Dysfunction in Early Modern Italian Books of Secrets." Here the author extends the focus to include problems afflicting women as well as men, examining erotic issues that were seen as being susceptible to treatment, from virile malfunction to the repair of lost virginity. In a period which saw the popularization of medical self-help literature, the *libro di segreti* (book of secrets) reveals a series of sexual dilemmas that could arise in the 16th-century household, while the tactful coding of certain entries opens a window onto the embarrassment threshold of the Renaissance reader. A backdrop of common attitudes towards impotence, cuckoldry and adultery emerge from the three essays in this section. Skepticism with regard to occult causes of impotence, comic topoi with regard to elderly swains and medicinal remedies for a variety of sexual dysfunctions were to be found not just in Renaissance Italy but in all of early modern Europe, where regional variations were minor compared to the pervasiveness of a shared sexual culture.

Part III: Horns and Visual Innuendo builds on the preceding sections by examining the ways in which painting, drawing and engravings used cuckoldry and impotence as a means to comment on religious, social and political issues. It begins with Francesca Alberti's "'Divine cuckolds': Joseph and Vulcan in Renaissance Art and Literature," where the late medieval tradition of representing the saintly carpenter as being endowed with horns gives way, in the early 16th century, to visual interest in the mythological blacksmith, cuckolded by the young and beautiful Venus. Figures of fun, these unfortunate husbands also provide a more serious commentary on theological doctrine, artistic identity and professional rivalry. Cuckolded by God, Joseph's sexual dishonor turns into a guarantee of Mary's immaculate virginity, while Vulcan's cuckoldry provides a pretext for Tintoretto to belittle his rival, Titian. Christiane Andersson's essay, "Niklaus Manuel and Urs Graf: Cuckolds, Impotence and Sex Workers in Swiss Renaissance Art (c. 1510–1517)," follows with a look at a cluster of drawings in which inconsequent and impotent men are juxtaposed with domineering and powerful women. The resulting vision of contemporary gender disorder acts as a vehicle for more generalized concerns. Both Niklaus Manuel and Urs Graf alternated an urban artisan practice with a part-time military career as Swiss mercenaries. The rapid changes that mercenary culture had brought about in Swiss cities such as Bern and Basel, with often unsettling effects on social and economic life, are brought to account in their satirical drawings. The third essay in this section looks at an enigmatic series of humorous drawings by a 17th-century Florentine artist. In "The Cuckoldries of Baccio del Bianco," Louise Rice examines whimsical sketches that were probably made to amuse the author's social entourage and testify to the use of graphic talent as a source of entertainment. Rice not only analyzes the various horns and snails of the cuckold *topos* in order to make sense of the various visual jokes, but also hypothesizes innovative connections with female rulers, unhappy Medici marriages and gossip networks within the city. In conclusion to this volume, an essay by Sara Matthews-Grieco examines a series of mid-17th-century engravings in relation to a contemporary surge in representations of cuckoldry, impotence and adultery. Her essay, entitled "Picart's Browbeaten Husbands in 17th-Century France: Cuckoldry in Context," accounts for this quantitative increase by contextualizing satirical images of domestic disorder with reference to legislative norms, theater culture and a prevailing political climate. In a period in which Paris was still smarting from having been brought to heel after the revolt known as the *Fronde*, satirical prints take a position in favor of both royal and patriarchal authority. The essays in this last section demonstrate the extent to which Renaissance and early modern visual culture relied upon commonly understood sexual metaphors, symbols and gestures to reflect upon current events. Be the content comic or religious, a social critique or a political commentary, references to cuckoldry, impotence and adultery provided a widely used and universally understood sexual code that could be employed to comment on contemporary affairs (pun intended).

The essays in this volume reveal the extent to which references to sexual transgression or dysfunction could be used as a diplomatic weapon, define a physical problem meriting medical intervention, serve as a pretext to evoke laughter while simultaneously reinforcing social norms or yet again function as a rhetorical tool to discuss wider issues, ranging from political legitimation to military rivalry. As a whole, the case studies examined throughout this volume testify to the importance of re-examining areas of the sexual culture of the past that have tended to be discounted as being self-evident. They confirm the value of looking more closely at specific erotic *topoi* in order to focus on neglected areas of social discourse and translate some of the coded signifiers that were in common use.

Of course, the essays that appear here are hardly exhaustive in terms of the specific moments in which attention to adultery, cuckoldry and impotence emerged in early modern European culture, neither do they explore all the possible ways in which references to the same could be used on a symbolic or metaphorical level. Yet, as this volume amply demonstrates, the culture of sexuality occupied a wide and very public arena, encompassing all levels of society and infiltrating every means of communication. The erotic was omnipresent in Renaissance and early modern Europe, both materially and metaphorically. Deployed simultaneously as a rhetorical device and as a negotiating strategy for personal, social or political ends, sexual culture deserves to be recognized as an essential piece of the puzzle that is the European past.

Notes

1 "Coquuz proprement ne sont pas ceulx/ qui hont femme ribaulde, mais au contraire/ ceulx qui couchent avec la femme d'aul-/ truy. Le mot prins sur la nature de L'oy-/ seau, qui pont ses oeufz au nid des aultres," Andrea Alciato, *Emblemes d'Alciat*, Lyons, Macé Bonhomme for Guillaume Rouille, 1549, 85. French translation by Barthélemy Aneau (my translation).

2 Research on the history of gender, marriage and sexuality has multiplied exponentially since the 1970s thanks to the innovative work by pioneer historians such as Jean-Louis Flandrin and Lawrence Stone. See, by Lawrence Stone, *The family, sex and marriage in England 1500–1800* (London: Weidenfeld & Nicolson, 1977), and by Jean-Louis Flandrin, *Families in former times: kinship, household, and sexuality* (Cambridge: Cambridge University Press, 1979 [Paris ©1976]) and *Sex in the Western World* (Philadelphia: Harwood Academic Publishers, 1991 [Paris ©1981]). A number of publications specifically on marriage and adultery appeared in the 1990s, such as Régine Beauthier's history of legislation *La répression de l'adultère en France du XVIème au XVIIIème siècle: de quelques lectures de l'histoire* (Brussels: E. Story-scientia, 1990), Lawrence Stone's examination of court cases in *Broken lives: separation and divorce in England, 1660–1857* (Oxford: Oxford University Press, 1993) and David M. Turner's study of literature and legal sources in *Fashioning Adultery: Gender, Sex and Civility in England, 1660–1740* (Cambridge: Cambridge University Press, 1998). This is not the place to provide an extensive historiographic survey of the

field, but it bears mention that more recently publications on the history of sexuality have moved the investigation into a more interdisciplinary arena. In the year 2010 alone, no less than three publications appeared: a collective volume edited by Allison Levy, *Sex Acts in Early Modern Italy* (Farnham, UK/Burlington, VT: Ashgate, 2010), where the term "sex acts" is interpreted broadly, from the acting out, or performing, of one's (or another's) sex to sexual activity, a collective volume edited by myself, *Erotic Cultures in Renaissance Italy* (Farnham, UK/Burlington, VT: Ashgate, 2010), which concentrates largely on the middle ranks of society in Renaissance Italy and focuses on new social subjects and inedited documents with particular attention to the ludic and ritual aspects of erotic culture, and a monograph exploring literary, philosophical and political approaches to the history of sexuality by Kathleen Crawford, *The Sexual Culture of the French Renaissance* (Cambridge: Cambridge University Press, 2010).

3 The pioneer study in this area was Keith Thomas's "The Double Standard," *Journal of the History of Ideas*, Vol. 20, No. 2 (Apr., 1959), 195–216.

4 On comic theatre, see the essays by Laura Giannetti and Sara Matthews-Grieco in this volume. On literary satire and misogyny, the bibliography is vast. For a recent overview see: Danielle Haase-Dubosc and Marie-Élisabeth Henneau (eds), *Discours sur l'égalité/inégalité des sexes, de 1600 à 1750*, St. Etienne, Publications de l'Université de Saint-Etienne, 2013. Some useful secondary sources (organized by historical period) are provided in Rinaldina Russell (ed.), *The Feminist Encyclopedia of Italian Literature* (Westport, CT: Greenwood Press, 1997). For the Renaissance, some of the earlier surveys of the debate on women remain useful: see Pamela J. Benson, *The Invention of the Renaissance Woman The Challenge of Female Independence in the Literature and Thought of Italy and England* (University Park: University of Pennsylvania Press, 1992); Katherine Henderson and Barbara F. McManus, *Half Humankind: Contexts and Texts of the Controversy about Women in England, 1540–1640* (Urbana/Chicago: University of Illinois Press, 1985); Marina Zancan, *Nel cerchio della luna: figure di donna in alcuni testi del XVI secolo* (Venice: Marsilio Editore, 1983); Madeleine Lazard, *Images littéraires de la femme à la Renaissance* (Paris: Presses Universitaires de France, 1985).

5 See for example Caroline P. Murphy, *Murder of a Medici Princess* (Oxford/New York: Oxford University Press, 2009); Antonia Fraser, *Love and Louis XIV: The Women in the Life of the Sun King* (London/New York: Doubleday Anchor Books; 2007); Diane Haeger, *The Secret Wife of King George IV* (New York: St. Martin's Press, 2001).

6 Jeffrey Merrick, "Impotence in Court and at Court," *Studies in Eighteenth Century Culture*, Volume 25 (1996), 187–202; Pierre Darmon, *Trial by impotence: Virility and marriage in pre-Revolutionary France* (London: Chatto & Windus, 1985). See also in this volume the essay by Molly Bourne.

7 Publications on public shaming rituals known as the *charivari*, or skimmington ride, seem to have peaked in the 1980s. See amongst the vast bibliography: Jacques Le Goff and Jean-Claude Schmitt (eds.), L. Charivari (EHESS-CNRS, 1981); Anthony Fletcher and John Stevenson, *Order and Disorder in Early Modern England* (Cambridge/New York: Cambridge University Press, 1987); Brown, Pamela Allen, *Better a Shrew than a Sheep: Women, Drama and the Culture of Jest in Early Modern England* (Ithaca, NY: Cornell University Press, 2003). More recently, the history of the English skimmington has been re-examined by the men's rights activist, M. J. George in "Skimmington Revisited," *The Journal of Men's Studies* 10:2 (Winter 2002): 111–27, and in a more scholarly vein in David Underdown, "'But the shows of their street': civic pageantry and charivari in a Somerset town, 1607," *Journal of British Studies* 50:1 (2011): 4–23. In terms of court records on disorderly households, see for example: Silvana Seidel Menchi and Diego Quaglioni (eds.), *Trasgressioni. Seduzione, concubinato, adulterio, bigamia (XIV–XVIII secolo), Serie: I processi matrimoniali degli archivi ecclesiastici italiani* (Bologna: Il Mulino, 2004); Laura Gowing, *Domestic Dangers Women, Words, and Sex in Early Modern London* (Oxford: Clarendon, 1996); and of course the ground-breaking book by Arlette Farge and Michel Foucault, *Le Désordre des familles, lettres de cachet des Archives de la Bastille* (Paris: Gallimard Julliard, 1982).

8 The *longue durée* is a notion launched by the *Annales* school of history in France, whose scholarly journal (*Annales d'histoire économique et sociale*, founded in 1929) was extremely influential in Anglo-American scholarship in the second half of the 20th century. The focus on long-term social patterns, mental constructs or widely-held systems of belief continues to be particularly useful for historians looking at social and cultural change.

9 See in particular the essays in this volume by Molly Bourne and Francesca Alberti.

PART I

Defamed Buildings and Shamed Bodies

1

Adultery, Cuckoldry and House-Scorning in Florence: The Case of Bianca Cappello[1]

Jacqueline Marie Musacchio

The Venetian noblewoman and later Florentine Grand Duchess Bianca Cappello (1548–1587) was the subject of gossip in her own lifetime and in the centuries to follow. Of course, Florentines were inclined to speculate about the foibles of their ruling family, and the Medici gave them ample reason to do so. In 1574, the admittedly anti-Medicean chronicler Bastiano Arditi described Florence as a violent city, the subtext being that the Medici did nothing to stop the many atrocities that occurred.[2] Perhaps even more scandalous, however, and certainly more titillating from a popular perspective, were the family's sexual improprieties, which allowed Florentines to expand their prurient interest to encompass a number of real and reputed Medici paramours. Cosimo I de'Medici had lovers and illegitimate children before, during and after his marriage to Eleonora of Toledo, and their four legitimate children who lived to adulthood had multiple extramarital affairs. The youngest son, Pietro, married his cousin, Dianora of Toledo, but the match was far from ideal and both took lovers; in 1576, Pietro murdered Dianora.[3] Although the next son, Ferdinando, was named a cardinal in 1562 at age 14, he had a long affair with Clelia, the married daughter of his colleague Cardinal Alessandro Farnese.[4] Cosimo and Eleonora's daughter, Isabella, was murdered by her husband, Paolo Giordano Orsini, for her affair with his cousin in 1576.[5] The murders of Dianora and Isabella were condoned by the eldest son and heir, Francesco, to protect Medici family honor. And Francesco, following the double standard of the time, willfully failed to make the connection to his own situation: he and Bianca Cappello had been lovers since 1564, though by the time they met, he was betrothed to Giovanna of Austria and Bianca was married to the Florentine clerk Piero Buonaventuri.[6]

Each one of these adulterous affairs provided immediate fodder for Florentine gossip and left a lasting mark on the historical record. This essay will look in particular at popular perceptions of Francesco and Bianca's adulterous relationship and Piero's resulting cuckoldry. Like so many cities during this period, Florence was a patrilineal society that placed enormous emphasis on a wife's chastity and ability to produce legitimate heirs.[7] This was critical at the elite level of the Medici, but it was also important in lesser strata of Florentine society, with families like that of Piero Buonaventuri, who had little hope of advancement but adopted many of the same attitudes as their social superiors, including the dual standard which indulged peccadillos on the part of a husband but frowned on those of a wife.

A wife's adultery thus created unacceptable doubt about the future of the family, and weakened the authority of the male head of house. A cuckolded husband was seen as incapable of controlling his wife and, by extension, anything else, be it family, business or political relationships. Cuckoldry rendered a man impotent, both sexually and metaphorically, and diminished his honor. As the essays in this volume indicate, the cuckold was a well-known topos of literary, visual and popular culture whose behavior was socially problematic and open to ridicule.[8]

Rams, Goats and Horns in Early Modern Europe

Since Antiquity, cuckolds had been represented in the guise of certain animals, most often rams and goats, or as men with the curving horns of either animal on their heads; indeed, seemingly little distinction was made regarding these horns, which would been interchangeable to most viewers. Rams and goats were synonymous with luxury and lasciviousness in Renaissance art and literature, and particularly in popular bestiaries, making them particularly appropriate in this connection. Rams were celebrated for their fierce possession of all females in their vicinity, emphasizing virility above all.[9] Goats, though equally lustful, allowed their mates to be mounted by others, thus contributing to their own cuckoldry.[10] As a result, a popular Italian term for a cuckold was *becco*, or goat. In perhaps the most widely-circulated bestiary of the Renaissance, Edward Topsell's *The History of Four-Footed Beasts and Serpents* (1608), which was essentially a translation of the first volume of Conrad Gesner's influential *Historiae Animalium* (1551)— itself an adaptation of the medieval *Physiologus*— it was noted that "There is no beast that is more prone and given to lust then is a Goat, for he joyneth in copulation before all other beasts."[11] A number of Italian bestiaries, both manuscript and printed, had long reinforced similar ideas to the increasingly literate population.[12] Anthropologists, folklorists and linguists have used sources such as these to explain this union of the seemingly powerless husband of a philandering wife and the powerful animal horn with its ironically but appropriately phallic shape.[13]

The horn became a widely recognized symbol of a wife's sexual misbehavior, even though it was grafted onto her husband as a mark of *his* shame rather than hers. Indeed, according to Giovanni Boccaccio's *Decamerone* (c. 1350), the fact that the shame was directed towards the husband was why women felt free to engage in adultery: "if every time [a woman committed adultery] a horn grew from her forehead as testimony of what happened, I believe few would do it" (II:9).[14] Cuckolds needed to hide these shameful horns to protect their honor. In the 15th century, the humanist bookseller Vespasiano da Bisticci related how Cosimo il Vecchio de'Medici recommended that a cuckold bury his horn to conceal it (and his wife's behavior) from those around him.[15] First, however, it had to be cut off: a 15th-century Florentine engraving attributed to Baccio Baldini shows a goat-like cuckold king and his fashionably dressed court, some assisting their colleagues by sawing off horns to hide evidence of their cuckolded state.[16] The inscriptions scattered around the engraving, antecedents of the modern speech bubble meant to represent the dialogue between the cuckolds in the scene, stress what was believed to be the inescapable fate of cuckoldom ("He who is not dead will die; he who is not a goat will become one") as well as the importance of removing and concealing the horns ("For charity's sake, help him saw").[17] Similar iconography appeared on at least two examples of 16th-century maiolica, both likely from Deruta, where men saw off each other's horns to escape the stigmatization associated with cuckoldry and thus restore their virile reputation in the public forum.[18] Like other maiolica painters, the artists responsible for these wares may have been working from popular prints as their source material, similar to the Florentine engraving cited above.[19] Certainly they were influenced by the increasing importance of humor, in both visual and literary media, during the Renaissance.[20]

Such a widespread understanding of cuckoldry continued well into the reign of the Medici as Dukes and then Grand Dukes of Tuscany. The Anglo-Italian author John Florio (1553–1625), a translator at the court of King James, published several Italian phrasebooks and an Italian–English dictionary as well as a collection of Italian proverbs entitled *Giardino di ricreatione* (1591). According to one of these proverbs, "Wretched is he who wears horns for his device; there is nothing more shameful for a man to have."[21] Shameful or not, misogynist attitudes about the inevitability of adulterous female behavior only made cuckold images increasingly more ubiquitous. Baccio del Bianco's early 17th-century drawings of a horn-crazed world, examined in further detail in Louise Rice's essay in this volume, ably demonstrate this.[22] As one of the artists closely involved with Medici court activities,[23] albeit several decades after Bianca Cappello's death, Baccio's insights into contemporary attitudes toward cuckoldry are revealing. His satirical representation of elite shoppers buying horns and sitting for horn-wearing portraits of themselves may depend in part on his background as the son of a textile merchant, and therefore his awareness of the vagaries of consumer behavior in relation to fashion. But it also reflects the perceived prevalence of cuckoldry at elite levels of Florentine society. While humorous representations like this both reveal and denounce the understanding of cuckoldry amongst the upper classes, an accusation of cuckoldry, truthful or not, still carried considerable weight as an affront to the husband. These images touched on issues relating to male honor, female sexuality, and social order, making their message particularly potent.[24]

Bianca Cappello and Celio Malespini

Bianca Cappello's much-discussed (though little understood) life provides a case study of the ways in which adultery and cuckoldry were both perceived and handled in late Renaissance Florence. Although her contemporaries seemed well aware of the details of her biography, albeit with some exaggerations, the earliest and most influential written source is Celio Malespini's *Ducento novelle* (1609). Malespini had a varied career as a soldier, forger, theatrical designer and courtier across Europe. Although he moved frequently (in part to escape prosecution for a series of petty crimes), he was resident in the Medici court in Florence from at least 1572 to 1578, where he apparently knew both Bianca and her first husband Piero Buonaventuri, as well as some of the Medici.[25] His *Ducento novelle* is a collection of short stories that provides considerable insight into late 16th-century attitudes about a wide range of topics, including adulterous wives, cuckolded husbands and sexual relations in general. Similar to Boccaccio's earlier *Decamerone*, Malespini's book began with the premise of a group of courtiers who fled their city for the countryside to escape a plague outbreak, and entertained themselves through storytelling. Also like Boccaccio, Malespini's rather scandalous volume was placed on the papal list of banned books, in Malespini's case by 1617.[26]

Although some of Malespini's stories were based on earlier sources (such as the 15th-century French *Les Cent Nouvelles Nouvelles*), others seem to be based on people and events from Malespini's lifetime. Internal evidence indicates that at least some of the tales were written while he was at the Medici court and it is therefore no surprise that Malespini references Bianca in at least seven of his stories.[27] In one of these, which will be examined in detail at the end of this essay, he only cites a "most important lady," but the context makes it clear that this lady is indeed Bianca (I:73).[28] He references a nameless Medici grand duchess in stories about the voyage of a secretary and his friend to Livorno (I:55) and a shifty medical man in Florence (II:93),[29] but circumstantial evidence again indicates that the grand duchess in question was Bianca. Malespini also cites her by name in four further stories. One describes a necromancer's spectacle in her gardens, interrupted by the news of the death of Giovanna of Austria in April 1578 (II:24),[30] and another centers on the author Mario Venieri, who enjoyed Bianca's palace and idyllic garden (II:90).[31] The final two, however, are particularly important, and informative, because they actually narrate Bianca's biography—as it was popularly understood at that time—in considerable detail.

The first of these, titled "How Bianca Cappello became Grand Duchess of Tuscany," describes Bianca's life prior to her marriage with Francesco (II:84).[32] The second, "How the death of Piero Buonaventuri, husband of Bianca Cappello, occurred," describes how Piero's pride, and his many love affairs, led to his violent death in 1572 (II:85).[33] Malespini, or perhaps his Venetian printer, seemed to be aware of the risks associated with disseminating this information during the reign of Francesco's brother, Ferdinando. The table of contents lists all but three of Malespini's two hundred tales by number, title and page. One of those omitted refers to sodomy (II:18), so its omission is perhaps understandable in the fervor of the post-Tridentine era. But the other two are these biographies of Bianca. This subterfuge was not particularly effective. Copies in the British Library and the Newberry Library have a manicule and a cross respectively sketched by prior owners or readers at the appropriate spots in the tables of contents, with the titles of both stories and their page numbers inserted.[34] A gloss in the Newberry copy further advises the reader that these worthy stories, of special interest as Medici history, are in the book but their omission from the table of contents was due to a respectful gesture on the part of the printer.[35]

Regardless of this omission, Malespini's two Bianca Cappello stories are the most frequently republished ones in the entire volume and they were translated almost verbatim into several languages over the ensuing centuries. In the 18th century, they were included in at least eighteen very similar Italian manuscripts of somewhat scandalous and oftentimes apocryphal biographies and documents spanning Medici history from Giovanni di Bicci to Gian Gastone.[36] These manuscripts, many of which were titled with some variation of *Origine e descendenza della casa Medici*, have been attributed to the early 17th-century courtier Cosimo Baroncelli (1569–1626), who did in fact write a biography of his employer, Giovanni de'Medici.[37] They have also been attributed to Bernardo Benvenuti (1634–1699), the antiquarian prior of Santa Felicità who compiled a history of illustrious Florentine families for Ferdinando II,[38] and to Antonio Benvenuti, an official who worked for Anna Maria Luisa de'Medici.[39] None of these attributions, however, are completely plausible. Given that the Bianca sections of these manuscripts are essentially copied from Malespini, it is more reasonable to assume that an anonymous compiler assembled all of the material from various sources, signaling considerable demand for Medici lore in the mid-18th century, after the end of their reign when disreputable tales could be disseminated without fear of reprisal.

Malespini's version of Bianca's biography, whether through his *Ducento novelle*, these manuscript sources, or later printed reiterations in Italian or another language, has become the basis for our understanding of her life.[40] Although there are certain obvious embellishments and inaccuracies, a significant proportion of Malespini's account seems plausible.[41] In fact, Malaspini was not the only one to record some of these details: the contemporary chroniclers Giuliano de'Ricci and Bastiano Arditi recounted the basic outline of Bianca's arrival in Florence, evidence that the relationship between Bianca and Francesco was hardly a secret from the start.[42] Ricci was relatively circumspect in his comments and merely noted that she was Francesco's favorite.[43] Arditi, however, maintained a running condemnation, referring to her at various points as Francesco's *meretrice* (whore) and *concubina* (concubine) and even stating that she had *mal franzese* (syphilis).[44] Clearly these strong accusations were due in part to Arditi's dislike of the

Medici, but Bianca's behavior was hardly spotless. An anonymous chronicler from this same period echoed Arditi's slurs, and noted that Francesco "was so drunk on this Bianca that he ruled the whole state on her advice and poor Giovanna [his wife] no longer received a crust of bread for the love of God."[45] Piero's extramarital activities, and their ultimately tragic outcome, were also outlined: both Ricci and Arditi described Piero's violent death, as did two other now lost manuscripts by members of the well-informed Ricci family.[46]

These additional sources confirm Malespini's overall narrative, even if some of his more vivid details seem improbable. In II:84, Malespini related how Piero and Bianca originally crossed paths in Venice because her home and the Salviati bank, where he was employed, were on the same canal. Her maidservant facilitated their relationship by making the necessary arrangements for their clandestine nighttime meetings. However, one evening in late 1563, a cautious baker closed the door that Bianca had left ajar to permit her return home and, fearing discovery and scandal, the couple fled to Florence and Piero's family. The Buonaventuri reluctantly took them in, dismissing their servant so they could afford to feed them, which obliged Bianca to take on the more menial household tasks. Her father, backed by the Venetian government, sought her return and Piero's incarceration, but since they had left Venetian territory he had little recourse. Meanwhile, the young Francesco de'Medici, at the time heir apparent to Grand Duke Cosimo I, became interested in the fugitives. He passed by the Buonaventuri home, glimpsed Bianca at a window, and instantly fell in love. His Spanish manservant set up a meeting between them, when Francesco purportedly confessed his love and vowed to protect her. Malespini concludes with the diplomatic observation that Bianca and Francesco were eventually married and enjoyed their great love until their untimely deaths.

Malespini left out one very important fact: while Bianca, Francesco and Piero engaged in what one 18th-century biographer referred to as a *triangolo equilatero* (equilateral triangle),[47] Cosimo was negotiating Francesco's marriage to Giovanna of Austria, which took place in late 1565. Giovanna was daughter and sister of Habsburg emperors and a valuable asset for Florentine political ambitions, so such a match was in the Medici's, and the city's, best interests. By not mentioning Giovanna in his narrative, Malespini made Francesco's portrayal much more positive: without a wife, he was not an adulterer, and this was certainly a more politic way to characterize the deceased brother of the current grand duke.

Cuckoldry and House-Scorning in the *Ducento Novelle*

Despite the careful recasting of history with regard to Francesco's marital status, Malespini did not dissimulate the circumstances leading up to Bianca's marriage to Piero. To Malespini and his readers, Bianca clearly committed adultery, and this undoubtedly added to the negative perception of her in the centuries following her death. Of course, Piero's behavior was not without fault. In addition to seducing and marrying Bianca without her father's approval, an act that went against all acceptable notions of behavior in Renaissance Venice, Piero became a notorious philanderer and Florence's most famous, and willing, cuckold. By February 1565, Francesco had given him a job in the Medici *Guardaroba* (the office which administered all family possessions), although that position may have been a pretense to supply Piero with an adequate income to support Bianca in the necessarily elevated manner of a Duke's mistress.[48] Piero's horns were therefore the price he had to pay for a comfortable life, ducal favor, and the freedom to carry on his own extramarital affairs in hospitable beds across the city while his wife was otherwise occupied.[49]

Piero was not alone in this situation, although his case was unusual in that it became particularly notorious. Ortensio Lando's satiric advice manual *Paradossi* (1543) advocated for adulterous wives since their lovers might be, as Francesco certainly was, socially and financially useful to their husbands.[50] A man who was content to go along with this was known as a "wittol" in early modern England, a popular though much derided character in plays by Thomas Middleton and others, emphasizing the profit the cuckold gained from his wife's sexual escapades.[51] Such a cuckold was later characterized as a stag, his massive rack of horns indicative of his wife's hard work in the bedchamber.[52] Throughout Europe, these contented cuckolds were seen as a threat to a social order that held the protection of wives' chastity (and husbands' honor) as a primary concern. Surely this is one reason why contemporary art and literature employed humor to ridicule these cuckolds. In Niccolò Machiavelli's comedic play about Florentine mores, *La Mandragola* (c. 1518), the credulous Messer Nicia is told by the scheming Callimaco and his accomplices that the only way he can have his hoped-for heir is to dose his wife with mandrake, which will make her fertile but will also kill the first man who sleeps with her. Messer Nicia frets over the need to arrange a sacrificial lover for his wife, and tells Callimaco, who will ultimately cuckold him, that "I am not the sort of man to turn my wife into a whore and put horns on my own head."[53] However, by the end of the play, he reconciles himself to exactly these circumstances' state of affairs.

Unlike Machiavelli's Messer Nicia, however, Piero Buonaventuri was not able to keep his wife's adultery secret, and the widespread knowledge of Bianca's relationship with Francesco impinged on Piero's virile reputation. Both Florentines and visitors to the Medici court would have understood Bianca's affair as a sign of Piero's sexual impotence, as an extramarital affair on the part of a wife was almost always seen as a strategy to compensate for her husband's poor performance in their marriage bed. Piero seems to have overcompensated by making no secret of his own lovers. In fact, Malespini's second Bianca story shifts the focus to Piero and his very public affair with Cassandra Bongiani, a beautiful widow whose family, shamed by her behavior, had allegedly killed two of her previous lovers to expunge the dishonor. Piero may have assumed Francesco's patronage would protect him from a similar fate, but Cassandra's family, led by her nephew Roberto de'Ricci, asked Francesco to intercede with Piero on their behalf. In Malaspini's account, Piero refuses to change his behavior and Francesco sees no alternative but to send him out of the city. This leads to an argument between Piero and Bianca; she tries to reason with him but Piero calls her a whore and threatens to cut off the *corna d'oro* (golden horn) she put on his head, recalling the imagery of the engravings and maiolica cited earlier in this essay. Soon after this argument, Francesco leaves for the countryside and his absence gives the Ricci opportunity to take their revenge. They assemble 12 men, among them apparently Malespini himself; his participation accounts for the detailed description of these events in his *Ducento novelle*.[54] They attack and kill Piero as he walks home from an assignation with Cassandra, and then kill Cassandra herself the following evening.[55] Piero's *corna d'oro* proved more than a symbol of his wounded pride; it was, ultimately, the cause of his death.

Even before his assassination, Piero's ineffectual attempts to salvage his virile reputation are clear in the seventh and final Bianca-related story in Malespini's volume (1:73).[56] This tale, which provides even greater insight into how Piero was mocked as a cuckold in the wider urban setting, identifies Bianca, as noted earlier, only as "a most important lady." But Malespini knew his readers would recognize her. In this story, a Genoese courtier from the Spinola family, newly arrived in the city to serve in the Medici court but still a bit unsure of social norms, walks through the Oltrarno early one morning on his way to the market to buy fish for a luncheon. According to Malespini,

> passing by the via Maggiore, [the courtier] saw hanging around the door of a most important lady, who in those times lived there (whose name, and family I do not like to tell you) more than twenty pairs of horns, with many big wether bellies, and spread all around the excrement of those animals."[57]

When the courtier returned later in the day, however, the palace was free of this debris.Malespini's description of a horn-bedecked façade was essentially a colorful anecdote to amuse his readers, an aside in a narrative about the foreign courtier's trip to an unfamiliar market. But Malespini also expected those readers to recognize the reference to the Bianca Cappello and her *palazzo*. In 1567, Piero Buonaventuri bought this building in the fashionable via Maggio, the Oltrarno street leading from the Ponte Santa Trinità to the Palazzo Pitti. The sumptuous palace had been renovated by court architect Bernardo Buontalenti, and the money to make this purchase must have come from Francesco, in another attempt to elevate Bianca to an appropriate level as his mistress.[58] This was the most famous building on via Maggio, with its extensive *sgraffito* and polychrome ornament, and it is still associated with Bianca today due to her arms over the portal and her swan symbol on the façade. Malespini's description of its defilement implies that this was both a recognizable ritual and a regular occurrence; judging by the way Bianca's servants rapidly eliminated the debris, they were accustomed to dealing with recurring public censure of Piero.

Elizabeth Cohen used the term house-scorning to refer to this kind of practice; it could be tangible or intangible, audible or visible, and was directed at the home of someone seen as needing censure, often, though not always, for perceived sexual improprieties.[59] It might take the form of loud or otherwise offensive noise that crossed the threshold into the domestic space.[60] Graffiti might be used to make a visual, and longer lasting, statement. Court documents reveal that targeted homes were painted with *cose dishoneste* (lewd things), such as graphic representations of sexual organs, in a tradition that went back to Ancient Rome.[61] House-scorning might also include the throwing of stones, animal parts, excrement and, in cases involving cuckolds like Piero, affixing horns.[62] Indeed, the placement of horns on a palace façade, as Malespini described, made the shame of cuckoldry impossible to hide from the larger community. Evidence for such an ephemeral practice is sparse, but Florentines apparently understood this use of horns and had for some time. Gene A. Brucker's examination of a mid-15th-century Florentine trial, for example, cites witnesses who testify that horns were nailed above the door of Lusanna and Andrea Nucci's home in the 1440s or 1450s as a way to mock Andrea and to alert all who passed of Lusanna's adulterous behavior.[63]

By the mid-14th century, several cities and towns on the Italian peninsula had laws regarding house-scorning, indicative of the rifts it created in the social fabric. According to legislation set forth by the Spanish Cardinal Álvarez Carrillo de Albornoz in 1357, in the papal states it was forbidden to place "the horn or horns of beasts, foul stinking excrement, or defamatory or disgraceful writing" on or before any doors at night.[64] A Bolognese law of 1454 described the punishment for "throwing mud or sand in front of any house doorway or under any portico, for affixing horns, writing, or painting, or throwing any urine or dirt against anyone."[65] Two decades later Ferrara followed, likewise condemning those who dirtied homes with obscene paintings or offensive substances.[66] Similar legislation was passed well into the period under discussion here; a Roman law of 1580, echoing a papal edict of 1566, punished those who threw "excrement, or horns, or similar things at the thresholds and doorways of houses, and whoever throws rocks or stones at their doors, windows, panes, and roofs, to inflict an insult, or befouls the walls."[67]

House-scorning was often directed at the victim's door or windows, the liminal zones between domestic and public.[68] Records of the Roman tribunal from 1565 to 1666 include 20 cases, with 13 of these involving ink, excrement or animal blood on doors and windows, and seven involving the placement of horns.[69] Such attacks let the perpetrators metaphorically penetrate the gendered space of the home itself, and effect a symbolic, sexual penetration of the women inside it.[70] This would have had particular relevance when the resident of the home was in fact a cuckold, but it is no coincidence that many of the known incidents of house-scorning were directed at prostitutes or adulterers.[71] It is likewise no coincidence that Malespini states that Bianca was first glimpsed by Francesco while she gazed out of the Buonaventuri window, an activity no virtuous woman should engage in precisely because of the threat of visual violation that would inevitably lead to even worse forms of dishonor. Women were living ornaments, of both their families and their homes, but when they looked out at the world through their doors or windows, or when they courted lovers through them, they risked not only their own loss of honor and reputation but also that of the entire household.[72] This behavior became so problematic that Grand Duke Cosimo III de'Medici issued legislation against it in 1691.[73] However, societal norms had long stipulated that women of all ages should remain chastely inside the home. Malespini's mention of Bianca's appearance at her in-laws' window would thus have been automatically understood as a coded comment on her lack of virtue.

In many of the documented incidents of house-scorning, and certainly in Malespini's description, the house was defaced at night, when no one was around to witness the perpetrator. Surely the nocturnal defiler who splattered blood on the increasingly ostentatious Palazzo Medici during its construction in mid-15th-century Florence was encouraged in part by his cloak of anonymity.[74] Those who hung horns or flung excrement on palaces while the inhabitants slept must have felt similarly protected. There had been laws against throwing stones at windows since the 14th century in Florence,[75] and while censure of cuckolds with horns was not specifically prohibited, Dukes Cosimo and Francesco did make some effort to control this sort of night-time marauding.[76]

The overall attention paid to the palace, whether to protect it via legislation or defile it via house-scorning, is important to note. The palace was the most tangible and public face of the family and, as Elizabeth and Thomas Cohen have demonstrated, honor resided particularly in these faces.[77] The defilement of Bianca Cappello's palace was also related to the practice of slashing a face with a knife, known as *sfregio,* which served as punishment for a real or perceived sexual indiscretion.[78] Indeed, the Cohens have characterized this kind of house-scorning as a metaphoric *sfregio*.[79] The sexual implications behind face slashing are well documented. For example, in 1638 the artist Gianlorenzo Bernini infamously arranged for a servant to slash his married lover Costanza Piccolomini after he learned that she was also sleeping with Bernini's own brother.[80] Bernini's honor—his metaphorical face—was at stake, and to reclaim it he had to visibly destroy Costanza's literal face. Slashing was also a traditional punishment for prostitutes carried out by jealous lovers, such as the 16th-century Roman courtesan Antea was known as Antea *Sfregiata,* in reference to the brutal cut she suffered at the hands of a former client.[81] The extent to which slashing was a common practice is also demonstrated by Pietro Aretino's infamous whore Nanna, who arranged an elaborate trick to extort money from one of her clients: an artist painted a slash on her face to simulate the damaging effects of such an attack, and she claimed she needed to pay one doctor to treat the painted wound and another to heal it.[82] Though the *sfregio* resulted in permanent damage to a woman's appearance—the disfiguring scar was something she would carry for life and was particularly detrimental to a prostitute who relied on her appearance—the ephemeral damage to a palace façade similarly scarred the reputation of the occupants by advertising their transgressions to the outside world.[83] In Piero's case, the presumably repeated placement of horns on his home served to mark him as a willing cuckold.

With Piero's death in 1572, the placement of these horns must have stopped. Widowhood, however, did little to improve Bianca's reputation. When Grand Duchess Giovanna of Austria died in childbirth in April, 1578, the anonymous chronicler cited earlier claimed that sorrow over Francesco's relationship with Bianca, rather than a difficult pregnancy, caused her death.[84] Bianca and Francesco married in secret two months later, but Florentines quickly learned of their wedding vows. In September of that year, Bastiano Arditi records Bianca leaving her own palace and moving into the ducal residence at the Pitti, a public gesture that suggests absolute secrecy was no longer necessary.[85] Nevertheless, their marriage was not announced until the following June, when both the anonymous chronicler and the cleric Agostino Lapini noted that Francesco and Bianca had wed, though Lapini added "this was the first time that the Duke said it, and that one knows it is true, even though many thought and guessed it."[86]

Like widowhood, this long-awaited marriage did not change public perception of Bianca Cappello. The French essayist Michel de Montaigne visited Florence in 1580 and dined with Francesco and Bianca. He clearly disapproved of Bianca, making special note of the fact that she, rather than the Duke, sat at the head of the table, and that she mixed very little water with her wine. Since watering wine was a sign of temperance, Montaigne implied that she was not only intemperate and gluttonous, but also a domineering lover who usurped the Duke's rightful place at table. He also described her as "beautiful in the Italian manner, with an agreeable and dignified face, large bosom, and breasts as they like. She managed to manipulate the duke to her will, and...she would be able to retain him at her feet for a long time."[87] Around this same time, Scipione Gonzaga, the Patriarch of Jerusalem and member of the ruling Mantuan family, described Bianca in his autobiography as low-born and of bad repute.[88] Florentines seemed to agree with these harsh assessments, and a verse allegedly sung in Florence's streets during this time capitalized on the rhyme between *veneziana* (Venetian woman) and *puttana* (whore):

Il granduca di Toscana
Ha sposato una puttana
Gentildonna venetiana.[89]

Even if the horns disappeared, the house-scorning apparently continued in another form. Both Arditi (or someone who later commented on Arditi's manuscript)[90] and the Duke of Urbino's agent in Florence[91] reported that the ducal couple, and particularly Bianca, was the subject of slanderous verses posted around the city. Neither source, however, describes these libelous comments in detail.[92]

Conclusion

By all accounts Bianca and Francesco remained devoted to each other for the rest of their lives. But their time together was limited. In October, 1587, Francesco died, apparently due to malaria contracted in the Tuscan countryside, and Bianca followed less than a day later.[93] She, however, may have been poisoned by, or by order of, her brother-in-law Ferdinando.[94] Rumors about this circulated almost immediately; the anonymous chronicler cited several times in this essay noted that her death was apparently due to poison.[95] Ferdinando's subsequent behavior was definitely self-serving; he quickly put aside Bianca and Francesco's 11-year-old son Antonio to claim the ducal throne for himself and, surely counting on the public's willingness to believe scurrilous gossip about Bianca, he forged documents that accused Bianca of faking Antonio's birth.[96] Given these circumstances, it is no surprise that both her contemporaries and even modern scholars have gravitated to the sensational and scandalous when discussing Bianca. Her biography provides a case study of the impact of adultery, cuckoldry and house-scorning in late Renaissance Florence; the horns on her palace, both metaphorical and literal, resulted in a long history of scandal and derision.

Works Cited

Early Printed Sources (pre-1900)

Anonymous. "Bianca Capello. An Historical Novel," trans. Lady Pomfret. *The New Novelist's Magazine* 1 (1787): 16–24.

Anonymous. "The History of Bianca Capello," trans. Offaria Cellini. *The Lady's Museum* 1 (1760): 344–52, 456–64, 529–37.

Anonymous. *The Lively Character of a Contented and Discontented Cuckold, ala-mode de Anglitere*. London and Westminster, 1760.

Brand, John and Sir Henry Ellis. *Observations on the Popular Antiquities Chiefly Illustrating the Origin of our Vulgar Customs, Ceremonies, and Superstitions*. London: Chatto and Windus, 1888.

Cantini, Lorenzo, ed. *Legislazione Toscana*. Florence: Pietro Fantosini e figlio, 1800–1808.

Correspondence between Frances, Countess of Hartford, (Afterwards Duchess of Somerset,) and Henrietta Louisa, Countess of Pomfret, between the years 1738 and 1741. London: Richard Phillips, 1806.

Florio, John. *Giardino di ricreatione nel quale crescono fronde, fiori e frutti, vaghe, leggiadri, e soavi, sotto nome di sei mila proverbii, e piacevoli riboboli italiani, colti e scelti da Giovanni Florio.* London: Thomaso Woodcock, 1591.

Galluzzi, Jacopo Riguccio. *Istoria del granducato di Toscana sotto il governo della casa Medici.* Florence: Gaetano Cambiagi, 1781.

Hove, Nicolaas ten. *Memoirs of the House of Medici, from its Origin to the Death of Francesco, the Second Grand Duke of Tuscany, and of the Great Men who Flourished in Tuscany within that Period,* trans. Sir Richard Clayton. Bath: G. G. and J. Robinson, 1797.

Landucci, Luca. *Diario fiorentino dal 1450 al 1516,* ed. Iodoco del Badia. Florence: Sansoni, 1883.

Malespini, Celio. *Ducento novelle del Signor Celio Malespini nelle quali si raccontano diversi avvenimenti così lieti, come mesti & stravaganti.* Venice: Al Segno dell'Italia, 1609.

Mazzuchelli, Giammaria. *Gli scrittori d'Italia cioe notizie storiche, e critiche intorno alle vite, e agli scritti dei letterati italiani.* Brescia: Giambatista Bossini, 1760.

Morbio, Carlo, ed. *Storie dei municipi italiani.* Milan: Coi torchi di Omobono Manini, 1838.

Moreni, Domenico. *Bibliografia storico ragionata della Toscana.* Bologna: Forni, 1805.

Moreni, Domenico. *Serie d'autori di opera risguardanti la celebre famiglia Medici.* Florence: Stamperia Magheri, 1826.

Potter, Louis Joseph Antoine de. *Vie et Mémoires de Scipion de Ricci.* Paris: J. Tastu, 1826.

Roscoe, William. *Illustrations, Historical and Critical, of the Life of Lorenzo de'Medici Called the Magnificent.* London: T. Cadell, 1822.

Roscoe, William. *The Life of Lorenzo de'Medici Called the Magnificent,* 3rd ed. London: A. Strahan, 1797.

Saltini, Guglielmo Enrico. *Bianca Cappello e Francesco I de'Medici.* Florence: Rassegna Nazionale, 1898.

Saltini, Guglielmo Enrico. "Della morte di Francesco I de'Medici e Bianca Cappello." *Archivio storico italiano.* 18 (1863): 19–81.

Saltini, Guglielmo Enrico. "Di Celio Malespini ultimo novelliere italiano in prosa del secolo XVI." *Archivio storico italiano.* Series 5, vol. 13 (1894): 35–80.

Siebenkees, Johann Philipp. *The Life of Bianca Capello, Wife of Francesco de' Medici, Grand-Duke of Tuscany,* trans. C. Ludger. Liverpool: J. M'Creery, 1797.

Topsell, Edward. *The History of Four-Footed Beasts and Serpents.* London: E. Cotes, 1608.

Trollope, Thomas Adolphus. *A Decade of Italian Women.* London: Chapman and Hall, 1859.

Secondary Sources and Modern Editions

Anonymous. *Dialogo dello Zoppino de la vita e genealogia di tutte le cortigiane di Roma,* ed. Gino Lanfranchi. Milan: Editrice del libroraro, 1922.

Arditi, Bastiano. *Diario di Firenze e di altre parti della cristianità*, ed. Roberto Cantaglli. Florence: Istituto Nazionale di Studi sul Rinascimento, 1970.

Aretino, Pietro. *I ragionamenti*. Bologna: Sampietro editore, 1965.

Barkan, Leonard. *Unearthing the Past*. New Haven/London: Yale University Press, 1999.

Barolsky, Paul. *Infinite Jest: Wit and Humor in Italian Renaissance Art*. Columbia: University of Missouri Press, 1978.

Baroncelli, Cosimo. *Il discorso del Sig.re Cosimo Baroncelli fatto a' suoi figliuli dove s'intende la vita di Don Giovanni Medici figlio naturale del Gran Duca Cosimo Primo con la morte di Concino Concini e Dianora sua mogle e della Sig.ra Livia Vernazzi moglie del suddetto Don Giovanni de' Medici*, ed. Marina Macchio. Florence: Nicomp, 2009.

Benefiel, Rebecca R. J. "Dialogues of Ancient Graffiti in the House of Maius Castricius in Pompeii." *American Journal of Archaeology* 114 (2010): 59–101.

Berti, Luciano. *Il principe dello studiolo. Francesco I dei Medici e la fine del Rinascimento fiorentino*. Pistoia: Maschietto & Musolino, 2002.

Blok, Anton. "Rams and Billy-Goats: A Key to the Mediterranean Code of Honour." *Man* 16 (September 1981): 427–40.

Boccaccio, Giovanni. *Decamerone*, ed. Mario Marti. Milan: Biblioteca Universale Rizzoli, 1990.

Brucker, Gene A. *Giovanni and Lusanna. Love and Marriage in Renaissance Florence*. Berkeley: University of California Press, 1986.

Burke, Peter. *The Historical Anthropology of Early Modern Italy*. Cambridge: Cambridge University Press, 1987.

Cantagalli, Roberto. "Cosimo Baroncelli." *Dizionario biografico degli italiani*. Rome: Istituto della Enciclopedia Italiana, 1964. http://www.treccani.it/enciclopedia/cosimo-baroncelli_%28Dizionario_Biografico%29/.

Cantagalli, Roberto. "Bianca Cappello e una leggenda da sfatare: la questione del figlio supposto." *Nuova rivista storica* 49 (1965): 636–52.

Celli, Giorgio, Annamaria Carrega and Giorgio Navone. *Le Proprietà degli animali*. Genova: Costa & Nolan, 1983.

Cohen, Elizabeth S. "Honor and Gender in the Streets of Early Modern Rome." *The Journal of Interdisciplinary History* 22 (Spring 1992): 597–625.

Cohen, Elizabeth S. and Thomas V. "Open and Shut: The Social Meanings of the Cinquecento Roman House." *Studies in the Decorative Arts* 9 (Fall–Winter 2001–2002): 61–84.

Cohen, Simona. *Animals as Disguised Symbols in Renaissance Art*. Leiden: Brill, 2008.

Cohen, Thomas V. and Elizabeth S. Cohen. *Words and Deeds in Renaissance Rome*. Toronto: University of Toronto Press, 1993.

Colleran, Kate. "Scampanata at the Widows' Windows: A Case Study of Sound and Ritual Insult in Cinquecento Florence." *Urban History* 36 (2009): 359–78.

Connell, William J. and Giles Constable. *Sacrilege and Redemption in Renaissance Florence: The Case of Antonio Rinaldeschi*. Toronto: Centre for Renaissance and Reformation Studies, 2005.

Dean, Trevor. "Gender and Insult in an Italian City: Bologna in the Later Middle Ages." *Social History* 29 (May 2004): 217–31.

DeBujanda, J. M., ed. *Index librorum prohibitorum 1600–1966*. Geneva: Librairie Droz, 2002.

di Maria, Salvatore. "Cecchi's *Assiuolo*, a Creative Imitation of the Old and a Telling Reflection of Contemporary Realities." *Forum Italicum* 45 (Fall 2011): 287–310.

Fitzgerald, William. *Catullan Provocations. Lyric Poetry and the Drama of Position*. Berkeley: University of California Press, 1995.

Fornaciari, Gino, Valentina Giuffra, Ezio Ferroglio, Sarah Gino and Raffaella Bianucci. "Malaria was the Killer of Francesco I de'Medici (1531–1587)." *The American Journal of Medicine* 123 (2010): 568–9.

Fornaciari, Gino, Valentina Giuffra, Ezio Ferroglio, Sarah Gino and Raffaella Bianucci. "Plasmodium Falciparum Immuno detection in Bone Remains of Members of the Renaissance Medici Family (Florence, Italy, Sixteenth Century)." *Transactions of the Royal Society of Tropical Medicine and Hygiene* 104 (2010): 583–7.

Giannetti, Laura and Guido Ruggiero, eds. and trans. *Five Comedies of the Italian Renaissance*. Baltimore: Johns Hopkins University Press, 2003.

Goldberg, Edward L. *Jews and Magic in Medici Florence: The Secret World of Benedetto Blanis*. Toronto: University of Toronto Press, 2011.

Gonzaga, Scipione. *Autobiografia*, ed. Dante Della Terza. Modena: Edizioni Panini, 1987.

Gowing, Laura. *Domestic Dangers: Women, Words, and Sex in Early Modern London*. Oxford: Oxford University Press, 1999.

Graber, Robert Bates and Gregory C. Richter. "The Capon Theory of the Cuckold's Horns: Confirmation or Conjecture?" *The Journal of American Folklore* 100 (January–March 1987): 58–63.

Graham-Dixon, Andrew. *Caravaggio. A Life Sacred and Profane*. New York: W. W. Norton & Co., 2011.

Guerzoni, Guido A. "The Erotic Fantasies of a Model Clerk: Amateur Pornography at the Beginning of the Cinquecento." In *Erotic Cultures of Renaissance Italy*, ed. Sara F. Matthews-Grieco. Farnham, UK/Burlington, VT: Ashgate, 2010. 61–88.

Hassig, Debra. "Sex in the Bestiaries." In *The Mark of the Beast. The Medieval Bestiary in Art, Life and Literature*, ed. Debra Hassig. New York/London: Garland Publishing, 1999. 71–93.

Hind, Arthur M. *Early Italian Engraving. A Critical Catalogue with Complete Reproduction of all the Prints Described*. London: Quaritch, 1938.

Hochmann, Michel, ed. *Villa Medici. Il sogno di un cardinale. Collezioni e artisti di Ferdinando de'Medici*. Rome: De Luca, 1999.

Ingram, Martin. "Ridings, Rough Music, and Mocking Rhymes in Early Modern England." In *Popular Culture in Seventeenth-Century England*, ed. Barry Reay. London: Croom Helm, 1985. 166–97.

Jackson, Margaret Hastings. *Catalogue of the Frances Taylor Pearsons Plimpton Collection of Italian Manuscripts in the Library of Wellesley College*. Cambridge, MA: Harvard University Press, 1929.

Jones, Malcolm. "The English Broadside Print, c. 1550–c.1650." In *A New Companion to English Renaissance Literature and Culture*, ed. Michael Hattaway. West Sussex: John Wiley & Sons, 2010. 478–526.

Jones, Robert C. "Italian Settings and the 'World' of Elizabethan Tragedy." *Studies in English Literature 1500–1900* 10 (Spring 1970): 251–68.

Katz, Dana E. "'Clamber not you up to the casements': On Ghetto Views and Viewing." *Jewish History* 24 (2010): 127–53.

Katz, Dana E. *The Jew in the Art of the Italian Renaissance*. Philadelphia: University of Pennsylvania Press, 2008.

Kent, Dale V. "The Importance of Being Eccentric: Giovanni Cavalcanti's View of Cosimo de'Medici's Florence." *Journal of Medieval and Renaissance Studies* 9 (1979): 101–32.

Klapisch-Zuber, Christiane. *Women, Family, and Ritual in Renaissance Italy*, trans. Lydia G. Cochrane. Chicago: University of Chicago Press, 1987. 261–82.

Lando, Ortensio. *Paradossi. Ristampa dell'edizione Lione 1543*, ed. Eugenio Canone and Germana Ernst. Pisa: Istituto editoriali e poligrafici internazionali, 1999.

Langdon, Gabrielle. *Medici Women. Portraits of Power, Love, and Betrayal*. Toronto: University of Toronto Press, 2006.

Lapini, Agostino. *Diario fiorentino di Agostino Lapini dal 252 al 1596*, ed. Giuseppe Odoardo Corazzini. Florence: Sansoni, 1900.

Lennox, Charlotte Ramsey. *The Life of Harriot Stuart, Written by Herself*, ed. Susan Kubica Howard. Cranbury: Associated University Presses, 1995.

Lombardi, Daniela. *Matrimoni di antico regime*. Bologna: Società editrice il Mulino, 2001.

Măgureanu, Ivana. "Baccio del Bianco and the Cultural Politics of the Medici Court." *Revue roumaine d'histoire de l'art* 48 (2011): 13–26.

Mari, Francesco Aldo Polettini, Donatello Lippi and Elisabetta Bertol. "The Mysterious Death of Francesco I de'Medici and Bianca Cappello: An Arsenic Murder?" *British Medical Journal* 333 (2006): 1299–301.

McEachern, Claire. "Why Do Cuckolds Have Horns?" *Huntington Library Quarterly* 71 (December 2008): 607–31.

McKenzie, Kenneth. "Unpublished Manuscripts of Italian Bestiaries." *PLMA* 20 (1905): 380–433.

McPhee, Sarah. *Bernini's Beloved. A Portrait of Costanza Piccolomini*. New Haven/London: Yale University Press, 2012.

Mezzalira, Francesco, et al. *Beasts and Bestiaries: The Representation of Animals from Prehistory to the Renaissance*. Turin: Allemandi, 2001.

Montaigne, Michel de. *Journal de voyage*, ed. Louis Lautrey. Paris: Librairie Hachette et Cie, 1906.

Mulryne, J. R. "Manuscript Source-Material for the Main Plot of Thomas Middleton's *Women Beware Women*." *The Yearbook of English Studies* 5 (1975): 70–74.

Murphy, Caroline P. *Murder of a Medici Princess*. Oxford: Oxford University Press, 2008.

Musacchio, Jacqueline Marie. *Art, Marriage, and Family in the Florentine Renaissance Palace*. New Haven/London: Yale University Press, 2008.

Neilson, Christina. *Parmigianino's Antea: A Beautiful Artifice*. New York: Frick Collection, 2008.

Novelli, Roberta Lencioni. *Celio Malespini tra biografia e novella*. Naples: Liguori Editore, 1983.

Nussdorfer, Laurie. "The Politics of Space in Early Modern Rome." *Memoirs of the American Academy in Rome* 42 (1997): 161–86.

Panek, Jennifer. "'A Wittall cannot be a Cookold': Reading the Contented Cuckold in Early Modern English Drama and Culture." *Journal for Early Modern Cultural Studies* 1 (Fall–Winter 2001): 66–92.

Pastoureau, Michel. *Bestiares du Moyen Age*. Paris, Seuil, 2011.

Quaife, G. R. *Wanton Wenches and Wayward Wives*. New Brunswick, NJ: Rutgers University Press, 1979.

Ricci, Giuliano de'. *Cronaca (1532–1606)*, ed. Giuliana Sapori. Milan: Riccardo Ricciardi editore, 1972.

Righetti, Maria. *Per la storia della novella italiana al tempo della reazione cattolica*. Teramo; Giovanni Fabbri Editore, 1921.

Rogers, Mary and Paola Tinagli, ed. and trans. *Women in Italy, 1350–1650 Ideals and Realities: A Sourcebook*. Manchester: Manchester University Press, 2005.

Romolo Caggese, ed. *Statuti della repubblica fiorentina. Statuto del podestà dell'anno 1325*. Florence: Tipografico E. Ariani, 1921.

Ruggiero, Guido. "'Più che la vita caro': Onore, matrimonio e reputazione femminile nel tardo rinascimento." *Quaderni storici* 66 (1987): 753–75.

Sella, Pietro, ed. *Corpus statutorumitalicorum*. Rome: Ermanno Loescher & C., 1912.

Siegmund, Stefanie Beth. *The Medici State and the Ghetto of Florence*. Stanford: Stanford University Press, 2006.

Taylor, Scott K. *Honor and Violence in Golden Age Spain*. New Haven/London: Yale University Press, 2008.

Turner, James. *Libertines and Radicals in Early Modern London: Sexuality, Politics, and Literary Culture 1630–1685*. Cambridge: Cambridge University Press, 2002.

Ugolini, Grazia Biscontini and Jacqueline Petruzzellis Scherer, eds. *Maiolica e incisione: Tre secoli di rapporti iconografici*. Vicenza: Neri Pozza, 1992.

Underdown, D. E. "The Taming of the Scold." In *Order and Disorder in Early Modern England*, ed. Anthony Fletcher and John Stevenson. Cambridge: Cambridge University Press, 1985, 116–36.

Vespasiano, da Bisticci. *The Vespasiano Memoirs. Lives of Illustrious Men of the XVth Century*, trans. William George and Emily Waters. Toronto: University of Toronto Press, 1997.

Verga, Marcello. "Pitti e l'estinzione della dinastia medicea. Materiali per una lettura politica della reggia di Firenze tra sei e settecento." In *Vivere a Pitti. Una reggia dai Medici ai Savoia*, ed. Sergio Bertelli et al. Florence: Olschki, 2006. 271–87.

Waldman, Louis. "A Satiric Image on a Maiolica Pharmacy Jar." *Burlington Magazine* 134 (June 1992): 375–8.

Weinstein, Donald. *The Captain's Concubine: Love, Honor, and Violence in Renaissance Tuscany*. Baltimore: Johns Hopkins University Press, 2001.

Wilson, Timothy. "Un 'intricamento' tra Leonardo ed Arcimboldo." *CeramicAntica* 15 (February 2005): 10–44.

Winspeare, Fabrizio. *Isabella Orsini e la corte medicea del suo tempo*. Florence: Olschki, 1961.

Zucker, Mark, ed. *The Illustrated Bartsch. Early Italian Masters*. New York: Abaris Books, 1980.

Notes

1 I am grateful to Molly Bourne, Touba Ghadessi and Sara Matthews-Grieco for advice and assistance, and Wellesley College's Committee on Faculty Awards for funding my research. Much of the material in this essay was presented at the 2011 and 2012 Renaissance Society of America conferences; it forms part of my larger biographical and historiographical study of Bianca Cappello.

2 Bastiano Arditi, *Diario di Firenze e di altre parti della cristianità*, ed. Roberto Cantaglli (Florence: Istituto Nazionale di Studi sul Rinascimento, 1970), 57.

3 Gabrielle Langdon, *Medici Women. Portraits of Power, Love, and Betrayal* (Toronto: University of Toronto Press, 2006), 171–93.

4 Michel Hochmann, ed., *Villa Medici. Il sogno di un cardinale. Collezioni e artisti di Ferdinando de'Medici* (Rome: De Luca, 1999), 304–5.

5 Fabrizio Winspeare, *Isabella Orsini e la corte medicea del suo tempo* (Florence: Olschki, 1961) and Caroline P. Murphy, *Murder of a Medici Princess* (Oxford: Oxford University Press, 2008).

6 Though often romantic in interpretation, the most reliably documented biography of Bianca Cappello is still Guglielmo Enrico Saltini, *Bianca Cappello e Francesco I de'Medici* (Florence: Rassegna Nazionale, 1898).

7 These ideas were emphasized in a wide range of contemporary treatises on the family and marriage; for an overview see Mary Rogers and Paola Tinagli, ed. and trans., *Women in Italy, 1350–1650 Ideals and Realities: A Sourcebook* (Manchester: Manchester University Press, 2005).

8 See, for example, the role of cuckoldry in Italian theater in Salvatore di Maria, "Cecchi's *Assiuolo*, a Creative Imitation of the Old and a Telling Reflection of Contemporary Realities," *Forum Italicum* 45 (Fall 2011): 287–310. It was similarly emphasized in British theater on Italian topics; see Robert C. Jones, "Italian Settings and the 'World' of Elizabethan Tragedy," *Studies in English Literature 1500–1900* 10 (Spring 1970): 258. References to the cuckold's horn extended to metaphorical marriages, too; Giovanni Boccaccio mentions the case of the lustful gardener Masetto who put horns on Christ's head by having sex with all the nuns in a convent (III:1): "Così adunque Masetto vecchio, padre e ricco, senza aver fatica di nutricare i figliuoli o spesa di quegli, per lo suo avvedimento avendo saputo la sua giovanezza bene adoperare, donde con una scure in collo partito s'era, se ne tornò, affermando che così trattava Cristo chi gli poneva le corna sopra il cappello" (Giovanni Boccaccio, *Decamerone*, ed. Mario Marti (Milan: Biblioteca Universale Rizzoli, 1990), I: 191–2.

9 Anton Blok, "Rams and Billy-Goats: A Key to the Mediterranean Code of Honour," *Man* 16 (September 1981): 428, and Debra Hassig, "Sex in the Bestiaries," in *The Mark of the Beast. The Medieval Bestiary in Art, Life and Literature*, ed. Debra Hassig (New York/London: Garland Publishing, 1999), 71–93.

10 Blok, 428. Peter Burke, *The Historical Anthropology of Early Modern Italy* (Cambridge: Cambridge University Press, 1987), 97. Michel Pastoureau, *Bestiares du Moyen Age* (Paris: Seuil, 2011), 113–19.

11 Edward Topsell, *The History of Four-Footed Beasts and Serpents* (London: E. Cotes, 1608), 181.

12 For Italian bestiaries, see, among other sources, Kenneth McKenzie, "Unpublished Manuscripts of Italian Bestiaries," *PLMA* 20 (1905): 380–433; Giorgio Celli, Annamaria Carrega and Giorgio Navone, eds. *Le Proprietà degli animali* (Genova: Costa & Nolan, 1983); Francesco Mezzalira et al., *Beasts and Bestiaries: The Representation of Animals from Prehistory to the Renaissance* (Turin: Allemandi, 2001); and Simona Cohen, *Animals as Disguised Symbols in Renaissance Art* (Leiden: Brill, 2008).

13 See for example Robert Bates Graber and Gregory C. Richter, "The Capon Theory of the Cuckold's Horns: Confirmation or Conjecture?" *The Journal of American Folklore* 100 (January–March 1987):

58–63 and Claire McEachern, "Why Do Cuckolds Have Horns?" *Huntington Library Quarterly* 71 (December 2008): 607–31.

14 Boccaccio, I:161 ("… se per ogni volta che elle a queste così fatte novella attendono, nascesse loro un corno nella fronte, il quale desse testimonianza di ciò che fatto avessero, io mi credo che poche sarebber quelle che v'attendessero.")

15 Vespasiano da Bisticci, *The Vespasiano Memoirs. Lives of Illustrious Men of the XVth Century*, trans. William George and Emily Waters (Toronto: University of Toronto Press, 1997), 226.

16 Arthur M. Hind, *Early Italian Engraving. A Critical Catalogue with Complete Reproduction of all the Prints Described* (London: Quaritch, 1938), I:73–4 and Mark Zucker, ed., *The Illustrated Bartsch. Early Italian Masters* (New York: Abaris Books, 1980): 24:1:265–7.

17 For the inscriptions see Zucker, 24:1:265–7 ("chinonemortomorira/cnnonemorira/cnnonebechovenghira" and "percharitaauti/gliuozegare").

18 Louis Waldman, "A Satiric Image on a Maiolica Pharmacy Jar," *Burlington Magazine* 134 (June 1992): 375–8. For another example of this kind of satirical and sexual iconography on maiolica see Timothy Wilson, "Un 'intricamento' tra Leonardo ed Arcimboldo," *CeramicAntica* 15 (February 2005): 10–44.

19 Grazia Biscontini Ugolini and Jacqueline Petruzzellis Scherer, eds., *Maiolica e incisione: Tre secoli di rapporti iconografici* (Vicenza: Neri Pozza, 1992).

20 On the role of humor see Paul Barolsky, *Infinite Jest: Wit and Humor in Italian Renaissance Art* (Columbia: University of Missouri Press, 1978).

21 John Florio, *Giardino di ricreatione nel quale crescono fronde, fiori e frutti, vaghe, leggiadri, e soavi, sotto nome di sei mila proverbii, e piacevoli riboboli italiani, colti e scelti da Giovanni Florio* (London: Thomaso Woodcock 1591), 155. ("Misero chi corna porta per insegna, che l'huomo non può haver cosa più indegna"); cited in Waldman, 376 note 14. For additional cuckold-related adages see Florio, 18 and 34.

22 See the essay in this volume by Louise Rice, "The Cuckoldries of Baccio del Bianco," chapter 9.

23 Ivana Măgureanu, "Baccio del Bianco and the Cultural Politics of the Medici Court," *Revue roumaine d'histoire de l'art* 48 (2011): 13–26.

24 For similar accusations of cuckoldry see, for example, Edward L. Goldberg, *Jews and Magic in Medici Florence: The Secret World of Benedetto Blanis* (Toronto: University of Toronto Press, 2011), 38, 142 and 151.

25 On Malespini's ties to the Medici and other princely courts see Guglielmo Enrico Saltini, "Di Celio Malespini ultimo novelliere italiano in prosa del secolo XVI," *Archivio storico italiano* series 5, vol. 13 (1894): 35–80, Saltini, 1898, 137–55 and Maria Righetti, *Per la storia della novella italiana al tempo della reazione cattolica* (Teramo; Giovanni Fabbri Editore, 1921), 101–40.

26 J. M. DeBujanda, ed., *Index librorum prohibitorum 1600–1966* (Geneva: Librairie Droz, 2002), 574.

27 Although it has been said that the stories about Bianca Cappello were declared false in Venice in 1572 and 1589, there is no evidence that they circulated in written form at such early dates; see Jacopo Riguccio Galluzzi, *Istoria del granducato di Toscana sotto il governo della casa Medici* (Florence: Gaetano Cambiagi, 1781), II:85 and Johann Philipp Siebenkees, *The Life of Bianca Capello, Wife of Francesco de' Medici, Grand-Duke of Tuscany*, trans. C. Ludger (Liverpool: J. M'Creery, 1797), xvi. Florence and the Medici were certainly on Malespini's mind during and after this period; he sent a number of obsequious letters to Francesco's brother and successor, Ferdinando, and Ferdinando's aide Belisario Vinta around the time of publication. For transcriptions of these letters see Saltini, 1894, 75–80. Ferdinando died in February 1609 and probably never saw Malespini's book, which was printed that same year; see Roberta Lencioni Novelli, *Celio Malespini tra biografia e novella* (Naples: Liguori Editore, 1983), 98–9.

28 Celio Malespini, *Ducento novelle del Signor Celio Malespini nelle quali si raccontano diversi avvenimenti così lieti, come mesti & stravaganti* (Venice: Al Segno dell'Italia 1609), I:200 verso–201 verso.

29 Malespini, I:148 verso–152 verso and II:299 recto–301 verso.

30 Malespini, II:80 verso–85 verso; for a partial English translation see Thomas Adolphus Trollope, *A Decade of Italian Women* (London: Chapman and Hall, 1859), 275–81 and, for further analysis, Zakiya Hanafi, *The Monster in the Machine: Magic, Medicine, and the Marvelous in the Time of the Scientific Revolution* (Durham: Duke University Press, 2000), 16–18.

31 Malespini, II:288 verso–293 verso.

32 Malespini, II:275 verso–278 recto ("Come pervenisse la Signora Bianca Capello Gran Duchessa di Toscana"); see note 40 below for early English translations of II:84 and 85.

33 Malespini, II:278 recto–280 verso ("Successo della morte di Pietro Buonaventura, marito della Signora Bianca Capello").

34 For these copies see Newberry Y712.M27 and British Library 89.b.4.

35 The gloss reads "Queste due novelle sono nel corpo del libro, per le quali si rende più preggevole e si sono tralasciate nella Tavola per degni rispetti dalla stampatore. Le averta chi legge, essendo curios[a] per la gran casa de'Medici."

36 These manuscripts are widely scattered. I know of three versions housed in the British Library (London), three in the Biblioteca Riccardiana (Florence), two in the Newberry Library (Chicago), two at Wellesley College (Wellesley, MA), and one each at Cornell University (Ithaca, NY), Harvard University (Cambridge, MA), Princeton University (Princeton, NJ), Syracuse University (Syracuse, NY), the Vatican Library (Rome), the Biblioteca Casanatense (Rome), the Biblioteca Nazionale Centrale (Florence) and in private hands (http://www.tuscany-toscana.info/medici_manuscript.htm); for a further six possible examples in the Biblioteca Nazionale Centrale in Florence, see J. R. Mulryne, "Manuscript Source-Material for the Main Plot of Thomas Middleton's *Women Beware Women*," *The Yearbook of English Studies* 5 (1975): 73. Some of these manuscripts incorporate an additional description of Francesco and Bianca's deaths at the end, which does not appear in Malespini's original text. This manuscript type was recognized as a useful source for Medici history by at least the late 18th century; see William Roscoe, *The Life of Lorenzo de'Medici Called the Magnificent*, 3rd ed. (London: A. Strahan, 1797), I:7 note a, Domenico Moreni, *Bibliografia storico ragionata della Toscana* (Bologna: Forni, 1805), I:87, and Domenico Moreni, *Serie d'autori di opera risguardanti la celebre famiglia Medici* (Florence: Stamperia Magheri, 1826), 30–31. Moreni allegedly owned one of these manuscripts; his library went to the Biblioteca Riccardiana but I have not been able to determine if his copy is one of the three listed above for that location; see William Roscoe, *Illustrations, Historical and Critical, of the Life of Lorenzo de'Medici Called the Magnificent* (London: T. Cadell, 1822), 79–80 note a.

37 For Baroncelli, see Cosimo Baroncelli, *Il discorso del Sig.re Cosimo Baroncelli fatto a' suoi figliuli dove s'intende la vita di Don Giovanni Medici figlio naturale del Gran Duca Cosimo Primo con la morte di Concino Concini e Dianora sua mogle e della Sig.ra Livia Vernazzi moglie del suddetto Don Giovanni de' Medici*, ed. Marina Macchio (Florence: Nicomp, 2009) and, negating the attribution of these manuscripts to Baroncelli, see Roberto Cantagalli, "Cosimo Baroncelli," *Dizionario biografico degli italiani* (Rome: Istituto della Enciclopedia Italiana, 1964), http://www.treccani.it/enciclopedia/cosimo-baroncelli_%28Dizionario_Biografico%29/.

38 For Benvenuti, see Giammaria Mazzuchelli, *Gli scrittori d'Italia cioe notizie storiche, e critiche intorno alle vite, e agli scritti dei letterati italiani* (Brescia: Giambatista Bossini, 1760), 885–6 and Marcello Verga, "Pitti e l'estinzione della dinastia medicea. Materiali per una lettura politica della reggia di Firenze tra sei e settecento," in Sergio Bertelli et al, *Vivere a Pitti. Una reggia dai Medici ai Savoia* (Florence: Olschki, 2006), 276.

39 Margaret Hastings Jackson, *Catalogue of the Frances Taylor Pearsons Plimpton Collection of Italian Manuscripts in the Library of Wellesley College* (Cambridge, MA: Harvard University Press, 1929), 398.

40 One example of the transmission of Bianca's biography, from Malespini to manuscript to popular magazines, involves Henrietta Louisa Jeffreys, Countess of Pomfret (1698–1761), who lived in Florence with her family from 1739 to 1741. She wrote to her friend the Countess of Hartford in April 1740 to say that Giovanni Battista Maria Uguccioni, who worked in what she described as the "office of records," loaned her a manuscript about Medici history that included a story about Bianca, which she translated and sent to the Countess; see *Correspondence between Frances, Countess of Hartford, (Afterwards Duchess of Somerset) and Henrietta Louisa, Countess of Pomfret, between the years 1738 and 1741* (London: Richard Phillips, 1806), I:233. Uguccioni's manuscript must have been one of these 18th-century compilations. Unfortunately, the anonymous editor of the Countess's correspondence did not include the translation in this publication, noting, "This history, from its being already well known to the public, is omitted here" (*Correspondence*, I:258). I have been unable to locate the original letter, though I thank Keith Overden at the Record Office for Leicestershire, Leicester and Rutland and Dennine Dudley for their efforts on my behalf. But it seems that the Jeffreys translation did circulate. An English translation of Malespini, with additional information on the deaths of Bianca and Francesco, was published in *The Lady's Museum* 1 (1760): 344–52, 456–64, 529–37. This was one of the earliest English women's magazines, founded by Charlotte Ramsey Lennox, the novelist and protégé of Samuel Johnson. Although the magazine attributed this translation to the improbably named Offaria Cellini, described as a Florentine woman married to a British man, recent scholarship attributes it to Lennox; see Charlotte Ramsey Lennox, *The Life of Harriot Stuart, Writen by Herself*, ed. Susan Kubica Howard (Cranbury: Associated University Presses, 1995), 14. However, Lennox and Jeffreys were acquaintances and it seems more likely to me that Lennox published her friend's translation under an Italian alias. In fact, an identical version, described as "translated from the Italian by Lady Pomfret," was then published as "Bianca Capello. An Historical Novel," *The New Novelist's Magazine* 1 (1787): 16–24, perhaps correcting the earlier Cellini attribution more than 20 years after Jeffreys's death.

41 For an account of some of these see Saltini, 1898, 67, note 1.

42 Giuliano de'Ricci, *Cronaca (1532–1606)*, ed. Giuliana Sapori (Milan: Riccardo Ricciardi editore, 1972), 58 and Arditi 20–21.

43 Ricci, 136 ("favoritissima per le sue belle qualità del nostro gran duca").

44 Arditi, 62, 198 and 34. Both men also accused Bianca of consorting with the Jewish population, a troublesome contention in a city that had established one of the earliest ghettos in Europe; see Ricci, 514 and Arditi, 62, 163 and 219, as well as Stefanie Beth Siegmund, *The Medici State and the Ghetto of Florence* (Stanford: Stanford University Press, 2006).

45 Carlo Morbio, ed., *Storie dei municipi italiani* (Milan: Coi torchi di Omobono Manini, 1838), IV:25–6 ("Il Gran Duca era tanto briaco di questa Bianca, che tutto lo stato si governava per suo consiglio, e la povera regina Giovanna non era più padrona di dare un tozzo dì pane per l'amor di Dio").

46 Ricci, 41–3 and 58, Arditi, 122 and 138, and Louis de Potter, *Vie et Mémoires de Scipion de Ricci* (Paris: J. Tastu, 1826), I:135–47. I have not been able to trace these manuscripts.

47 Nicolaas ten Hove, *Memoirs of the House of Medici, from its Origin to the Death of Francesco, the Second Grand Duke of Tuscany, and of the Great Men who Flourished in Tuscany within that Period*, trans. Sir Richard Clayton (Bath: G. G. and J. Robinson, 1797), 509.

48 According to Arditi, however, he was paid six *scudi* a month, hardly a princely sum (Arditi, 136).

49 For verses allegedly sung in the Florentine streets about Piero's philandering habits see Saltini, 1898, 138.

50 Ortensio Lando, *Paradossi. Ristampa dell'edizione Lione 1543*, ed. Eugenio Canone and Germana Ernst (Pisa: Istituto editoriali e poligrafici internazionali, 1999), 89–97.

51 It is no coincidence that one of Middleton's plays, *Women Beware Women* (c. 1621), was based on Bianca Cappello's biography, which Middleton seems to have known through Malespini. For wittols in general, see Jennifer Panek, "'A Wittall cannot be a Cookold': Reading the Contented Cuckold in Early Modern English Drama and Culture," *Journal for Early Modern Cultural Studies* 1 (Fall–Winter 2001): 66–92. Early modern England was rife with horn symbolism; Shakespeare endowed many of his characters, including Othello and Falstaff, with cuckold horns and an annual carnivalesque Horn Fair took place in Kent, near a site known as Cuckold's Point. For English horn lore see John Brand and Sir Henry Ellis, *Observations on the Popular Antiquities Chiefly Illustrating the Origin of our Vulgar Customs, Ceremonies, and Superstitions* (London: Chatto and Windus, 1888), 417–22.

52 Anonymous, *The Lively Character of a Contented and Discontented Cuckold, ala-mode de Anglitere* (London and Westminster, 1760), unpaginated. Surely this idea was popular earlier; a 17th-century French engraving entitled "Le Cornard Contant" ("The Counting Cuckold")—a pun on "Le Cornard Content" (The Contented Cuckold)— as well as a slightly later British engraving based on it, shows a cuckolded husband wearing expensive clothing and counting the loot garnered from the large and bejeweled horns on his head while, in the British version, his wife earns even more for him in the next room; see Malcolm Jones, "The English Broadside Print, c. 1550–c. 1650," in *A New Companion to English Renaissance Literature and Culture*, ed. Michael Hattaway (West Sussex: John Wiley & Sons, 2010), 490.

53 Niccolò Machiavelli, "La Mandragola," in *Five Comedies of the Italian Renaissance*, ed. and trans. Laura Giannetti and Guido Ruggiero (Baltimore: Johns Hopkins University Press, 2003), 87; see also the essay by Laura Giannetti in this volume: "*The Satyr in the Kitchen Pantry*," chapter 5.

54 On Malespini's participation see Saltini 1898, 142–56.

55 In the interest of maintaining order several of the weapons Malespini describes as used in this fight had been outlawed in previous years; see, for example, Lorenzo Cantini, ed., *Legislazione Toscana* (Florence: Pietro Fantosini e figlio, 1803), 7:401–3 and 7:405–6.

56 Malespini, I:200 verso–201 verso.

57 Malespini, I:200 verso ("… passando egli per via Maggiore, vide appese d'intorno la porta di una gentildonna principalissima, che a que'tempi vi habitava, (Il cui nome, e famiglia non mi piace à dirti) più di venti paia di corni, con molti ventroni di castrato, & versatore d'inttrno sterco infinito di quei animali …"). I am grateful to Sergio Parussa and Allen Grieco for assistance with this passage. Capons, too, had a role in cuckold imagery and above all verbal puns, but they were useless in defamatory rituals that employed animal parts; see Graber and Richter.

58 Saltini, 1898, 120–22.

59 Elizabeth S. Cohen, "Honor and Gender in the Streets of Early Modern Rome," *The Journal of Interdisciplinary History* 22 (Spring 1992): 597–625.

60 See, for examples, Kate Colleran, "Scampanata at the Widows' Windows: A Case Study of Sound and Ritual Insult in Cinquecento Florence," *Urban History* 36 (2009): 359–78 and Christiane Klapisch-Zuber, *Women, Family, and Ritual in Renaissance Italy*, trans. Lydia G. Cochrane (Chicago: University of Chicago Press, 1987), 261–82.

61 Colleran, 376 note 70; for Ancient examples see William Fitzgerald, *Catullan Provocations. Lyric Poetry and the Drama of Position* (Berkeley: University of California Press, 1995), 66–7 and Rebecca R. J. Benefiel, "Dialogues of Ancient Graffiti in the House of Maius Castricius in Pompeii," *American Journal of Archaeology* 114 (2010): 59–101. Such graphic representations were relatively common in Renaissance Italy. They might even pair with a sensitively written love letter; for a letter with a sketch of the author as an enormous dripping penis staring at his beloved in the form of a vulva, see Donald Weinstein, *The Captain's Concubine: Love, Honor, and Violence in Renaissance Tuscany* (Baltimore: Johns Hopkins University Press, 2001), 132–3. Similarly explicit images appear as essentially doodles in administrative documents; see Guido A. Guerzoni, "The Erotic Fantasies of a Model Clerk: Amateur Pornography at the Beginning of the Cinquecento," in *Erotic Cultures of Renaissance Italy*, ed. Sara F. Matthews Grieco (Farnham, UK/Burlington, VT: Ashgate, 2010), 61–88.

62 Burke, 103–4 and Trevor Dean, "Gender and Insult in an Italian City: Bologna in the Later Middle Ages," *Social History* 29 (May 2004): 228. The use of horns was recorded in Spain (Scott K. Taylor, *Honor and Violence in Golden Age Spain* [New Haven/London: Yale University Press, 2008], 46–7) and England (Laura Gowing, *Domestic Dangers: Women, Words, and Sex in Early Modern London* (Oxford: Oxford University Press, 1999), 72 and 102, Martin Ingram, "Ridings, Rough Music, and Mocking Rhymes in Early Modern England," in *Popular Culture in Seventeenth-Century England*, ed. Barry Reay (London: Croom Helm, 1985), 166–97, G. R. Quaife, *Wanton Wenches and Wayward Wives* (New Brunswick, NJ: Rutgers University Press, 1979), 199–200, and D. E. Underdown, "The Taming of the Scold," in *Order and Disorder in Early Modern England*, ed. Anthony Fletcher and John Stevenson (Cambridge: Cambridge University Press, 1985), 128.

63 Gene A. Brucker, *Giovanni and Lusanna. Love and Marriage in Renaissance Florence* (Berkeley: University of California Press, 1986), 28, 85, and 89.

64 Pietro Sella, ed., *Corpus statutorumitalicorum* (Rome: Ermanno Loescher & C., 1912), I:181. ("De deponentibus ad domum alicuius habitationis cornua vel aliam rem iniuriosam et diffamatoriam. Rubrica. Si quis de nocte studiose posuerit ad domum vel ostium alicuius sive ante domum alicuius cornum sive cornua bestiarum, feces fetidas vel aliquod valde turpe aut scripturam sive cedulam continentem aliquod diffamatorium vel obbrobriosum domino vel habitatori domus, in vigenti florenis auri puniatur; et, si de die, in decem florenis auri puniatur.") This was partly transcribed in Klapisch-Zuber, 269, note 40.

65 Dean, 229.

66 Dean, 229, note 69.

67 Cohen, 606.

68 The portal was also potent on sacred buildings; for messages affixed to the door of the Florentine Duomo in response to a 1581 sermon see Morbio, IV:42.

69 Burke, 103–4; see also Andrew Graham-Dixon, *Caravaggio. A Life Sacred and Profane* (New York: W. W. Norton & Co., 2011), 287–8 and Elizabeth S. and Thomas V. Cohen, "Open and Shut: The Social Meanings of the Cinquecento Roman House," *Studies in the Decorative Arts* 9 (Fall–Winter 2001–2002): 77.

70 For this gendered distinction see Cohen and Cohen, "Open and Shut," 61–84, Laurie Nussdorfer, "The Politics of Space in Early Modern Rome," *Memoirs of the American Academy in Rome* 42 (1997): 161–86, and Guido Ruggiero, "'Più che la vita caro': Onore, matrimonio e reputazione femminile nel tardo rinascimento," *Quaderni storici* 66 (1987): 761.

71 Cohen, 610 and Dean, 228.

72 For this practice also see my *Art, Marriage, and Family in the Florentine Renaissance Palace* (New Haven and London: Yale University Press, 2008), 79–85, Diane Wolfthal, "The Woman in the Window: Licit and Illicit Sexual Desire in Renaissance Italy," in *Sex Acts in Early Modern Italy. Practice, Performance, Perversion, Punishment*, ed. Allison Levy (Farnham, UK/Burlington, VT: Ashgate, 2010), 57–75, and, in regard to the Jewish population of 16th-century Venice, see Dana E. Katz, "'Clamber not you up to the casements': On Ghetto Views and Viewing," *Jewish History* 24 (2010): 127–53.

73 Lorenzo Cantini, ed., *Legislazione Toscana* (Florence: Pietro Fantosini e figlio, 1800), 20:242–3 and Daniela Lombardi, *Matrimoni di antico regime* (Bologna: Società editrice il Mulino, 2001), 182–4.

74 Dale V. Kent, "The Importance of Being Eccentric: Giovanni Cavalcanti's View of Cosimo de'Medici's Florence," *Journal of Medieval and Renaissance Studies* 9 (1979): 130–31.

75 Romolo Caggese, ed., *Statuti della repubblica fiorentina. Statuto del podestà dell'anno 1325* (Florence: Tipografico E. Ariani, 1921), 2:200 (III:XXXV. De puniendo qui proiecerit lapides vel rombolaverit. Si michi clarum fuerit quod aliquis proiecerit lapides de nocte in domo vel pariete alicuius in civitate, burgis et suburgis, tollam ei libras quinquaginta, et plus et minus, ad arbitrium Potestatis, specta qualitate personarum et facti, et tenea[n]tur investigare et inventare hoc convicini. Et nullo modo posit proici vel debeat ad domos alicuius admoglaccum vel alio modo; et hoc faciam banniri, sub pena librarum decem, primo mense mei regiminis. Et cappellani populi in quo proiceretur admoglaccum teneantur denuntiare proicientes, et contra facientes puniam in solids quadraginta f.p.) and 201 (III:XXXVII: De puniendo qui percusserit fenestras. Si quis de die vel de nocte percusserit fenestras vel columnas alicuius in civitate, burgis vel suburgis cum aliquot genere ferramenti ad dedecus alterius, ita quod percussion appareat, vel si quis cadaver vel aliquam turpitudinem aliam prohici fecerit vel posuerit ad domum alterius et mihi clarum fuerit, tollam ei libras vigintiquinque. Qui vero extraxerit hostium de domo alterius de nocte puniam eum in libris quinquginta.)

76 For a 1537 law against nocturnal disorder see Cantini I:170–71.

77 Thomas V. Cohen and Elizabeth S. Cohen, *Words and Deeds in Renaissance Rome* (Toronto: University of Toronto Press, 1993), 100 as well as their "Open and Shut," 61–84.

78 The connection between damaged faces and palaces was likewise made by Sarah McPhee, *Bernini's Beloved. A Portrait of Costanza Piccolomini* (New Haven/London: Yale University Press, 2012), 45–6.

79 Cohen and Cohen, "Open and Shut," 70.

80 For an analysis of this incident see McPhee, 44–8.

81 Anonymous, *Dialogo dello Zoppino de la vita e genealogia di tutte le cortigiane di Roma*, ed. Gino Lanfranchi (Milan: Editrice del libroraro, 1922), 71. For the problematic association of the prostitute with the painting of the same name see Christina Neilson, *Parmigianino's Antea: A Beautiful Artifice* (New York: Frick Collection, 2008). For a similar practice in England see James Turner, *Libertines and Radicals in Early Modern London: Sexuality, Politics, and Literary Culture 1630–1685* (Cambridge: Cambridge University Press, 2002), 24–6.

82 Pietro Aretino, *I ragionamenti* (Bologna: Sampietro editore, 1965), 135–6.

83 In some ways, using a palace for popular expression was like the placement of notes on or around the Ancient fragmentary statue known as Pasquino in Rome; see Leonard Barkan, *Unearthing the Past* (New Haven/London: Yale University Press, 1999), 209–31 and Rose Marie San Juan, *Rome A City Out of Print* (Minneapolis: University of Minnesota Press, 2001), 1–21. Incidents of sacred defilement served a similar purpose. The Florentine chronicler Luca Landucci cited two examples with evident fascination; for the 1493 case see Luca Landucci, *Diario fiorentino dal 1450 al 1516*, ed. Iodoco del Badia (Florence: Sansoni, 1883), 66 and Dana E. Katz, *The Jew in the Art of the Italian Renaissance* (Philadelphia: University of Pennsylvania Press, 2008), 99–103, and for the 1501 incident see Landucci, 233–4 and William J. Connell and Giles Constable, *Sacrilege and Redemption in Renaissance Florence: The Case of Antonio Rinaldeschi* (Toronto: Centre for Renaissance and Reformation Studies, 2005).

84 Morbio, IV:28.

85 Arditi, 193.

86 Morbio, IV:38–9 and Agostino Lapini, *Diario fiorentino di Agostino Lapini dal 252 al 1596*, ed. Giuseppe Odoardo Corazzini (Florence: Sansoni, 1900), 200 ("questa fu la prima volta che sua Altezza lo dicessi, e che per cosa certa si sapessi, ancor che quasi ciascuno se lo pensassi et indovinassi").

87 Michel de Montaigne, *Journal de voyage*, ed. Louis Lautrey (Paris: Librairie Hachette et Cie, 1906), 193 ("Cete Duchesse est belle à l'opinion Italienne, un visage agreable et imprieux, le corsage gros, et de tetins à leur souhait. Elle lui sambla bien avoir la suffisance d'avoir angeolé ce Prince, et de le tenir à sa devotion long-tamps").

88 Scipione Gonzaga, *Autobiografia*, ed. Dante Della Terza (Modena: Edizioni Panini, 1987), 70 ("… nec Franciscus aut ex Joanna, aut ex Blanca Capella, quam deinde, impotenti amore victus, neque Principum genere ortam, neque integra fama, uxorem duxit, liberum praeterea sustulit quemquam").

89 Although this verse is widely quoted, the earliest reference to its use I can find is ten Hove, 2:510.

90 Arditi, 182 and 184; according to Roberto Cantagalli, the editor of the published version of Arditi's manuscript, the comment about these slanderous verses was added later.

91 Luciano Berti, *Il principe dello studiolo. Francesco I dei Medici e la fine del Rinascimento fiorentino* (Pistoia: Maschietto & Musolino, 2002), 44.

92 This apparently continued after their deaths, according to Guglielmo Enrico Saltini, "Della morte di Francesco I de'Medici e Bianca Cappello," *Archivio storico italiano* 18 (1863): 75–6; however, Saltini does not provide contemporary sources for the verses he cites.

93 Gino Fornaciari, Valentina Giuffra, Ezio Ferroglio, Sarah Gino and Raffaella Bianucci, "Plasmodium Falciparum Immuno detection in Bone Remains of Members of the Renaissance Medici Family (Florence, Italy, 16th Century)," *Transactions of the Royal Society of Tropical Medicine and Hygiene* 104 (2010): 583–7 and Gino Fornaciari, Valentina Giuffra, Ezio Ferroglio, Sarah Gino and Raffaella Bianucci, "Malaria was the Killer of Francesco I de'Medici (1531–1587)," *The American Journal of Medicine* 123 (2010): 568–9.

94 See, for example, Francesco Mari, Aldo Polettini, Donatello Lippi, and Elisabetta Bertol, "The Mysterious Death of Francesco I de'Medici and Bianca Cappello: An Arsenic Murder?" *British Medical Journal* 333 (2006): 1299–301.

95 Morbio, IV:47 ("parimente di veleno").

96 It says something about the poor opinion of Bianca that such improbable rumors were able to flourish for so long, only to be finally proven false in 1965; see Roberto Cantagalli, "Bianca Cappello e una leggenda da sfatare: la questione del figlio supposto," *Nuova rivista storica* 49 (1965): 636–52. However, even now, almost half a century after Cantagalli's well-documented study, both popular and scholarly sources continue to repeat these accusations.

2

Vincenzo Gonzaga and the Body Politic: Impotence and Virility at Court[1]

Molly Bourne

Florence, 19 February 1584: For the first born [Eleonora de'Medici], betrothal was strictly negotiated with the Prince of Mantua [Vincenzo Gonzaga], whose first wife had been a daughter of the Prince of Parma. And they were divorced on account of her impotence, something that rarely happens to women. And because the Farnese factions went about denying the thing, our Most Serene Patrons [the Medici] wanted to clarify the situation with extraordinary diligence.[2]

Giuliano de' Ricci, Cronaca (1532–1606)

On October 9, 1583, Cardinal Carlo Borromeo pronounced the annulment of the marriage of Vincenzo Gonzaga, crown prince and future Duke of Mantua, with Margherita Farnese, whom he had wed two years earlier when she was just thirteen years old.[3] The reason for the annulment, according to evidence from extensive medical examinations of the young princess, was a congenital deformation that prevented her from consummating the union.[4] Margherita's clinical diagnosis as an "unbreachable gate" rendered her perfect for the cloister, to which she was offered no alternative. Still and forever destined to be a virgin, Margherita entered a convent in Parma, where she spent the rest of her long life under the religious name of Maura Lucenia, and died there in 1643 at the age of 75. After this first fiasco in the princely marriage market, Vincenzo's family lost no time in proceeding with negotiations for a second and hopefully more successful marriage, this time to Eleonora de' Medici, eldest daughter of Grand Duke Francesco I. The future of the Gonzaga state depended upon the ability of Vincenzo (Duke Guglielmo's only son), to generate a male heir. Dynastic continuity was at stake, and procreation was, of course, critical for this purpose.

Deeply offended by Margherita's repudiation by the Gonzaga, the Farnese fomented rumors that the failure to consummate the marriage was due not to any physical "defect" of the princess, but rather the impotence of prince Vincenzo. Accusations of impotence were a powerful threat to a man's honor and identity, and when the man in question was a dynastic prince, the stakes were raised even higher. The Farnese knew this well, and were therefore unleashing a powerful weapon when they spread rumors about the Gonzaga prince, whose youthful escapades were already earning him a reputation as a pleasure-seeker who reveled in women, luxury goods, fine foods and a dashing lifestyle.[5]

As the epigraph from the Florentine chronicle of Giuliano de' Ricci points out, it wasn't long before suspicions of Vincenzo's impotence had spread beyond the princely circles of Mantua and Florence, threatening this match as well with the shameful taint of sexual inadequacy. Consequently, the Medici decided to demand proof of Vincenzo's virility as a pre-condition for granting Eleonora's hand in marriage. Thus, in March, 1584, the Gonzaga heir was obliged to demonstrate his ability to deflower an orphan girl in a carefully orchestrated test carried out in Venice. Present were political and medical eye-witnesses from both the Medici and Gonzaga courts, who meticulously described these events in documents conserved in the State Archives of both Florence and Mantua.[6]

This extraordinary episode has provided sensationalist fodder for popular 20th-century novelists like Maria Bellonci and Roger Perfitte, while filmmaker Pasquale Festa Campanile made it the focus of his 1965 feature-length film, *A Virgin for the Prince,* starring Vittorio Gassman and Virna Lisi.[7] Only a handful of scholars—amongst them Valeria Finucci, Davide Galesi and Nicholas Terpstra—have examined the affair with any sort of academic rigor, but none have as yet analyzed the sexual culture and social context in which rumors about Vincenzo's impotence circulated, nor examined the logic behind the procedures adopted for dispelling them.[8] As my essay will argue, an investigation of Vincenzo's virility test provides valuable insights into period attitudes and approaches to male impotence, demonstrating that it was considered not only a threat to family lineage, but also an integral, intangible component of how the body was implicated in the construction of a man's social identity. Moreover, the criteria according to which this test was conducted support the notion that the ability to generate offspring was not considered essential to early modern definitions of male virility. Rather, a man's sexual identity was based primarily upon his capacity to penetrate and ejaculate within a woman's body.[9]

Male and Female Impotence in the Early Modern Period

Evolving Western conceptions of gender and sexuality have influenced the ways impotence has been perceived throughout history. In the ancient world, Greek and Roman men were expected to be potent, but not excessively virile, since they also needed to exercise self-control. Although ideal penis size was debated in medical literature, men shared a preoccupation with penetrative capacity and emission, whereas procreation was not necessarily a central concern.[10] For the Western Church, penetrative sex was almost always considered immoral outside of procreative purposes, although premarital and extra-conjugal concourse were never brought entirely under its moral control.[11] Advances in scientific and medical knowledge during the early modern period demonstrate a growing preoccupation with the sexual functions of the body and the mechanics of reproduction.[12] In turn, medical theory provided new information upon which canonical doctrine and jurisprudence could base definitions of impotence, while religious leaders dedicated much time delineating what consummation was, and drafting texts to define it.[13]

An important source for definitions of sexual impotence in this period is the early 17th-century work of Paolo Zacchia (1584–1659), a medical jurist and pioneer of forensic medicine in Italy. Consisting of nine books published between 1621 and 1650, with a complete edition published in 1654, Zacchia's lengthy treatise, *Quaestiones medico-legales,* drew upon current medical knowledge and copious legal evidence. Because it scientifically clarified and summarized the Church's stance on sexual impotence and impediments to the consummation of marriage more than previous texts had done, this cornerstone of modern legal medicine soon became the standard authority for judges and advocates alike in impotence cases. The *Quaestiones* is thus a useful point of reference when considering the case of Margherita Farnese and Vincenzo Gonzaga.[14]

In post-Tridentine Italy, what we might call performative impotence was defined as the inability to perform the sexual act (*impotentia coeundi*), a condition that both ecclesiastical and civil jurisprudence clearly distinguished from another type of impotence, namely sterility (*impotentia generandi*). Only the first of these could render a marriage null, provided that the condition was permanent and predated the marriage,[15] for a marriage that had not been consummated was considered invalid by canon law. As Joanne Ferraro has shown in her work on Venetian society in this period, the term "impotence" could be applied equally to both women and men, and, in keeping with canon law, signified "the incapability to have the sexual relations necessary for reproduction."[16] Doctors agreed that, for a man, the ability to perform the sexual act from which generation could follow was defined by the presence of three elements: the erection of the genital organ, penetration inside the woman's vagina and ejaculation therein; for a woman, she must possess a vagina capable of receiving the man's genital organ.[17] According to Zacchia, sexual impotence could have either natural or functional causes. "Functional" impotence for both genders could be caused by frigidity (including *eiaculatio praecox* or erection without ejaculation for men), or by witchcraft (*maleficium*). For men, "functional" impotence could also result from emotional impediments such as timidity or repulsion, as well as from disease or a wound.[18] For women, "natural" causes of impotence were linked almost exclusively to the condition of a narrow or closed vagina that prevented the male member from entering; in most cases this involved a malformation of the vagina or the hymen, and sometimes both.[19] The "natural" causes of male impotence boasted a longer list of symptoms and potential causes, the vast majority of which concern either testicular anomalies (large or atrophied testicles; lack of testicles; testicles out of place, etc.) or malformations of the penis (long, short, slender, twisted, etc.), although according to Zacchia, most of these conditions could not be considered an impediment to marriage.[20] While Margherita Farnese's sexual impotence was a textbook case of "natural" impediment, caused by her narrow and impenetrable vagina, the accusations of impotence brought against Vincenzo were more varied, and included both "natural" and "functional" causes.

Margherita Farnese's Hymen

Less than two weeks after their wedding in Piacenza on March 2, 1581, leading medical experts were summoned urgently to Parma to examine Margherita and Vincenzo, who despite repeated attempts had not yet succeeded in consummating the marriage. For Marcello Donati, a Gonzaga court physician and tutor of Vincenzo Gonzaga who would later become secretary of state, the young Margherita had not yet reached puberty ("ne ancor le è fiorito il maggio"), although in his opinion neither her youth, nor the generous dimensions of Vincenzo's member—which was examined both erect and at rest—would have represented impediments for successful sexual relations between the couple.[21] According to Donati, it was, however, a fleshy excrescence (*una escrescenzia di carne*) that prevented Margherita from being able to receive Vincenzo's member; he recommended its surgical removal by following Arab medical lore, although he warned her entourage of the potentially fatal consequences of such a procedure.[22] The noted anatomy professor Girolamo Fabrici d'Acquapendente, who had been called from the University of Padua to examine Margherita, found that "that membrane called hymen (*quella membrana chiamata himen*), which all virgins have, … in this one is inordinately fleshy, and besides her nature is small because of her young age."[23] Rather than surgery, Acquapendente recommended the dilation of Margherita's vagina by inserting custom-made cones of increasing dimensions until a cone corresponding to the precise size of Vincenzo's penis could be easily introduced. Put into practice, this painful "therapy" was quickly suspended due to the blood-curdling screams that Margherita produced when she was subjected to it.[24]

For more than a year and a half, attempts to determine the root cause for the non-consummation of Margherita and Vincenzo's marriage continued, generating escalating tensions between the Farnese and the Gonzaga. Finally, in February 1583, Pope Gregory XIII dispatched to Parma the Milanese Archbishop and future saint, Cardinal Carlo Borromeo, in the hopes of resolving the delicate state affair once and for all: because Borromeo was respected by the Farnese and Gonzaga alike, his decision would be accepted by all parties concerned. Borromeo's role was to represent the Pope in a potential case for annulment but also to serve as a referee in the evaluation of medical testimony provided by an extraordinary deployment of doctors, surgeons, ladies-in-waiting and even a nun. At least 15 people had been called in from across the Italian peninsula to examine the genitalia of the princely couple. This examination involved not only an inspection of the Farnese princess's *pudenda,* but also a comparison with the hymens of four certified virgins, all roughly the same age as Margherita, who were brought in for the occasion from a Parmese convent and promised dowries in return.[25] As for Vincenzo, his member in erection was examined by the medical team in order to "make a secure judgment as to whether there is proportion between his member and the nature of the Most Serene Princess," although when asked how much of it he had introduced into Margherita, his answer was "none."[26] In the end, Borromeo convinced Margherita to embrace her unbreachable body by becoming a nun. She ended up following Borromeo to Milan where, at the end of May, 1583, she entered a convent for her novitiate, eventually transferring to the aristocratic convent of San Paolo in Parma. On October 9, 1583, Margherita's marriage to Vincenzo was officially annulled, and on October 30, she took her vows and the name Maura Lucenia. The Gonzaga, meanwhile, took delight in being able to retain 100,000 ducats of her dowry (one third of the original sum) since the "impediment" was determined to have been caused by the bride's impotence, and not by that of Vincenzo.[27]

Vincenzo Gonzaga's Member and the Rumor Mill

Notwithstanding Borromeo's judgment, suspicions about Vincenzo's member continued to circulate. Speculation about the crown prince's impotence first emerges in the correspondence of Cardinal Pierdonato Cesi, Papal Legate in Bologna and a key informant to the Medici court, who suspected physical problems due to a particularly enlarged penis size and to the presence of various diseases affecting the genital area. In May, 1583, Cesi shared with Grand Duke Francesco I information obtained from his own medical doctor, a certain "Beato" who also served the Gonzaga court.[28] Recently returned from Mantua, this "Beato" had informed Cesi of a rumor that Prince Vincenzo was becoming increasingly "impotent" on account of his enormous penis and erectile dysfunction: "[…] his 'material' (*materia*) is huge, and in addition to its size, it becomes flaccid and incapable of an erection that could penetrate a woman's *natura.*"[29] Moreover, the informant asserted that Vincenzo's ability was further compromised by a "fistula … located close to certain 'nerves' (*membretti*) that provide the vigor and spirit needed to achieve an erection," as well as by the prince's often excessive behavior (*disordini*).[30] Finally, there was suspicion that Vincenzo suffered from syphilis, a condition that would have further rendered him "impotent to achieve an erection or to penetrate."[31] According to Cesi, by the end of the summer the prince was still having trouble "getting it up" as a combined result of his immaturity (Vincenzo was by then 20 years of age),[32] the disadvantage of his "immense member" and "that fistula."[33]

However, the specter of Vincenzo's libertine reputation continued to loom large in the rumor mill, for in the same letter, Cesi informed the Medici Grand Duke that only a few months earlier Vincenzo, in an effort to dispel suspicions of his impotence, had attempted to "demonstrate his ability with a virgin, showing himself to be so virile that he mistreated her, and she needed to be medicated."[34]

Gonzaga-Medici marriage prospects had been fraught even without issues of impotence being brought into the fray. Back in 1580, Vincenzo's cousin Eleonora de' Medici had been a leading prospect for his first marriage, but had been passed over in favor of the more lucrative dowry offered by the Farnese.[35] Even before the union between Vincenzo and Margherita Farnese had been officially dissolved, marriage negotiations between the Gonzaga and Medici courts were resumed, but with pre-conditions. Grand Duke Francesco I, encouraged by his second wife and former mistress, Grand Duchess Bianca Cappello, was firm: the marriage between his eldest daughter and the Gonzaga crown prince would proceed only on condition that reports of Vincenzo's impotence which had been "so assertively spread by the Farnese, and upon which everything depends" be dispelled once and for all.[36] Only if the Gonzaga duke could provide assurances that his son "is potent to consummate a marriage with a young virgin" could the Gonzaga-Medici engagement be publicly announced to other European heads of state "so that ... there is no need for differences or loathing to arise."[37] Bianca Cappello had good reason to want to force the issue. Before she married Francesco I to become Grand Duchess of Tuscany, the Gonzaga had been among Bianca's most severe and outspoken critics, denouncing her as a courtesan and inappropriate match for the Grand Duke. Requiring the Gonzaga court to undergo a humiliating and widely followed test of their crown prince's virility provided a golden opportunity for her to obtain revenge at the expense of some of her most vociferous detractors.[38]

Meanwhile, embarrassing rumors of Vincenzo's impotence continued to spread dangerously. The Gonzaga chancery and diplomatic network was among the most sophisticated of those used by Europe's princely rulers, providing widespread, efficient and—in this case—potentially seditious conduits for the rapid transmission of information.[39] As recent studies have demonstrated, early modern rumors and gossip could also travel by more popular, less institutionalized means, enjoying swift diffusion via oral transmission in taverns, brothels, piazzas and other public meeting places.[40] Consequently, it wasn't long before news of Vincenzo's purported impotence had reached the papal court. Writing from Rome in early February, 1584, Aurelio Zibramonti, Bishop of Casale and a trusted advisor to the Duke of Mantua, noted that "the aforementioned difficulty [in concluding the betrothal] is very public here,"[41] although he had earlier acknowledged that Pope Gregory XIII—a promoter of the Gonzaga-Medici union—considered the notion of the Prince's impotence with virgins to be a joke (*una burla*).[42] According to Cardinal Cesi, by November, 1583, "all of Lombardy" was aware of the situation, and he advised the Grand Duke that it was "necessary to clarify this suspicion of impotence."[43] Casual demonstrations of virility were not sufficient to waylay doubts at the highest ranks of society; the scent of scandal had spread throughout the entire peninsula.

The Virility Test

By the late 16th century, impotence trials in Europe had become a standard means by which men or, somewhat less commonly, women accused of a supposedly deficient sexuality were expected to demonstrate their sexual potency or viability. As we have seen, for men this meant performing the standard trifold operation of erection, penetration and ejaculation. The test that crown prince Vincenzo needed to pass, therefore, was not designed to verify his capacity to successfully impregnate a woman, but rather his physical ability to have intercourse and emit seed in the appropriate vessel.

Impotence trials, which in terms of contemporary jurisprudence were typically marital (ecclesiastical) as opposed to criminal (civil) suits, could range from small-scale, local proceedings tried by Episcopal courts to highly publicized affairs when the accused was someone of particular note.[44] In the case of Vincenzo Gonzaga, his princely status and elevated dynastic stakes meant that the "trial" [*prova*] to ascertain his potency would be held not in a judicial court, for no marriage had yet been celebrated, but rather as a formal demonstrations in a place and according to terms that had been carefully negotiated between the Medici and Gonzaga courts, with high-ranking witnesses from each providing ocular testimony. The first proposal for dispelling these rumors of princely impotence was relatively discreet: Cardinal Cesi recommended that Don Cesare d'Este, cousin of Duke Alfonso II and friend of Vincenzo Gonzaga, provide sworn testimony that the prince was capable of having complete sexual relations with a virgin. Don Cesare had been Vincenzo's frequent companion on nocturnal adventures in Ferrara, where the crown prince often visited his beloved sister Margherita, consort of the Estense duke. Cesare promptly signed an autograph oath, dated December 11, 1583, and sent it to both the Medici and Papal courts with the following declaration: "I swear and affirm that His Highness [Vincenzo] can have an erection (*si rizza il membro*) like any other man, and that His Highness can use it carnally with any woman, virgin or not, as readily as any other man."[45] During this period, Vincenzo was also required to undergo various physical examinations. In one, "tests were made to determine whether he could support a reasonable (*onesto*) weight with his erect member and if he could thrust sufficiently against the palm of a hand so as to be able to pass through a maiden. Moreover, a model was made in the shape of his member to see whether it was so deformed as to cause impotence."[46]

The Medici, however, were not satisfied by the evidence, and after lengthy deliberations it was decided that the crown prince's successful and performative deflowering of a carefully selected virgin would constitute the most appropriate way to determine his virility and primary qualification for marriage. A successful defloration would certainly trump any moral, legal or religious scruples: the defilement of a virgin (necessarily of low social status) was considered entirely preferable to accusations of Vincenzo's impotence. This time the Medici demanded that Vincenzo demonstrate his sexual ability to deflower a virgin in a test to be held in Ferrara in the presence of Don Cesare d'Este or his father, Alfonso, both considered to be trustworthy eyewitnesses by the Medici court. This same test and pre-condition was also stipulated in the provisional marriage agreement drawn up in January, 1584.[47] Medici ambassador Orazio Urbani outlined three conditions for the test: first, that the girl's virginity be confirmed in a physical examination by a doctor and midwife; second, that she be vigilantly guarded until the test was carried out; and third, that Don Cesare attend the test and be allowed not only to watch, but "to touch with his hands as much as he can."[48] The Medici were tapping into ancient traditions here, since the use of tactile witnesses who touched the genitals can be found in oath-taking rituals in the Bible as well as in papal inspections.[49]

One of the proposed candidates for the requisite virgin in Ferrara was a daughter of the Este court antiquarian Pirro Ligorio, whose recent death had left his wife and daughters in precarious financial conditions.[50] In the end, however, the test was never carried out in Ferrarese territory. When the Gonzaga demanded that Vincenzo be granted more than one night to perform, rumors of his impotence were further amplified and, for reasons not entirely clear, both the Gonzaga heir and Cesare d'Este withdrew from the trial. Subsequently, Venice was chosen as a more neutral proving ground.[51]

It was agreed that the virgin for the Venetian test would be selected in Florence by Medici minister Belisario Vinta and approved by Marcello Donati, *medico* and trusted Gonzaga secretary, who had been instructed by Prince Vincenzo to ensure that the girl possess "the appropriate age, ability and other qualities that you know to look for," rejecting any virgins that did not conform to the crown prince's specifications and "demanding that another be found who is perfectly good, in conformity with the plan that the aforementioned S. Carlo [Gonzaga] says he has been given."[52] One of the best places to find a respectable virgin without family ties that might complicate matters was in a charitable institution such as a home for destitute girls or an orphanage. Girls from orphanages were respectable, as they were cared for by an institution that served *in loco parentis*, but at the same time they were easier to dispose of at the whims of the civic and religious authorities who ran such philanthropic services.[53] After surveying numerous orphanages, Vinta reported that the girls were "all so wretched, scabby and of such bad flesh and figure as to make you nauseous," with the exception of one found at the *Casa della Pietà* (a home for indigent girls) named Giulia, who was "twenty-one years old, tall, of fine complexion, neither thin nor fat, and with a pleasant face … modest and shy but also lively and astute, giving good likelihood that she will allow herself to be trained."[54] Although it was probably out of convenience that Vinta decided to select a virgin in Florence, the choice of a test-case virgin from the same city as Vincenzo's intended bride would not have been without significance. The fact that the final candidate was from a Florentine welfare institute would have insured both compliance on the girl's part as well as a geographic provenance that would have made her even more "similar" to the Medici girl. Although when founded in Borgo Ognissanti in 1554 this shelter for abandoned girls housed some of the city's poorest young women, who were also most sexually at risk, following its 1568 relocation to an area near Piazza SS. Annunziata the social status of the girls it took in began to improve. By 1584, when Vinta and Donati were scouring Florentine orphanages to find an "appropriate" virgin for Vincenzo's test, the Casa della Pietà may have been one of the city's more respectable homes for destitute or orphaned girls.[55]

After being subjected to a physical exam by both Donati and Medici surgeon Piero Galletti to confirm her virginity, Giulia was approved for the test and transported in secrecy to Venice by Vinta, reaching their destination on the 7th of March, 1584.[56] The following night, Vincenzo, who had arrived a few days earlier, looked Giulia over and announced that he "wished to assault here then and there" (*mostrando gran risentimento di volontà per assaltarla allhora*). However, the prince was asked to wait, both because the girl was menstruating (*le havevano cominciato le sue purghe*) and because the following day was Friday, a day deemed inappropriate for intercourse for reasons of religious decorum.[57]

In the preceding weeks, conditions for the test had been meticulously negotiated and stipulated. In exchange for conducting it in a Venetian residence occupied by the Medici envoys and not on "Gonzaga turf," prince Vincenzo was to be allowed a total of 24 hours, potentially spread over a period of a few days. A log of hours would be kept, with the clock ticking only while he was in the room with Giulia, who was to be constantly chaperoned by the unnamed *guardadonna* who had accompanied her from Florence. Each time Vincenzo came into the room, he was to be wearing only "a long robe over his nightshirt" (*una roba lunga della notte su la camicia*) and be examined by a Medici representative to ensure that he was not carrying with him "anything but his natural instrument, and that it was well made and proportioned."[58] The Medici Grand Duke accepted these conditions but reminded Vinta that it was his responsibility to "clarify as much as possible the [prince's] virility, and what is happening, providing detailed accounts of everything."[59] The first test on the night of March 10 was a disaster: while Belisario Vinta lay awake on a couch in an adjacent room, Vincenzo purportedly fell asleep on top of Giulia and later burst from the room, clutching his stomach and crying "*Cavaliere*, alas, I am sick!" The prince, evidently a victim of food poisoning from oysters (perhaps overly indulged in due to their supposed aphrodisiac effect?), quickly departed by gondola to undergo a sweet almond-oil enema, while Vinta, assisted by the *guardadonna*, confirmed that Giulia's virginity was still intact.[60] This was a major setback for members of the Gonzaga camp, who voiced concern that witchcraft (*malefici*)[61] may have played a role in the prince's embarrassing performance, and attempted to offset his initial failure by both religious and practical means: with pious orations and the application of "*morselli* to help make the penis erect."[62] Although it is not clear exactly what these "morselli" were, they may have been a medicinal electuary meant to be eaten, or a rub applied topically.[63]

On the night of Wednesday, March 14, a restored and confident Vincenzo returned to the Medici headquarters, where he undressed Giulia before disrobing in front of Vinta for the requisite inspection. Vinta then left the couple alone in the bedroom and but not fifteen minutes had passed when, according to his report, the prince called out: "*Cavaliere, Cavaliere,* come here: touch and feel it with your hand," at which point the Medici minister—who later confessed to some embarrassment—entered the room and placed his hand in between the conjoined couple to ensure that everything was exactly where, and as, it was supposed to be, and that the breached virgin was appropriately weeping. Vincenzo then curtly told Vinta: "Now that you have touched and removed all doubt, leave me to finish my business."[64]

Although the prince claimed to have "assaulted" Giulia and "broken three lances" (*disse di aver rotto tre lancie*) that night,[65] when Vinta and the Medici surgeon Piero Galletti subjected the girl to a follow-up interrogation and physical exam the next morning, she said she was not sure if she was still a virgin, confirming that seed had been emitted during their rapport but claiming that Vincenzo had not entered her completely, thus leaving the impotence question still unresolved.[66] Consequently, on the morning of March 15, with Vincenzo still in his nightshirt, Galletti thoroughly examined Vincenzo's penis. Although satisfied that his member and testicles were of normal size, Galletti reported that "because the animal was not erect, I wasn't fully convinced that he could get it inside" (*perchè l'animale non era ritto, non mi ci pareva d'aver drento* [*sic*] *il pieno della mia sodisfattione*). On the morning of March 16, however, when Vincenzo, still in bed, invited Galletti to inspect and handle his member, Galletti reported that this time it was "erect and hard like a spindle, pointed and very well proportioned" (*mostrommi il membro ritto e sodo come un fuso, appuntato, et proportionatissimo*). He added that it had not inflicted injuries on the girl despite its generous but not disproportionate size (*la grossezza et la lunghezza del membro assai grande, ma non però fuor di natura*), and that the fistula, which Vincenzo invited him to touch, while located close to the penis "had nothing to do with the instruments of coitus" (*con li instrumenti del coito non ha a far nulla*).[67] For good measure, that night Vincenzo arranged an impromptu visit to Giulia under the same secure conditions, and once again emerged victorious as we learn from a letter of March 17 to Duke Guglielmo Gonzaga from one of his envoys: "[...] you should know that last night his Lordship the Prince returned to the girl, and it was carried out so that neither she, nor Ser Vinta, nor their doctor, wishes to repeat it. This morning I spoke to everyone and they are all extremely satisfied, along with the midwife. I wanted to tell this to Your Highness so that You may know that in this test there remains not a single doubt in the world."[68]

With the virility test successfully passed, including repeat performances, preparations for the Gonzaga-Medici marriage proceeded apace. The following month, Vincenzo and Eleonora exchanged vows in Florence before traveling to Mantua for their wedding there on April 29, 1584. Vinta, who accompanied Eleonora as a member of her entourage, jubilantly reported the next day to the Medici Grand Duke that the couple "had been seen all happy, with confirmation that the marriage had been consummated, trampling for once and all the false rumors that surrounded the affair."[69] Even Grand Duchess Bianca Cappello, stepmother of Eleonora and a key orchestrator of the test, coyly expressed particular satisfaction that in this new union "his Lordship the Prince has got off to such a valorous start."[70] Giulia, on the other hand, seems to vanish from the documentary record. Unsubstantiated accounts claim that she was sent, pregnant, back to Florence, where versions of her fate vary: according to one, she was married off to Giulio Caccini of the musical group the Camerata de' Bardi, while according to another she faced life begging as a single mother.[71] While neither of these outcomes can be documented, it is certainly more probable that Giulia's tribulations would have been dealt with in a manner considered honorable at this time. The amount of publicity that accompanied this impotence trial would not have permitted the Gonzaga to abandon a deflowered virgin who may have also been pregnant (although conception is unlikely in the first couple of days following *menses*). Post-Tridentine court cases between social unequals awarded dowries to virgins who could prove the identity of the man who took their honor, through force or by seduction, and generally the penalty included care of the mother through pregnancy and childbirth, although the fate of the child was often uncertain. If not abandoned to a foundling home, illegitimate children might be cared for at the expense of their biological father until weaned, and even until seven or eight years of age (when they could begin to work); even in court circles, where illegitimate offspring were seldom a cause for moral concern or economic abandonment, their future was not necessarily assured.[72] Given the fact that Giulia was taken from a Florentine *Casa della Pietà*, her successful albeit dolorous service to the Gonzagas (and indirectly to the Medici) would have earned her a dowry, and thus the coveted future reserved to the most "fortunate" orphan girls as a respectably married woman.[73]

Conclusion

Over and above the theatricality of the impotence trial and the orchestration of its participants, this episode raises some significant issues with respect to the perception of the early modern body. The bodies and intimate anatomy of the unfortunate Margherita Farnese, of the (ex)virgin Giulia and of the randy prince Vincenzo Gonzaga were so extensively and repeatedly probed and examined that there is no question as to fact that they did not belong to the individuals who inhabited them. Neither did they belong to their families, but rather to the apparatus of the State. Sergio Bertelli's analysis of the rituals that surrounded the ruler's body during the early modern period, such as the touching of genitals during papal coronations, or the *ostentatio genitalium* of newborn male royals, reminds us that during this period, virility was an essential and non-negotiable part of a ruler's rightful claim to office.[74] Similarly, Kantorowicz's classic model of the King's two bodies is neatly illustrated by Vincenzo's *prova di virilità*, a case where the body politic became fused with the body natural—quite literally—in the performative virile member of the Gonzaga prince.[75]

A larger-than-life reputation would accompany Vincenzo until his death in 1612. After succeeding his father Guglielmo to the ducal throne in 1587, Vincenzo's reign was characterized by both political and physical excess, carried out within a context of conspicuous consumption. He fathered six children with Eleonora de' Medici and sired numerous illegitimate offspring. A profligate spender on magnificent ceremonies, music and the arts, he successfully recruited to his Court high-profile figures like Claudio Monteverdi and Peter Paul Rubens, and enriched the Gonzaga collections with important additions by the finest European artists.[76] Awarded the Order of the Golden Fleece in 1589, Vincenzo lead three costly but ultimately unsuccessful campaigns against the Ottoman Turks in Hungary in 1595, 1597 and 1601, following which he founded his own equestrian "Order of the Redeemer" in 1608. That same year, at the age of 46, Vincenzo dispatched an apothecary on a lengthy and covert journey to the New World in search of the fabled *gusano*, a worm or insect believed to possess Viagra-like powers.[77] Despite the duke's advancing age, and although recurrent arthritis prompted him to seek relief at thermal spas across Europe, Vincenzo was determined to continue his legendary lifestyle of sexual promiscuity and had no plans of slowing down. In 1608, he engaged in yet more extramarital affairs and marched as Cupid's slave in a Petrarchan "Triumph of Love" procession for the wedding festivities of his only son, Francesco.[78]

We do not know if Vincenzo's adventurous apothecary succeeded in his mission, for he had not yet returned when the duke died on February 9, 1612. Vincenzo's final Testament, written less than a week before his death, specified that his body was to be displayed for 40 hours, sitting upon a throne with his sword, and then buried in this position in the crypt of the Mantuan church of Sant'Andrea, next to the body of his consort Eleonora, who had been interred there (in the conventional supine position) the previous year.[79] By requesting burial in this unusual manner, Vincenzo may have been emulating Byzantine emperors or the patriarchs of Constantinople, rulers for whom this ancient custom was traditionally reserved.[80] Whatever the reason, it seems that—even in death—Vincenzo was determined to remain eternally erect.

Works Cited

Early Printed Sources (pre-1900)

Benzi, Ugo, *Regole della sanità et della natura de cibi. Di Vgo Benzo medico, & filosofo Sanese. Con le annotationi di Gio. Lodouico Bertaudo … Opera vtile, ornata di varie storie, et arricchita d'vn trattato nuouo della ebbrietà, & dell'abuso del tabaco.* In Torino – per gli heredi di Gio. Domenico Tarino, 1618.

Conti, Giuseppe, ed. *Altri documenti inediti sul parentado fra la Principessa Eleonora de' Medici e il Principe Don Vincenzio Gonzaga e i cimenti a cui fu costretto il detto Principe per attestare la sua Potenza virile. Tratti dal R. Archivio di Mantova e pubblicati con una nota storica.* Bibliotechina Grassoccia: Capricci e curiosità letterarie inedite o rare raccolte da F. Orlandi e G. Baccini. Florence, *Il giornale di erudizione* 26–7 (1893): 7–170.

Durante, Castore da Gualdo, *Il tesoro della sanità, di Castor Durante da Gualdo, medico, et cittadino romano. Nel quale s'insegna il modo di conservar la sanità … Et si tratta Della Natvra De' Cibi & de' Rimedij de' nocumenti loro …* Venezia, appresso Andrea Muschio, 1588.

Il Parentado fra la Principessa Eleonora de' Medici e il Principe Don Vincenzio Gonzaga e i cimenti a cui fu costretto il detto Principe per attestare come egli fosse abile alla generazione. Documenti inediti tratti dal R. Archivio di Stato di Firenze. Bibliotechina Grassoccia: Capricci e curiosità letterarie inedite o rare raccolte da F. Orlandi e G. Baccini. Florence, *Il giornale di erudizione* 5 (1886): 3–96; 6 (1887): 97–192; 7 (1888): 193–292.

Morbio, Carlo, ed. *Storia dei municipi italiani: illustrate con documenti inediti.* Vol. 4. Milan: Omobono Manini, 1838.

Secondary Sources and Modern Editions

Bajada, Joseph. *Sexual Impotence: the Contribution of Paolo Zacchia (1584–1659).* Rome: Editrice Pontificia Università Gregoriana, 1988.

Behrend-Martinez, Edward. "Manhood and the Neutered Body in Early Modern Spain." *Journal of Social History* 38:4 (2005): 1073–93.

Behrend-Martinez, Edward. "Female Sexual Potency in a Spanish Church Court, 1673–1735." *Law and History Review* 24:2 (Summer 2006): 297–330.

Behrend-Martinez, Edward. *Unfit for Marriage: Impotent Spouses on Trial in the Basque Region of Spain 1650–1750.* Reno: University of Nevada Press, 2007.

Bell, Rudolph. *How to Do It: Guides to Good Living for Renaissance Italians.* Chicago: University of Chicago Press, 1999.

Bellonci, Maria. *A Prince of Mantua: The Life and Times of Vincenzo Gonzaga,* trans. Stuart Hood. New York: Harcourt Brace and Company, 1956. First published as "Il duca nel labirinto" in *Segreti dei Gonzaga.* Milan: A. Mondadori, 1947.

Berriot-Salvadore, Évelyne. *Un Corps, Un Destin. La Femme Dans La Medecine De La Renaissance.* Paris: Honore Champion, 1993.

Bertelli, Paolo. "Appunti sulla ritrattistica di Vincenzo I Gonzaga," in *Scritti per Chiara Tellini Perina,* ed. Daniela Ferrari and Sergio Marinelli. Mantua: G. Arcari Editore, 2011. 229–49.

Bertelli, Sergio. *The King's Body: Sacred Rituals of Power in Medieval and Early Modern Europe,* trans. R. Burr Litchfield. University Park: Pennsylvania State University Press, 2001. First published as *Il corpo del Re: sacralità del potere nell'Europa medievale e moderna*. Florence: Ponte alle Grazie, 1990.

Berti, Luciano. *Il principe dello Studiolo: Francesco I dei Medici e la fine del Rinascimento fiorentino.* Florence: Edam, 1967.

Boutry, Philippe, ed. *Enfance abandonnée et société en Europe, XIVe–XXe siècle: Actes du Colloque international organisé par la Società italiana di demografia storica.* Rome: École Française de Rome, 1991.

Brundage, James A. *Law, Sex, and Christian Society in Medieval Europe*. Chicago: University of Chicago Press, 1990.

Capp, Bernard. *When Gossips Meet: Women, Family, and Neighbourhood in Early Modern England*. Oxford: Oxford University Press, 2004.

Chambers, David and Jane Martineau, eds. *Splendours of the Gonzaga.* Exhib. cat., London, November 4, 1981–January 31, 1982. Milan: A. Pizzi, 1981.

Cipolla, Costantino and Giancarlo Malacarne, eds. *El più soave et dolce et dilectevole et gratioso bochone: amore e sesso al tempo dei Gonzaga.* Rome: FrancoAngeli, 2006.

Colantuono, Anthony. *Titian, Colonna and the Renaissance Science of Procreation: Equicola's Seasons of Desire*. Farnham, UK/Burlington, VT: Ashgate, 2010.

Consiglio, Alberto, ed. *Una prova di matrimonio: Medici e Gonzaga.* Rome: Canesi editore, 1961.

Cowan, Alexander. "Gossip and Street Culture in Early Modern Venice," in *Cultural history of early modern European streets*, ed. Riitta Laitinen and Thomas V. Cohen. Leiden: Brill, 2009. 119–40.

Cristellon, Cecilia. "Public Display of Affection: The Making of Marriage in the Venetian Courts before the Council of Trent (1420–1545)" in *The Erotic Cultures of Renaissance Italy*, ed. Sara F. Matthews-Grieco. Farnham, UK/Burlington, VT: Ashgate, 2010. 173–97.

Darmon, Pierre. *Trial By Impotence: Virility and Marriage in pre-Revolutionary France,* trans. Paul Keegan. London: Chatto & Windus, 1985. First published in 1979 as *Le Tribunal de l'Impuissance.*

Eisenach, Emlyn. *Husbands, Wives, and Concubines: Marriage, Family, and Social Order in Sixteenth-Century Verona*. Kirksville, MO: Truman State University Press, 2004.

Ferrari, Daniela. "La cancelleria gonzaghesca tra Cinque e Seicento. Carriere e strategie parentali al servizio dei duchi," in *Gonzaga. La celeste galeria. L'esercizio del collezionismo*, ed. Raffaella Morselli. Milan: Skira, 2002. 297–318.

Ferraro, Joanne. *Marriage Wars in Late Renaissance Venice*. Oxford: Oxford University Press, 2001.

Ferraro, Joanne. *Nefarious Crimes, Contested Justice Illicit Sex and Infanticide in the Republic of Venice, 1557–1789*. Baltimore, MD: Johns Hopkins University Press, 2008.

Finucci, Valeria. *The Manly Masquerade: Masculinity, Paternity, and Castration in the Italian Renaissance*. Durham, NC/London: Duke University Press, 2003.

Finucci, Valeria. "Devianza sessuale e imperative genealogici: il caso di Margherita Farnese." *Acta Histriae* 15 (2007): 385–98.

Finucci, Valeria. "There's the Rub: Searching for Sexual Remedies in the New World." *Journal of Medieval and Early Modern Studies* 38.3 (2008): 523–57.

Finucci, Valeria. "The Virgin's Body and Early Modern Surgeons," in *Masculinities, Childhood, Violence: Attending to Early Modern Women—and Men*, ed. Amy E. Leonard and Karen L. Nelson. Newark: University of Delaware Press, 2011. 195–222.

Finucci, Valeria. *The Prince's Body: Vincenzo Gonzaga and Renaissance Medicine*. Cambridge, MA: Harvard University Press, forthcoming.

Flandrin, Jean-Louis. *L'Église et le contrôle des naissances*. Paris: Flammarion, 1970.

Franchini, Dario, et al. *La scienza a corte. Collezionismo eclettico, natura e imagine a Mantova fra Rinascimento e Manierismo*. Rome: Bulzoni Editore, 1979.

Galesi, Davide. "L'eros politico del principe Vincenzo," in Cipolla and Malacarne, *El più soave*, 245–63.

Gavitt, Philip. *Charity and Children in Renaissance Florence: The Ospedale degli Innocenti, 1410–1536*. Ann Arbor: University of Michigan Press, 1990.

Hacke, Daniela. *Women, Sex and Marriage in Early Modern Venice*. Aldershot, UK/ Burlington, VT: Ashgate, 2004.

Horodowich, Elizabeth. "The gossiping tongue: oral networks, public life and political culture in early modern Venice." *Renaissance Studies* 19:1 (2005): 22–45.

Kantorowicz, Ernst. *The King's Two Bodies: A Study in Medieval Political Theology*. Princeton, Princeton University Press, 1957.

Kümin, Beat. *Drinking Matters: Public Houses and Social Exchange in Early Modern Central Europe*. Basingstoke: Palgrave Macmillan, 2007.

Laqueur, Thomas. *Making Sex: Body and Gender from the Greeks to Freud*. Cambridge, MA: Harvard University Press, 1990.

Lepri, Nicoletta. "Nuovi documenti sulle nozze di Vincenzo Gonzaga e Margherita Farnese (1581)." *Civiltà Mantovana* 124 (2007): 167–93.

McClive, Cathy. "Masculinity on Trial: Penises, Hermaphrodites and the Uncertain Male Body in Early Modern France." *History Workshop Journal* 68 (2009): 45–68.

McLaren, Angus. *Impotence: A Cultural History*. Chicago: University of Chicago Press, 2007.

Merrick, Jeffrey. "Impotence in Court and at Court." *Studies in Eighteenth Century Culture* 25 (1996): 187–202.

Pazzini, Adalberto. "La medicina alla corte dei Gonzaga a Mantova," in *Mantova e i Gonzaga nella civiltà del rinascimento*, Acts of Congress held in Mantua, 6–8 October 1974. Verona: A. Mondadori, 1977. 291–351.

Perfitte, Roger. *The Prince's Person*, trans. Peter Fryer. London: Secker & Warburg, 1964. First published as *La Nature du Prince*. Paris, 1963.

Piccinelli, Roberta. "Le facies del collezionismo artistico di Vincenzo Gonzaga," in *Gonzaga. La celeste galeria. L'esercizio del collezionismo*, ed. Raffaella Morselli. Milan: Skira, 2002, 341–47.

Pullan, Brian. "Orphans and Foundlings in Early Modern Europe" in *Poverty and Charity: Europe, Italy, Venice, 1400–1700*. Aldershot, UK: Variorum, 1994. III: 5–28.

Quazza, Romolo. *La diplomazia gonzaghesca.* Milan: Istituto per gli studi di politica internazionale, 1941.

Ricci, Giuliano de'. *Giuliano de' Ricci, Cronaca (1532–1606)*, ed. Giuliana Sapori. Milan: Riccardo Ricciardi, 1972.

Satta, Fiamma. "Margherita Farnese." *Dizionario Biografico degli Italiani* 45 (1995): 106–8.

Scansani, Stefano. *L'amor morto.* Milan: Mondadori, 1991.

Seidel Menchi, Silvana and Diego Quaglioni, eds. *Trasgressioni. Concubinato, adulterio, bigamia (secoli XIV–XVIII). Processi matrimoniali degli archivi ecclesiastici italiani.* Bologna: Il Mulino, 2004.

Severi, Rita. "'Mantova porto bramato.' Viaggio, morte e fama di James Crichton, scozzese." *Quaderni di Palazzo Te* (n.s.) 3 (1996): 55–65.

Signorini, Rodolfo. "Gonzaga Tombs and Catalfalques," in Chambers and Martineau, *Splendours.* 3–13.

Simons, Patricia. *The Sex of Men in Premodern Europe: A Cultural History.* Cambridge: Cambridge University Press, 2011.

Taddei, Illaria. *Fanciulli e giovani: Crescere a Firenze nel Rinascimento.* Florence: Leo S. Olschki, 2001.

Terpstra, Nicholas. *Lost Girls: Sex and Death in Renaissance Florence.* Baltimore, MD: Johns Hopkins University Press, 2010.

Trexler, Richard. "The Foundlings of Florence, 1395–1455." *History of Childhood Quarterly* 1 (1973): 259–84.

Venturelli, Paola. *Vincenzo I Gonzaga 1562–1612. Il fasto del potere.* Exh. cat. Mantua, February 18–June 10, 2012. Mantua: Publi Paolini, 2012.

Viazzo, Pier Paolo, Maria Bartolotto and Andrea Zanotto. "Five Centuries of Foundling History in Florence: Changing Patterns of Abandonment, Care, and Mortality," in *Abandoned Children*, ed. Catherine Panter-Brick and Malcom T. Smith. Cambridge: Cambridge University Press, 2000. 70–91.

Vivo, Filippo de. *Information and Communication in Venice: Rethinking Early Modern Politics.* Oxford: Oxford University Press, 2007.

Wiesner-Hanks, Merry. *Christianity and Sexuality in the Early Modern World: Regulating Desire, Reforming Practice.* Cambridge: Cambridge University Press, 1999.

Zanca, Attilio. *Notizie sulla vita e sulle opera di Marcello Donati da Mantova (1538–1602) medico, umanista, uomo di stato.* Pisa: Casa Editrice Giardini, 1964.

Notes

1 I wish to thank Laura Gianetti, Sara Matthews-Grieco, Anne MacNeil, Jacqueline Musacchio and Nick Terpstra for helpful discussions during my preparation of this essay. Unless indicated otherwise, all translations are my own.

2 "Firenze. Addì 19 di febbraio 1583 al fiorentino … Per la primogenita si è trattato strettamente parentado con il principe di Mantova, quale prima havea hauto per moglie una figliola del principe di Parma. Et feciono divorzio per la inpotenzia di lei, cosa di rado suole alle donne avvenire. Et perché da i satellite de'Farnesi si andava bociando la cosa altrimenti, li nostri serenissimi patroni si volsono con strasordinarie [*sic*] diligentie assai ben chiarire" (Giuliano de' Ricci, *Cronaca (1532–1606)*, ed. Giuliana Sapori [Milan: Riccardo Ricciardi, 1972], 404). While the chronicler Giuliano de' Ricci (1543–1606), a highly educated member of a Florentine mercantile family, was not opposed to Medici rule, like many fellow citizens he did not approve of the union

between Francesco I and Bianca Cappello. I thank Jacki Musacchio for suggesting that I examine this chronicle for comments concerning Vincenzo Gonzaga's virility test.

3 Margarita Farnese, born in Parma on November 7, 1567, was 13 in March 1581 when she married Vincenzo Gonzaga on March 2, 1581; Vincenzo, born September 21, 1562, was 18 at the time.

4 Valeria Finucci, "The Virgin's Body and Early Modern Surgeons," in *Masculinities, Childhood, Violence: Attending to Early Modern Women—and Men*, ed. Amy E. Leonard and Karen L. Nelson (Newark: University of Delaware Press, 2011), 195–222; eadem, "Devianza sessuale e imperative genealogici: il caso di Margherita Farnese," *Acta Histriae* 15 (2007): 385–98. On the March 1581 wedding of Vincenzo Gonzaga and Margherita Farnese, see Nicoletta Lepri, "Nuovi documenti sulle nozze di Vincenzo Gonzaga e Margherita Farnese (1581)," *Civiltà Mantovana* 124 (2007): 167–93.

5 This is a reputation Vincenzo would maintain throughout his life. The popular novelist Maria Bellonci memorably describes the young Vincenzo as the physical and moral opposite of his father: "Guglielmo was deeply religious and so after a fashion—a highly elaborate one—was Vincenzo. He liked the beauty of the church services, the altars with their silver statues, the great storied pictures; but instead of choosing churchmen for his friends and secretaries, as his father did ... Vincenzo picked as his companions the most degenerate of youths, abnormal libertines. His dress was of extreme elegance. He always wore jewels and velvets and rich brocades. Across his breast he carried silken sashes stiff with symbolical embroidery, and at his wrists, cuffs sewn by his mistresses ... He drank great goblets of Greek wine and ate heartily; he danced and leapt into the saddle and jousted and enjoyed women, with whom he was proving tender, fervent, and very fickle" (Maria Bellonci, *A Prince of Mantua: The Life and Times of Vincenzo Gonzaga*, trans. Stuart Hood [New York: Harcourt Brace and Company, 1956], 10–11, first published as "Il duca nel labirinto" in *Segreti dei Gonzaga* [Milan: A. Mondadori, 1947]). In July 1582 Vincenzo famously murdered the young Scottish scholar James Crichton, who was visiting Mantua as a guest of the court; see Rita Severi, "'Mantova porto bramato.' Viaggio, morte e fama di James Crichton, scozzese," *Quaderni di Palazzo Te* (n.s.) 3 (1996): 55–65; Dario Franchini et. al, *La scienza a corte. Collezionismo eclettico, natura e imagine a Mantova fra Rinascimento e Manierismo* (Rome: Bulzoni Editore, 1979), 31–3.

6 Complete transcriptions of the copious relevant correspondence was first published in the late 19th century. For the Florentine documents, see *Il Parentado fra la Principessa Eleonora de' Medici e il Principe Don Vincenzio Gonzaga e i cimenti a cui fu costretto il detto Principe per attestare come egli fosse abile alla generazione. Documenti inediti tratti dal R. Archivio di Stato di Firenze,* "Bibliotechina Grassoccia: Capricci e curiosità letterarie inedite o rare raccolte da F. Orlandi e G. Baccini," Florence, *Il giornale di erudizione* 5 (1886): 3–96; 6 (1887): 97–192; 7 (1888): 193–292, republished verbatim by Alberto Consiglio, ed. *Una prova di matrimonio: Medici e Gonzaga* (Rome: Canesi editore, 1961). A selection of these documents, edited by Giancarlo Malacarne, were republished by Costantino Cipolla and Giancarlo Malacarne, eds., *El più soave et dolce et dilectevole et gratioso bochone: amore e sesso al tempo dei Gonzaga* (Rome: FrancoAngeli, 2006), 421–37. For the Mantuan documents, see Giuseppe Conti, ed. *Altri documenti inediti sul parentado fra la Principessa Eleonora de' Medici e il Principe Don Vincenzio Gonzaga e i cimenti a cui fu costretto il detto Principe per attestare la sua Potenza virile. Tratti dal R. Archivio di Mantova e pubblicati con una nota storica,* "Bibliotechina Grassoccia: Capricci e curiosità letterarie inedite o rare raccolte da F. Orlandi e G. Baccini," Florence, *Il giornale di erudizione* 26–7 (1893): 7–170.

7 Bellonci, *Prince of Mantua*; Roger Perfitte, *The Prince's Person*, trans. Peter Fryer (London: Secker & Warburg, 1964), first published as *La Nature du Prince* (Paris, 1963). While not a novel, see also Stefano Scansani's, *L'amor morto* (Milan: Mondadori, 1991), which is similarly characterized by a largely sensationalist approach to Vincenzo's sexuality.

8 Valeria Finucci, "The Virgin's Body," esp. 202–13, and eadem "Devianza sessuale," esp. 390–95; see also Finucci's book, *The Prince's Bodyl: Vincenzo Gonzaga and Renaissance Medicine* (Cambridge, MA, Harvard University Press, forthcoming); Davide Galesi, "L'eros politico del principe Vincenzo," in *El più soave et dolce et dilectevole et gratioso bochone. Amore e sesso al tempo dei* Gonzaga, eds. Costantino Cipolla and Giancarlo Malacarne (Rome: FrancoAngeli, 2006), 245–63; Nicholas Terpstra, *Lost Girls: Sex and Death in Renaissance Florence* (Baltimore, MD: Johns Hopkins University Press, 2010), esp. 183–90. The dissolution of the Gonzaga-Farnese marriage and Vincenzo's virility test are also discussed from a medical point of view by Adalberto Pazzini, "La medicina alla corte dei Gonzaga a Mantova," in *Mantova e i Gonzaga nella civiltà del rinascimento*, Acts of Congress held in Mantua, 6–8 October 1974 (Verona: A. Mondadori, 1977), 291–351 (at 324–31).

9 My findings support the "penetration-with-emission" construction of early modern male virility as presented by Patricia Simons, *The Sex of Men in Premodern Europe: A Cultural History* (Cambridge: Cambridge University Press, 2011), esp. 5–6, 25–51, 189–90. For the alternative model of virility based on a man's ability to engender progeny, see Valeria Finucci, *The Manly Masquerade: Masculinity, Paternity, and Castration in the Italian Renaissance* (Durham, NC: Duke University Press, 2003), esp. Chapter 6, 225–80; for a fascinating discussion of how messages of dynastic procreation were embodied in artistic projects at the Estense court during this period, see Anthony Colantuono, *Titian, Colonna and the Renaissance Science of Procreation: Equicola's Seasons of Desire* (Farnham, UK/Burlington, VT: Ashgate, 2010).

10 Simons, *The Sex of Men*, Part II, "Projecting male sex: models and metaphors."

11 On Church attitudes towards sexuality see, for example: Jean-Louis Flandrin, *L'Église et le contrôle des naissances* (Paris: Flammarion, 1970); James A. Brundage, *Law, Sex, and Christian Society in Medieval Europe* (Chicago: University of Chicago Press, 1990); Merry Wiesner-Hanks, *Christianity and Sexuality in the Early Modern World: Regulating Desire, Reforming Practice* (Cambridge: Cambridge University Press, 1999).

12 See for example: Thomas Laqueur, *Making Sex: Body and Gender from the Greeks to Freud* (Cambridge, MA: Harvard University Press, 1990); Évelyne Berriot-Salvadore, *Un Corps, Un Destin. La Femme Dans La Medecine De La Renaissance* (Paris: Honore Champion, 1993); Rudolph Bell, *How to Do It: Guides to Good Living for Renaissance Italians* (Chicago: University of Chicago Press, 2000).

13 A useful overview of the history of impotence in the western world from classical times up to the present is given by Angus McLaren, *Impotence: A Cultural History* (Chicago: University of Chicago Press, 2007).

14 Joseph Bajada, *Sexual Impotence: the Contribution of Paolo Zacchia (1584–1659)* (Rome: Editrice Pontificia Università Gregoriana, 1988).

15 Ibid., 15.

16 Joanne Ferraro, *Marriage Wars in Late Renaissance Venice* (Oxford: Oxford University Press, 2001), 70. For discussions of impotence and its implications, see esp. 69–103.

17 Bajada, *Sexual Impotence*, 75–7, 129–32.

18 Ibid., 107–28; 149–59.

19 Ibid., 129–48.

20 Ibid., 81–105.

21 "Insomma il membro del maschio è più grossa di quello che possa comportare la natura della femmina che è picciola fuor di l'ordinario, per quanto mi dice il Sig.r Principe … né ancor le è fiorito Maggio" (Donati to duke Guglielmo Gonzaga, 11 March 1581, Attilio Zanca, *Notizie sulla vita e sulle opera di Marcello Donati da Mantova (1538–1602) medico, umanista, uomo di stato* [Pisa: Casa Editrice Giardini, 1964, 14]).

22 "Se bene sono molte le cagioni che possono impedire la donna a vicinarsi il membro dell'huomo, non dimeno io, lasciate l'altre, mi restringerò a quella che nel caso nostro con la fede dell'occhio è stata giudicata propria et particolare cioè che sia una escrescenzia di carne; questa Signor mio è necessaria che sia levata perché essendo forata concludono tutti i nostri dottori che in tutto et impedisca l'entrata del membro dell'huomo … bisogna essere benissimo avvertiti nel tagliare che non si tocchi parte della matrice, altrimenti sopravvengono dolori spasmosi, flussi di sangue pericolosissimi, ulcere et apostemi della matrice effetti tutti mortali. Il modo dell'aministrare quella operazione è descritto minutissimamente da nostri autori Arabi poiché da Greci poco o nulla è stato scritto in qualle [*sic*] materia …" (Marcello Donati to Gonzaga secretary Aurelio Zibramonti, 15 March 1581; Zanca, *Notizie sulla vita*, 15–16; see also the discussions by Finucci, "Devianza," 390–95; eadem "Virgin's Body," 203–4).

23 The opinion of Acquapendente is recounted in Marcello Donati's letter of 8 April 1581 to Zibramonti: "quella membrana chiamata himen che si trova in tutte le vergini che in questa è carnosa più del ordinario et che anco la natura è piccola per la poca età" (Zanca, *Notizie sulla vita*, 16; translation from Finucci, "Virgin's Body," 204). Acquapendente had studied in Padua under Gabriele Fallopio, one of the earliest members of the medical profession to recognize the hymen and understand that it broke in the case of complete sexual relations. See Finucci, "Virgin's Body," 200.

24 Finucci, "Devianza sessuale," 391.

25 The episode is recounted by Finucci, "Devianza sessuale," 393–5; eadem, "Virgin's Body," 206–8.

26 "Bisogna ch'il membro sia erretto per far giudicio sicuro si vi sia proportione fra esso et la natura della Ser.ma S.ra Principessa. Nella visita hanno li sopradetti medici dimandato a S.A. quanta parte della gianda ella ha introdotto con essa Ser.ma S.ra, et S.A. ha risposto che non ne ha introdotto niente" (letter of Aurelio Zibramonti in Reggio Emilia, 15 February 1583, Archivio di Stato di Mantova, Archivio Gonzaga b. 201, cc. 344–5, Cipolla and Malacarne, *El più soave*, 422 doc. A/I).

27 Fiamma Satta, entry for "Margherita Farnese," *Dizionario Biografico degli Italiani* 45 (1995): 106–8, at 107.

28 Valeria Finucci identifies this "Beato" as the "well-known Bolognese doctor Gabriello Beato," a figure about whom I have been unable to locate further information. Finucci, "Virgin's Body," 209.

29 "Ha la materia grandissima, la quale oltre che per la grandezza, diventi fiacca et impotente a erigersi per posser penetrare in la natura della donna" (Cardinal Cesi in Bologna to Grand Duke Francesco I de' Medici, 31 May 1583; Consiglio, *Una prova*, 30 [doc. 1]).

30 "[la materia] diventa ancora tanto più fiacca et impotente per quella fistula che V. Altezza scrive, essendo vicina a certi membretti quali soglion dar forza et spirito di far erigere la materia, oltra poi che per infiniti disordini che fa, il Beato tiene che ogni dì si augmenta questa impotentia; dice bene che stando il Principe con donne, si corrompe et *emictit semen*; ma non crede che possa poi eriger da penetrar dentro come saria per posser ingravidare, et tutto questo detto Beato lo sa per haverlo intese diverse volte segretemente a Mantua …" (ibid.). In his 1564 treatise, the noted professor of anatomy at the University of Padua, Prospero Borgarucci, attempted to define the anatomical nature of the male member. Excluding the possibility that it was made of nerve, membrane, muscle or cartilage, he argued that it consisted of fatty ligament, with arteries and nerves extending to the tip of the penis that served to enable an erection. See Rudolph Bell, *How to Do It: Guides to Good Living for Renaissance Italians* (Chicago: University of Chicago Press, 1999), 55–7.

31 "Si che il Beato conclude che per quest'accidente et altro che il Principe di Mantua ha ancora il mal francese, oltre li sopra detti difetti et per questo lui tiene più si debbia render impotente a eriger et penetrar" (Cardinal Cesi in Bologna to Grand Duke Francesco I de' Medici, 31 May 1583; Consiglio, *Una prova*, 31 [doc. 1]).

32 At age 20 Vincenzo would have been considered an immature youth. On the stages of male adolescence and youth in Renaissance Italy see Illaria Taddei, *Fanciulli e giovani: Crescere a Firenze nel Rinascimento* (Florence: Leo S. Olschki, 2001).

33 "Et dice che il non posser eriger più che tanto et che in questo, essendo giovane, mostra debolezza, procede dal membro smisurato che ha et da quella fistula che ha" (Cardinal Cesi in Bologna to Grand Duke Francesco I de' Medici, 21 August 1583; ibid., 32 [doc. II]).

34 "[il Beato] ha ben inteso ragionar et discorrere tra quelli della Corte che veramente il Principe è potente, e tanto più con donne che non siano vergini, anzi ha inteso ancora che volse provare con una vergine alcuni mesi sono, et si mostrò tanto potente che la trattò male e bisognò medicarla" (ibid.).

35 Lepri, "Nuovi documenti," 169–70.

36 "Purchè mi si levi lo scrupolo, che importa il tutto, della voce, che così asseverantemente è stata sparsa dai Farnesi, dell'impotentia di quel Principe" (Grand Duke Francesco I in Poggio a Caiano to Cardinal Cesi, 30 October 1583; Conti, *Altri documenti*, 51 [doc. IV]).

37 "Se ne lasciasse intendere al S.r Duca, che assicurando, che suo figlio sia potente a consumar matrimonio con giovane Vergine, che il parentado non haverà difficultà, et pigli anco V.S. Ill.ma appuntamento, che concludendosi la pratica si rimanga di darne conto in un medesimo tempo di concerto all'Imperatore, al Re Cattolicissimo, alli Archiduchi, et a chi convenga, affinchè prevenendo in questo complimento l'una delle parti l'altra, non ci havesse a nascere disgusti et alterazioni" (ibid., 51–2).

38 On Bianca Cappello's motivations for demanding and orchestrating the terms of Vincenzo's virility test, see the introduction to Consiglio, *Una prova*, 21–4.

39 The classic study of the Gonzaga chancery remains Romolo Quazza, *La diplomazia gonzaghesca* (Milan: Istituto per gli studi di politica internazionale, 1941). See also Daniela Ferrari, "La cancelleria gonzaghesca tra Cinque e Seicento. Carriere e strategie parentali al servizio dei duchi," in *Gonzaga. La celeste galeria. L'esercizio del collezionismo*, ed. Raffaella Morselli (Milan: Skira, 2002), 297–318.

40 Elizabeth Horodowich, "The gossiping tongue: oral networks, public life and political culture in early modern Venice," *Renaissance Studies* 19.1 (2005): 22–45; Filippo de Vivo, *Information and Communication in Venice: Rethinking Early Modern Politics* (Oxford: Oxford University Press, 2007); Alexander Cowan, "Gossip and Street Culture in Early Modern Venice," in *Cultural History of Early Modern European Streets*, ed. Riitta Laitinen and Thomas V. Cohen (Leiden: Brill, 2009), 119–40. See also Bernard Capp, *When Gossips Meet: Women, Family, and Neighbourhood in Early Modern England* (Oxford: Oxford University Press, 2004); Beat Kümin, *Drinking Matters: Public Houses and Social Exchange in Early Modern Central Europe* (Basingstoke: Palgrave Macmillan, 2007).

41 "La suddetta difficultà è assai pubblica qui, et come sono varie le passioni, così vari anco sono li pareri; alcuni danno torto al Gran Duca che procuri di far procedere un peccato ad un Sacramento, et non si fidi della parola del S.mo Principe, altri gli danno ragione a volere chiarezza, essendo insospettito per tante vie, et massime dei primi medici che intervennero alla cura della S.ra D. Maura Lucenia [Margherita Farnese]" (Aurelio Zibramonti in Rome to Duke Guglielmo Gonzaga, 4 February 1584; Conti, *Altri documenti*, 82–3 [doc. XVIII]).

42 "Sua Santità ... desidera che questo matrimonio riesca, nè sa intendere che cosa lo possa impedire, nè differire, essendovi tanta ragione dall'una et l'altra parte di farlo, et che il dubbio dell'impotenza del S.r Principe con vergini è una burla" (Aurelio Zibramonte in Rome to Duke Guglielmo Gonzaga, December 19, 1583; ibid., 64–5 [doc. IX]).

43 "In conclusione il prefato Vescovo [Zibramonti] restò sodisfattissimo di quanto V.A. [Francesco I] scriveva, et mi disse che teneva per certo che il sig. Duca di Mantua ancora restaria sodisfattissimo, perché era necessario chiarir questo dubio dell'impotentia, et tanto più, essendosi già pubblicato tal dubio per tutta Lombardia da quelli stessi che V.A. scrive, et che questo non solo lo sapeva il sig. Duca, ma il principe ancora" (Cardinal Cesi in Rome to Grand Duke Francesco I de' Medici, 11 November 1583; Consiglio, *Una prova*, 33 [doc. III]).

44 Much work on impotence trials has been done for early modern France; see Pierre Darmon's classic "*Trial By Impotence: Virility and Marriage in pre-Revolutionary France*, trans. Paul Keegan (London: Chatto & Windus, 1985), first published in 1979 as *Le Tribunal de l'Impuissance*. See also Cathy McClive, "Masculinity on Trial: Penises, Hermaphrodites and the Uncertain Male Body in Early Modern France," *History Workshop Journal* 68 (2009): 45–68; Jeffrey Merrick, "Impotence in Court and at Court," *Studies in Eighteenth Century Culture* 25 (1996): 187–202. On impotence trials in Spain, see Edward Behrend-Martinez, "Manhood and the Neutered Body in Early Modern Spain," *Journal of Social History* 38:4 (2005): 1073–93; idem, *Unfit for Marriage: Impotent Spouses on Trial in the Basque Region of Spain 1650–1750* (Reno: University of Nevada Press, 2007); idem, "Female Sexual Potency in a Spanish Church Court, 1673–1735," *Law and History Review* 24,2 (Summer 2006): 297–330. On the relative responsibility of civil and ecclesiastical courts in Italy see Cecilia Cristellon, "Public Display of Affection: The Making of Marriage in the Venetian Courts before the Council of Trent (1420–1545)" in Sara F. Matthews-Grieco (ed.), *The Erotic Cultures of Renaissance Italy* (Farnham, UK/Burlington/VT: Ashgate, 2010) 173–97.

45 "Non potendo io per debito di conoscienza mancare d'affirmare quello ch'io so dell'attitudine del serenissimo Sig. Principe di Mantova, dico et affermo che all'A.S. si rizza il membro come a qual si voglia altro huomo, et che so che S.A. può usare carnalmente con ogni donna vergine o non vergine così prontamente quanto qualunque altro che sia, et in fede del vero ho fatto la presente di mia mano et sottoscritta il dì soprascritto," Affidavit of Don Cesare d'Este, 11 December 1583 (Consiglio, *Una prova*, 40–41 [doc. VII]).

46 These tests are described in an *avviso* from Milan (undated but probably from December 1583) conserved in the Florentine State Archives: "Dicono anco essersi fatto prova se può reggere peso honesto con il membro ritto, et se può aspettare incontro fattoli col palmo delle mani tanto che potesse una cittella. Et di più fatto una misura in forma di natura per veder se il membro suo è tanto disforme che causi l'impotentia" (Archivio di Stato di Firenze, Mediceo del Principato, filza 3255, n.n. in Documentary Sources for the Arts and Humanities [Medici Archive Project, Inc.], doc. ID 10834; translation from Finucci, "Virgin's Body," 209).

47 The amendment to the provisional marriage agreement, signed in Florence by Gonzaga agent Carlo Gonzaga on 6 January 1584 (modern dating), stated: "Quanto alla potentia et attitudine del Sig. Principe di Mantova al matrimonio con fanciulla vergine, o il Sig. Don Alfonso d'Este, o il Sig. Don Cesare suo figliuolo, a' quali si presterà indubitata fede, debbano testificarlo per altra pruova vistane innanzi in qualche vergine, et ciò habbia da precedere all'essecutione d'ogni altra cosa et non ci essendo questa, non sia fatto nulla, perché importa il tutto, et non è conveniente haver poi a fare dire di sé, né fare una inimicitia in cambio di quel parentado et cordiale unione, che si desidera da amendue le parti" (Consiglio, *Una* prova, 49 [doc. XI]). A similar amendment, signed by Grand Duke Francesco I de'Medici and dated 12 January 1584 (modern dating), is transcribed by Conti, *Altri documenti*, 45–7 [doc. I]).

48 "Il negotio insomma si restringa a tre capi: l'uno che si trovi fanciulla securamente vergine e che sia sana; il secondo che trovatala si mantenga sotto la debita custodia fin che si faccia la prova, et il terzo avvertire che l'amico [Vincenzo] la svergini nel modo che si conviene e non con violenza di mano o altro artifizio. Quanto al primo si farà vedere et tochare e disaminare al medico et a una comare, alla presentia del Sig. Don Alfonso e mia; circa al second l'Ecc. S. dice che s'obbliga, e dà la parola sua, di custodirla sicurissima e lontana da ogni sospetto; per il terzo finalmente procurerà che l'amico non parli alla fanciulla fuori della sua presentia. Sarà presente insieme col Sig. Don Cesare alla fazione, né solalmente vorrà vedere, ma tochare con le mani al più che potrà" (Orazio Urbani in Ferrara to Grand Duke Francesco I de' Medici, 16 January 1584 (modern dating); Consiglio, *Una prova*, 58–9 [doc. XXII]).

49 Simons, *Sex of Men*, 106.

50 "Io allora le proposi alcune figliole di M. Pirro Ligorio antiquario, il quale è pocho che morì avendo lassato la moglie che è non ferrarese ma romana, donna di buona vita, e similmente molte figliuole con pochissima facultà da recapitarle" (Urbani in Ferrara to Francesco I, 16 January 1584 [modern dating], Consiglio, *Una prova*, 58 [doc. XXII]).

51 "Restiamo fortemente meravigliati, et insospettiti per la recusatione che ha fatta il Principe, et quello che non fa in tutta una notte un giovane di 21 anno, che poteva ancho tirare quella notte in lugno [*sic*] sino a qualche hora del giorno, secondo il suo comodo, meno si deve sperare che lo faccia in più notti, né mai più sentito, che una prova tale si allunghi per più notti, sicché non sappiamo che ci dire, se non ringratiare affettuosamente il Sig. Don Alfonso et sempre più meravigliarci di questa ritirata, con accusarcisi il timore della impotentia, della quale havendo noi sospettato per quelle monellate, et per quella pubblica fama che sapete, dal principio al mezzo alla fine habbiamo sempre posta questa conditione dello esserne prima innanzi ad ogni altra cosa certificati" (minutes of letter from Grand Duke Francesco I de' Medici to Orazio Urbani, 21 January 1584; ibid., 72–3 [doc. XXIX]). See also the letter of Urbani in Ferrara to Francesco I de' Medici, 6 February 1583: "Quanto al Sig. Principe … questa sua disdetta della pruova per una notte, si son tanto in universale achresciuti i circolamenti, et il solito sospetto di qualche sua impotenzia, che anche da molti si specifica hora la causa di tale impotentia essere che per quella sua fistola gli fu dato un bottone di fuoco, il quale venne ad offendere qualche nerbetto o cosa simile" (ibid., 84 [doc. XXXIX]).

52 "Andando dunque collà colle lettere nostre credenziali vederete la giovane preparata per questo, et avvertirete che in lei siano le qualità convenienti, dell'età, abilità et altre che sapete ricercarsi. Et caso che il soggetto che ne preparano alla prima non vi paia a proposito, farete instanza che se ne trovi altra compitamente buona conforme all'intentione che il suddeto S.r Carlo [Gonzaga] scrive esserle stata data" (Vincenzo Gonzaga in Mantua to Marcello Donati, 10 February 1584; Conti, *Altri documenti*, 88–9 [doc. XX]).

53 On foundling homes and charitable institutions for girls in Renaissance Italy see: Richard Trexler, "The Foundlings of Florence, 1395–1455." *History of Childhood Quarterly* 1 (1973): 259–84; Philip Gavitt, *Charity and Children in Renaissance Florence: The Ospedale Degli Innocenti, 1410-1536* (Ann Arbor: University of Michigan Press, 1990); Philippe Boutry (ed.), *Enfance abandonnée et société en Europe, XIVe–XXe siècle: Actes du Colloque international organisé par la Società italiana di demografia storica* (Rome: École Française de Rome, 1991); Brian Pullan, "Orphans and Foundlings in Early Modern Europe" in *Poverty and Charity: Europe, Italy, Venice, 1400–1700* (Aldershot, UK: Variorum, 1994) III: 5–28; Pier Paolo Viazzo, Maria Bartolotto and Andrea Zanotto, "Five Centuries of Foundling History in Florence: Changing Patterns of Abandonment, Care, and Mortality" in *Abandoned Children*, ed. Catherine Panter-Brick and Malcom T. Smith (Cambridge: Cambridge University Press, 2000), 70–91; Nicholas Terpstra, *Lost Girls*.

54 Vinta informed the Grand Duke that he and Piero Cappelli had spent the entire day surveying Florentine orphanages, but that "nelli [Ospedale degli] Innocenti et in più altri spedali non habbiamo trovato cosa buona, essendo tutte sgratiate, rognose, et di così male carni et fattezze da far nausea. Solamente nelle *Abbandonate*, che stanno dove stavano le monache del Ceppo [*sic*], n'habbiamo trovate due che non ci dispiaceno a fatto" (Belisario Vinta in Florence to Grand Duke Francesco I de' Medici, 21 February 1584; Consiglio, *Una prova*, 86 [doc. XLI]). The following day Vinta sent the Grand Duke his description of one of the two girls, named Giulia: "Questo dì 22 verso la sera in cocchio ho fatto venir la fanciulla in casa. Il nome è Giulia, è in 21 anno, è grande, ha cera nobile, né magra, né grassa; ha viso da piacere, al mio giuditio, et fuori m'è riuscita più bella che non pareva nello spedale, ma allevata bene, però modesta e vergognosa; pure par desta, di conoscimento et di spirito, et di speranza che l'ha s'habbia a lasciare ammaestrare" (Vinta to Grand Duke Francesco I de' Medici, 22 February 1584; ibid., 93 [doc. XLIV]). According to Nicholas Terpstra, the place "where the nuns of the Ceppo once stayed" can be identified as either S. Niccolò or S. Maria Vergine. However, because other contemporary sources confirm that Giulia was in fact from the Casa della Pietà, it is likely that Vinta—a native of Volterra—was confused after a long day surveying Florentine orphanages. See Terpstra, *Lost Girls*, 218n2.

55 Dominican friars were given responsibility for the reform and management of the Casa della Pietà as of its relocation from Borgo Ognissanti to via Mandorlo in 1568. Correspondingly, the criteria for accepting girls in need became more stringent with regard to their family of origin, moral reputation and general health. Ibid., 134–41.

56 "Tanto mi sono adoperato, partecipando sempre il tutto con M. Piero [Galletti], che questo giorno il segretario et medico Donati, et egli, hanno vista et rivista, et maneggiata alla presenza di una donna, che sarà quella che anderà secco, la fanciulla. Et il mantovano, presente M. Piero, ha affermato, che sebbene l'haverebbe desiderata, anche un po' più bella, che nondimeno se ne sodisfà, et finalmente con la mano et con l'occhio il mantovano si è chiarito, che non vi è alcun impedimento, et l'ha del tutto, insieme con M. Piero, approvata per idonea alla pruova" (Belisario Vinta in Florence to Grand Duke Francesco I de' Medici, 23 February 1584; Consiglio, *Una prova*, 97 [doc. XLVII]). For the date of Vinta's arrival to Venice, see his letter to Francesco I of 10 March 1584 (ibid., 108 [doc. LVI]).

57 "A due hore della medesima notte delli VIII [Vincenzo] volse venire alla medesima compagnia a veder la giovane, et ne rimase molto sotisfatto, mostrando gran risentimento di volontà per assaltarla allhora, ma io non volsi, perché appunto alli V le havevano cominciato le sue purghe, et era anchora un po' dibattuta del viaggio. La sera de IX ritornò il Principe accompagnato nel

medesimo modo a riveder la giovane, et sempre gli è piaciuta più, et fece forza, ma gentilmente, di haverla, et io non acconsentii respetto al giorno del venerdì, et perché il paese durava anchora piovoso et lo reputavano nostro disvantaggio. Si è ferma la giornata per questa prossima notte, se il paese sarà rasciutto a bastanza, come si spera" (ibid., 112–13). Religious etiquette is given as the reason for not holding the test on Friday by Luciano Berti, *Il principe dello Studiolo: Francesco I dei Medici e la fine del Rinascimento fiorentino* (Florence: Edam, 1967), 216n22. On Renaissance menstrual phobias, including the belief that it was dangerous to have sex while a woman had her period, see Bell, *How to Do It*, 63–70.

58 "[Carlo Gonzaga and Marcello Donati] erano convenuti che la pruova si facesse drento allo spatio di 24 hore, ma che, per andare ancho più al sicuro per la parte del Principe, non fusse obbligato a star tutto quel tempo riserrato con la giovane ... Mi hanno ben detto, che concedendo l'A.V. questo tempo in questo modo, che si contentano et promettono che quanto al modo della pruova la si faccia in una camera assegnata, preparata et custodita dalli huomini di V.A.; che il Principe vi habbia da entrare solo con una roba lunga della notte su la camicia, et che nell'entrare si habbia a mostrare alli medesimi huomini di lei per chiarirgli, che non porti seco altri istrumenti, che naturali, et che quel naturale sia ben fatto et proportionato, et che nel medesimo modo vi habbia da rientrare ogni volta" (Belisario Vinta in Florence to Grand Duke Francesco I de' Medici, 25 February 1584; Consiglio, *Una prova*, 102–3 [doc. LI]).

59 "Usate voi ogni diligentia et industria di chiarirvi più che potete della potentia et di quello che passi, dandosi minuto ragguaglio di tutto" (Grand Duke Francesco I de' Medici in Florence to Belisario Vinta, 26 February 1584; ibid., 105–6 [doc. LII]).

60 "Ecco sonar le VII et quasi in un tempo medesimo uscire il Principe della camera con lamento e con la mano allo stomaco, et sento dirmi: 'Cavaliere, oimé, sto male' ... Si risolse d'andarsene, et io l'accompagnai sino alla gondola, et disse che voleva farsi un clistero, che haverebbe ricorso all'unico suo rimedio, all'olio di mandorle dolci. Partita S.A., subito chiamai la guardadonna, et la ricondussi dalla giovane, per non ritrovarmi solo con sola ... Con l'intervento della guardadonna l'essaminai, et alle mie interrogationi, tutta la sustantia della sua risposta fu questa: Son vergine come prima" (Belisario Vinta in Venice to Grand Duke Francesco I de' Medici, 11 March 1584; ibid., 117–18 [doc. LVIII]). In his report of 16 March to Francesco I, Vinta noted that "in tutti questi giorni [Vincenzo] si haveva aggravato lo stomaco con disordini, et massime con cattivo nutrimento di ostriche" (ibid., 123 [doc. LXII]). On the aphrodisiac effects commonly attributed to oysters in this time period see, for example: Castore Durante da Gualdo, *Il tesoro della sanità*, Venezia 1588, p. 281, as well as Ugo Benzi, *Regole della sanità et della natura dei cibi*, Torino, 1618, p. 461 (earlier editions exist of both of these self-help manuals). I thank Allen J. Grieco for these references.

61 On the widespread belief that witchcraft could cause impotence—especially in the case of bridegrooms who failed in deflowering their bride—see the essay by Matteo Duni, "Impotence, Witchcraft, and Politics " in this volume.

62 "Poichè non era meraviglia se in così puoco tempo, et con principio di dolori, non li era venuto fatto quello che si desiderava, et che non mancavano rimedi di provedere così al difetto naturale come al maleficio, quando ce ne fosse. Con questi et molti altri ragioni, che sarebbe longo il scriverle, si concluse di far orazioni et pigliare morselli che aiutassero l'eretione della carne, et di già si sono cominciati ad usare, et col mezzo di certo frate, proposto dal P. confessore del S.mo S. nostro, quale dicono essere compagno del P. commissario Generale dato ordine, poichè le celebrano per valentissimo homo in quello fatto, di far buone provisioni a' malefici quali potessero essere stati fatti, per non mancare a tutti i rimedi possibili" (Marcello Donati in Venice to Cavaliere Teodoro S. Giorgio, 14 March 1584; Conti, *Altri documenti*, 107–8 [doc. XXX]).

63 Perhaps these *morselli* were a variant of the "morselletti da eccitare Venere," apparently a sort of rub that included the satyrion root described in Stefano Rosselli's late 16th-century recipe book, conserved in manuscript copies in Florence (Marucelliana MS C.145) and Seville (Biblioteca Zayas, MS C-IV-15); however, the fact that Vincenzo Gonzaga is described as "taking (*pigliare*) morselli" may indicate instead that his were something taken orally. On such remedies for impotence, see the essays by Laura Giannetti and Meredith Ray in this volume. I thank Laura Gianetti for generously sharing and discussing this information on *morselletti* with me.

64 "'Cavaliere, cavaliere, vien qua, tocca et palpa con la mano.' Et io, se bene con un poco di vergogna et di respetto, non potendo metterla fra le loro intrecciate gambe et coscie, la posi di sopra tutta spianata, che a pena vi entrava, et anche S.A. si sollevò alquanto, reggendosi su le braccia per darmi luogo, et la condussi fra l'uno et l'altro pettignone, sino che con essa toccai la pube et urtai nel membro duro, che la fanciulla haveva in corpo, et ben si conosceva ch'ella ve l'havesse, havendola io trovata et lasciata con espresso pianto, ma sotto voce, misto, credo io, di dolore e di dolcezza. Et dissemì il Principe: 'Hor che hai tocchò et chiaritoti, lasciami finire i fatti miei'; et si lasciò ire sopra la giovane" (Belisario Vinta in Venice to Grand Duke Francesco I de' Medici, 16 March 1584; Consiglio, *Una prova*, 124 [doc. LXII]). See also Marcello Donati's account in his letter from Venice to Teodoro S. Giorgio of 15 March 1584: "Alle cinque della notte passata il S.r Principe S.mo accompagnato da me si corcò colla giovane, colla quale non stette più di un quarto d'ora che chiamò il Sig.r Cav. Vinta, il quale entrato nella camera toccò con mano che il membro dell'A.S. virile, era entrato nella natura della fanciulla poichè il petenechio di uno et dell'altra erano

congiunti, et egli stesso trovò il membro duro et in quell punto la giovane piangeva ed dolevasi, ciò fatto se ne usci il S.r Vinta, et in fatti et parole mostrò di restar sodisfatto et senza dubio, perciò egli et io si corcassimo vestiti sopra il letto dell'anticamera ove stessimo fin vicino al giorno, che levandosi doppo alle 14 hore S.A., disse di aver rotto tre lancie et che sarebbe passato alla 4 se la giovine fosse stata salda" (Conti, *Altri documenti*, 111–12 [doc. XXXII]).

65 Ibid. On the Renaissance metaphor of "broken lances" to signify performative sexual action, especially that of defloration, see Simons, *Sex of Men*, 38–45.

66 Giulia was subjected to an extensive interrogation after the *prova* during which, when asked if she believed she had been deflowered, she replied: "'la prima volta non mi pare che non l'habbia messo troppo dentro.' Domandata a quello che se ne fusse avvista—disse, 'perché nel cavarlo lo tirava su presto.' Domandata un'altra volta del parere d'essere sverginata o no—disse, che non se n'intendeva, et ficcava il capo in seno." An earlier portion of the interrogation focused on the emission of seed, asking the girl "se haveva sentito il Principe soffiare—disse, due volte. Se tutte le volte che egli gliene messe, ella lo sentì duro—disse di si. Se se il Principe ve l'haveva tanto drento che non potesse versar fuore—disse di si. Se ella havesse buttato seme—disse che la seconda volta che il Principe glie ne fece, poco doppo che l'hebbe cavato, si sentì gocciolare giù per la natura, et che poi anche alla terza volta ne uscì, et che ha tutta la camicia di dreto imbrattata, et che ella dubitava che fusse sangue. Se ella habbia sentito piacere nel buttare seme—disse che alquanto le era parso di sentirne due volte" (Interrogation of Giulia on 15 March 1584, Consiglio, *Una prova*, 130–31 [doc. LXIII]). See also the letter of Marcello Donati in Venice to Teodoro di S. Giorgio on 15 March 1584: "Disse [Vinta] che la giovane affermava di non essere sverginata, dicendo che era vero che S.A. le aveva dato in vari tempi quattro assalti, ma che non haveva intromesso se non poca parte del membro" (Conti, *Altri documenti*, 113 [doc. XXXII]).

67 "La mattina delli XV ... il Principe mostrommi ogni cosa. Considerai il tutto et tocchai et parvemi il membro in quello stato, ché era chinato, membro ordinario ma ben fatto, et così i due testicoli in ogni lor parte, et messa la mano sotto d'ogni lato dei testicoli, non vi trovai male, né impedimento nessuno; ma perché l'animale non era ritto, non mi ci pareva d'haver drento il pieno della mia sodisfattione. Però questa mattina andatomene di sua volontà nell'anticamera del Sig. Principe, mi fece chiamare ben presto che diaceva in letto, et mostrommi il membro ritto et sodo come un fuso, appuntato, et proportionatissimo et lo maneggiai, et lo scappellai con la mia mano, et così maneggiai li testicoli et rimasi contentissimo, parendomi la grossezza et la lunghezza del membro assai grande, ma non però fuor di natura, et le forme della fanciulla che l'hanno ricevuto non hanno patito lesione. Volse anche il Sig. Principe con molta sicurtà et domestichezza che io gli toccassi il luogo della fistola, che è dalla chiappa sinistra, vicinissima al sesso verso il di dreto, larga quanto una veccia nell'orifizio, ma che con li instrumenti del coito non ha a far nulla" (Piero Galletti in Venice to Grand Duke Francesco I de' Medici, 16 March 1584; Consiglio, *Una prova*, 131–2 [doc. LXIV]).

68 "Oltre a quello che potrà V.A. intendere dal S.r Marcello [Donati], ella saprà che il S.r Principe Ser. mo questa notte ha voluto ritornare alla giovane, et si è portato in modo, che nè lei nè il S.r Vinta nè il loro medico hanno che replicarle, et io questa mattina ho parlato a tutti che sono rimasti soddisfatissimi, e sono allegrissimi insieme colla comadre. Di ciò ho voluto dar conto all'A.V. acciò sappia che in questa prova non è rimasto un scrupolo al mondo" (Carlo Gonzaga in Venice to duke Guglielmo Gonzaga, 17 March 1584; Conti, *Altri documenti*, 118 [doc. XXXIII]).

69 "Li serenissimi sposi se n'andarono a dormire et questa mattina si son rivisti tutti lieti, con voce ed affermatione che si sia consumato il matrimonio, et che restino del tutto abbattute per terra le maligne falsità ch'erano andate attorno" (Belisario Vinta in Mantua to Grand Duke Francesco I de' Medici, 30 April 1584; Consiglio, *Una prova*, 178–9 [doc. LXXXV]).

70 "Se bene io ho inteso da altri l'arrivo et lo sposalitio della Ser.ma Principessa, m'è stato però di doppio contento l'aviso che vi è piaciuto de darmene voi, col quale io mi rallegro della sodisfatione ch'ha data S.A. a que' S.mi Sig.ri, et che il S.r Principe si sia portato così valorosamente in questo principio da sperarne sicuramente la felitică che io desidero per intera consolatione di tutti" (Bianca Cappello in Pratolino to Marcello Donati, 4 May 1584; Conti, *Altri documenti*, 161–2 [doc. XLIV]).

71 For the suggestion that Giulia was married off to Giulio Caccini and that their child—conceived during the virility test in Venice—grew up to be the musician Pompeo Caccini, see Timothy McGee, "Pompeo Caccini and *Euridice*: New Biographical Notes," *Renaissance and Reformation* 26, 2 (1990): 81–2, 90–93, 98–9 (cited by Terpstra, *Lost Girls*, 189–90). McGee's theory is based in part on a claim made in the anonymous introduction to the original nineteenth-century publication of the Florentine documents concerning Vincenzo's virility test, *Il parentado* (republished by Consiglio, *Una prova*, 20). Here, citing the early 18th-century Florentine diaries of Niccolò Susier, the author claims that "in quanto alla fanciulla che fu il soggetto della prova, il Susier nel suo Diario, che si conserva inedito nella Moreniana, dice che trovatasi gravida fu rimandata a Firenze per far fede di una sì indecente esperienza. Dopo che ella ebbe partorito fu data per moglie ad un Giuliano, musico romano, con dote di tremila scudi." As Terpstra points out, however, McGee's theory is flawed, not least by the fact that Giulio Caccini's wife was named "Lucia." Another anonymous source, clearly related to the one excerpted above, gives a more sober version of Giulia's destiny:

"era in Firenze un luogo di fanciulle detto della Pietà, ne cavorno una delle più belle, e con false lusinghe la mandorno a Mantova per far prova con detto principe, e saputo ciò da questa fanciulla ne fece gran pianto; nondimeno trovata gravida fu rimandata a Firenze per far fede d'una si indecente esperienza; mendicava di porta in porta un tozzo di pane" (Carlo Morbio, ed. *Storia dei municipi italiani: illustrate con documenti inediti*, vol. 4 [Milan: Omobono Manini, 1838], 46). Although correct in its identification of Giulia's orphanage as the Casa della Pietà, this account is also problematic because it states that the "prova" took place in Mantua, not Venice.

72 On such cases see, for example: Silvana Seidel Menchi and Diego Quaglioni (eds.), *Trasgressioni. Concubinato, adulterio, bigamia (secoli XIV–XVIII). Processi matrimoniali degli archivi ecclesiastici italiani* (Bologna: Il Mulino, 2004); Emlyn Eisenach, *Husbands, Wives, and Concubines: Marriage, Family, and Social Order in Sixteenth-Century Verona* (Kirksville, MO: Truman State University Press, 2004); Daniela Hacke, *Women, Sex and Marriage in Early Modern Venice* (Aldershot, UK/Burlington, VT: Ashgate, 2004); Joanne Ferraro, *Nefarious Crimes, Contested Justice Illicit Sex and Infanticide in the Republic of Venice, 1557–1789* (Baltimore, MD: Johns Hopkins University Press, 2008).

73 See *Supra* note 53.

74 Sergio Bertelli, *The King's Body: Sacred Rituals of Power in Medieval and Early Modern Europe*, trans. R. Burr Litchfield (University Park: Pennsylvania State University Press, 2001), esp. 151–70, 177–90. Bertelli's study was first published as *Il corpo del Re: sacralità del potere nell'Europa medievale e moderno* (Florence: Ponte alle Grazie, 1990).

75 Ernst Kantorowicz, *The King's Two Bodies: A Study in Medieval Political Theology* (Princeton: Princeton University Press, 1957).

76 Overviews of Vincenzo's cultural patronage are given by Paola Venturelli, *Vincenzo I Gonzaga 1562–1612. Il fasto del potere*, exh. cat. Mantua, 18 February–10 June 2012 (Mantua: Publi Paolini, 2012); Roberta Piccinelli, "Le facies del collezionismo artistico di Vincenzo Gonzaga," in *Gonzaga. La celeste galeria. L'esercizio del collezionismo*, ed. Raffaella Morselli (Milan: Skira, 2002), 341–7; eds. David Chambers and Jane Martineau, *Splendours of the Gonzaga*, exh. cat. London, 4 November 1981–31 January 1982 (Milan: A. Pizzi, 1981), 223–43. For a survey of portraits of Vincenzo I, see Paolo Bertelli, "Appunti sulla ritrattistica di Vincenzo I Gonzaga," in *Scritti per Chiara Tellini Perina*, ed. Daniela Ferrari and Sergio Marinelli (Mantua: G. Arcari Editore, 2011), 229–49.

77 For an excellent analytical account of this extraordinary journey, see Valeria Finucci, "There's the Rub: Searching for Sexual Remedies in the New World," *Journal of Medieval and Early Modern Studies* 38.3 (2008): 523–57.

78 Ibid., 525–6.

79 Vincenzo's Will of 1608 stipulated that he was to be buried not in a recumbent position but "sitting on a specially-prepared marble throne" (*non quidem, ut moris est, iacendo, sed sedendo super cathedra marmorea ad hoc parata*), a condition repeated in his final Will of 3 February 1612: "seated with his sword upon a marble throne" (*sedendo cum suo ense apposito super cathedra marmorea*). Rodolfo Signorini, "Gonzaga Tombs and Catalfalques," in Chambers and Martineau, 7–8.

80 Vincenzo may have learned of this practice through a more recent example from closer to home: when Pier Maria Rossi, count of San Secondo, died in 1482, his embalmed body was displayed seated in a throne in this manner. Later, in the early 18th century, the deceased body of Cosimo III de' Medici was also buried this way (Bertelli, *King's Body*, 49–51).

Historical and Literary Contexts for the Skimmington: Impotence and Samuel Butler's *Hudibras*[1]

M. A. Katritzky

Introduction: Cuckoldry and Popular Culture

This chapter draws on historical and cultural sources to examine the skimmington or riding, an English variant of the European charivari. It interrogates the specifics of this social shaming ritual and its impact on print culture. Its primary focus is the lengthiest skimmington account, in the "authorized" second part of Samuel Butler's three-part burlesque poem *Hudibras*, first published in 1664.[2] The central pair of this mock-heroic Augustan poem are the Presbyterian antihero Sir Hudibras and his Sectarian Independent squire Ralpho (or Ralph), a humble tailor whose occult medical skills enabled him to diagnose magical impotence and other causes of cuckoldry.[3] So obsessed was the early modern period with cuckoldry that, according to Douglas Bruster, "it is difficult to overestimate the predominance of cuckoldry in the popular drama of the period."[4] No level of society was exempt, and increasingly, parallels were drawn between cheating and betrayal in the private marital sphere and public political arena, especially in the aftermath of the Civil War, when Butler confronts England's monarch with his court's incontinence:

Cuckolds so cow'rdly and so base,
Lascivious wives so void of grace.
[…] Such stars could surely never shine,
O Charles! round any throne but thine;
Thy great example prompts each spouse
To make a jest of marriage-vows.[5]

Skimmingtons target marital transgression, especially cuckoldry. Their performative highpoint is a proxy couple (or, more rarely, a single stand-in), chosen from among the shamed couple's nearest male neighbors, to enact the transgressing pair. Their aggressively theatrical neighborly contribution is,

I here suggest, informed by responses to perceived mismatches between canon law, civil legislation and peasant traditions relating to marital infertility and paternity issues. English common law protected the paternity and birthright of children born to husbands abroad; requiring husbands to prove themselves legal cuckolds in courts of law before being permitted to disinherit children born within wedlock. Butler's contribution to the controversy surrounding this legislation is typically sharp:

To give the cheats the eldest hand
In foul play, by the laws o' th' land;
For which so many a legal cuckold
Has been run down in courts, and truckled.
[...] 'Tis we [wives] that can dispose alone,
Whether your heirs shall be your own,
To whose integrity you must,
In spite of all your caution, trust;
And, 'less you fly beyond the seas,
Can fit you with what heirs we please;
And force you t'own 'em, though begotten
By French valets, or Irish footmen.[6]

Brazenly turning common law to his advantage and proclaiming "Ile teach a Cuckold how to hide his horns," the pragmatic sailor hero of John Webster and William Rowley's early 17th-century play, *A cure for a cuckold* (first published only in 1661), successfully sues a wealthy childless merchant and his barren wife to win back custody of his wife's baby son, born shortly before his return from several years at sea.[7]

Potent husbands in childless marriages had the legal right to divorce their barren spouse, a right extended by canon law to the fertile wives of impotent men.[8] The previously unrecognized relevance of certain ancient regulations and traditional rules, governing the rights and duties of members of peasant groups, is also significant in the context of the skimmington. The authoritative legal historian (and collector of folk and fairy tales) Jacob Grimm published several volumes of "wisdoms" transcribed from 17th- and 18th-century vernacular German dialect manuscripts, whose references to outmoded weaponry and concepts such as longbows and spears, or crop damage by bears, suggest much earlier origins. The extent, if any, of their legal status or use in early modern law courts, is unclear.[9] Perhaps they are akin to the complex punishment rituals and other traditions practiced by early modern occupational groups such as game-keepers, miners or freemasons.[10]

Grimm's publications include four "wisdoms" exhorting impotent husbands to embrace the status of wittol, or compliant cuckold, and ensure an heir by requesting male neighbors to stand in for their marital duty. All elaborate on an impotent peasant farmer's right or duty to "call on his neighbors to help him with his wife's mortal peril" (*Hattinger landfeste*), "take her to his neighbor" (*Bockumer landrecht*), "deliver his wife to someone capable of taking care of her needs" (*Wendhager bauernrecht*) or "ask his nearest neighbor to help his wife" (*Benker heidenrecht*).[11] If that doesn't work, some advise the peasant to dress her in best or new clothes, fill her moneybag and send her to the nearest annual fair to sort out the problem herself, and, if that still doesn't solve it, to let her go to the devil, or even a thousand devils. Garbled overlaps between these ritualized stipulations suggest venerable oral transmission. Most instruct the impotent peasant to convey his wife, on his back, across his own boundary fence onto a neighbor's land, and exhort him to treat her gently, or not to be rough with her or hurt her in any way. According to the *Benker heidenrecht,* he must also carry her back home and provide her with a roast chicken and a jug of wine after her ordeal. Some authorities agree with Grimm in accepting these four "wisdoms" as a legitimate way of providing for an heir,[12] others classify them as ritual rape.[13] Although practice of this very public custom is known to Grimm only from legend and fable, there is evidence of some early modern childless couples' more discreet involvement of male neighbors in their attempts to secure heirs, a practice supported by Martin Luther.[14] From the 12th century onwards, canon law attempted to clarify the conundrum of whether binding marriage was established by consensual contract (the exchange of vows), or by a point of law (sexual consummation), and whether couples prevented by impotence from consummating their marriage could be regarded as legally married.[15] Concerned to minimize divorce, and apparently attempting to replace both Catholic canon law and peasant "wisdoms," Luther's anti-Papist sermon of 1522 directly addresses the fertile wife of an impotent husband.[16] Informing her that unconsummated childless marriages are not recognized by God, he advises her to seek her husband's explicit permission to provide him with an heir, by agreeing to be cheated by her "secret marriage" with his brother or closest relative.[17]

A Swiss visitor to London in 1599, the physician Thomas Platter the Younger, records the performative heart of the English skimmington not as the shamed couple, but their nearest neighbors:

> In England ... women have much more freedom than in other places, and also know well how to make good use of it. They often go for walks or coach-rides extremely impressively dressed, and their husbands just have to put up with this, and are not permitted to punish them for it. Instead, wives often beat their husbands, and when one hears about this, the very nearest of their neighbors is placed on a cart and paraded around the whole town in order to make fun of the beaten man, while proclaiming that this is his punishment for not having come to the aid of his neighbor while his wife was beating him.[18]

This practice was also confirmed by a Frenchman living in London:

> I have sometimes met in the Streets of *London* a Woman carrying a Figure of Straw representing a Man, crown'd with very ample Horns, preceded by a Drum, and follow'd by a Mob, making a most grating Noise with Tongs, Grid-irons, Frying-pans, and Saucepans: I ask'd what was the Meaning of all this; they told me, that a Woman had given her Husband a sound beating, for accusing her of making him a Cuckold, and that upon such Occasions some kind Neighbour of the *poor innocent injur'd Creature*[19] generally perform'd this Ceremony.[20]

This account highlights the centrality to the skimmington of horns, the ancient symbol of cuckoldry, of discordant noise and of mockery targeting the couple as a whole: in this case, the virago wife no less than her cuckolded husband.

Since Violet Alford's ground breaking article of 1959 on "Rough music or charivari," anthropologists and social historians such as Natalie Zemon Davis, Martin Ingram, EP Thompson and David Underdown have contributed greatly to our understanding of street theatre intended to shame couples who transgress sexual and social mores.[21] They examine the mythic origins and history of European charivaris and English skimmingtons, their relationship to regional variants such as "riding the stang," wheel-barrowing, hussitting, ritual hunts or the Welsh *ceffyl pren*, and overlaps with diverse rituals and "rough music" at official civic punishments, unofficial land closure and other occasions for public riots. Some skimmingtons involved little more than the public taunting of quarrelling couples, as in the case of Mary Hall of Cameley. In 1616, when neighbors learned that she had beaten their blacksmith (her husband John), on the back with a frying pan, they "had one to Ryde upon mens shoulders by the name of Skymerton without any hurt don or misdemeanours otherwise at all."[22] Although primarily, skimmingtons publicly shamed cuckolds or bawds, some mocked other types of antisocial transgressors. In 1691, one hundred Warwickshire villagers, led by a cross-dressed smith and a farmer crowned with a pair of horns, marched to the house of a local couple. Maligning them as a "cuckoldy dog" and a stealing "whore," they loudly broadcast the details of their petty thieving of timber and chickens.[23] Other skimmingtons, such as those staged as enclosure protests, targeted social rather than individual transgressions.

Hudibras

Interpretation of the domestic and political dimensions of Butler's skimmington account is necessarily informed by the convoluted book history of *Hudibras*. Dated 1663, the anonymously published first edition of Part I was an immediate bestseller. It was in the bookshops by December 26, 1662, when Samuel Pepys, hearing about "a new book of drollery in use, called *Hudebras*," rushed to buy it at the Temple. Pronouncing it "so silly ... that I am ashamed of it," he sold it on to a friend that same evening. However, determined to give this fashionable publication another go, he rebought it in February: "it being certainly some ill humour to be so against that which all the world cries up to be the example of wit; for which I am resolved once more to read him, and see whether I can find it or no."[24] Within a year, Part I was anonymously re-issued in five authorized and four pirated editions. Multiple editions of an "unauthorized" Part II (1663)[25] were followed by an entirely differently worded anonymous "authorized" Part II (1664), authenticated as Butler's by its later incorporation into all combined editions. Part III, also anonymous, followed in 1674. Pepys borrowed Part II[26] in November 1663: "to see if it be as good as the first, which the world cry so mightily up, though it hath not a good liking in me, though I had tried by twice or three times reading to bring myself to think it witty." A fortnight later, he bought: "*Hudibras*, both parts, the book now in greatest fashion for drollery, though I cannot, I confess, see enough where the wit lies"; this even though Pepys's colleague Sir William Petty reckoned *Hudibras* among the "three books … most esteemed and generally cried up for wit in the world," and the staunch "Parliament-man" Mr. Seymour quoted it "in a serious discourse."[27] By 1668, when Pepys and his wife invited Samuel Butler to dine at their house with the portraitist Samuel Cooper and others, they appreciated the company of the writer they now knew to be the author of *Hudibras*.[28] In August 1683, three years after Butler's death, and having finally been won over by his poem, Pepys "read over the first two books of *Hudibras*" while voyaging to Tangier on Navy business.[29]

Although critics dismiss the 1663 "unauthorized" Part II as a derivative work of little literary merit by some unidentifiable hack, Butler's authorial involvement cannot be excluded. Passages openly attacking religious and political belief systems with powerful supporters would have discouraged any writer with pretensions to court patronage from admitting to its authorship during the 1660s. Published barely a year after the anonymous Part I, the unauthorized Part II refers knowingly to "Butlero,"[30] and matches some of Butler's innovative literary quirks in ways that go beyond mere derivation or parody. Perhaps not coincidentally, *Hudibras* followed *Don Quixote* in inspiring an unauthorized sequel that both promoted and profited from the original work's commercial success.[31]

Magical Impotence

One pervasive leitmotif of *Hudibras* is the principle protagonist's virility. Although Sir Hudibras is a bachelor, his fear of impotence and cuckoldry is reflected in constant references to horns and tails (or lack thereof). The plot tracks his rambling quest to prove himself "no *Gelding*" in order to avoid the professed cure for folly and impotence (also featured in *Don Quixote*): being whipped with the dried penis of a bull.[32] Impotence was closely associated with cuckoldry; the occult practice of magical impotence, thought to render a bridegroom impotent with his new wife but not with other women, was regarded as a major cause of cuckoldry. Magical impotence thus threatened newlyweds with childlessness, and other couples with cuckoldry's complex legal, moral and economic dangers. Its roots are ancient and transnational. On mainland Europe, magical impotence rituals were integral to a continuous tradition of domestic witchcraft.[33] In early modern England, by contrast, their popular practice was all but obsolete.

Magical impotence rituals entered Jacobean theatre culture through the influence of practices owing less to indigenous traditions than to classically inspired necromancy of the type then flourishing at European courts. This revival of interest was fueled by a high-profile court scandal surrounding

Frances Howard, daughter of Thomas Howard, Earl of Suffolk. In 1606, 13-year-old Frances married 14-year-old Robert Devereux, Earl of Essex; in 1613, she filed for annulment of her marriage. Her successful case rested on proving her virginity and Essex's magically-induced impotence to an ecclesiastical commission chaired by George Abbott, Archbishop of Canterbury, whose vehement rejection of witchcraft as a cause of impotence was over-ruled by King James I.[34] Howard's case greatly influenced plays such as Thomas Middleton's *The Witch* (c. 1616), in which the garrulous chief witch Hecate renders clients' unwanted lovers magically impotent by dispensing knotted charms.[35] Similar magical knots feature in the anti-masque of Ben Jonson's *Masque of Queenes*, performed at court in 1609. Referencing demonological tracts, classical authors and dictionaries, Jonson notes of his witches that "the vntying of their knots is, when they are going to some fatall businesse."[36]

Magical impotence rituals involving knots were an ongoing occult practice in many European regions. Thomas Platter's account of them in Languedoc in 1598 is the earliest known detailed record of the performative sequence whereby occult practitioners enacted magical impotence rituals during the actual marriage ceremony of their intended victims. It notes that they involved knotting a point (a reinforced leather lace of the type used to lace up codpieces), during a specific part of the wedding ceremony itself.[37]

Although central to European magical impotence, knots had evidently fallen into disuse in 17th-century England. While Jonson's chief witch alludes to knots on stage, her fellow witches pierce effigies, proclaiming: "With pictures full, of waxe, and of wooll / Their liuers I sticke, with needles quicke."[38] Jacobean occult practitioners and dramatists, evidently unfamiliar with continental magical impotence rituals, seem to have pieced together their details from classical literary sources and European demonological tracts.

Alluded to in *Masque of Queenes* and *The Witch*, magical impotence is central to Thomas Heywood and Richard Brome's play *Late Lancashire Witches* (1634), featuring a simple country couple. Before their wedding ceremony, a jealous local witch (and former lover of the bridegroom) presents him with a knotted codpiece point. This renders him impotent with his new wife. Eventually, after much grief, including their public shaming in a skimmington, the newlyweds realize that the knotted point is a bewitched "charme."[39] Only by burning this "Inchauntment" does the couple finally restore the husband's potency and their marital harmony. While *Late Lancashire Witches* could still serve up a plot dependent on codpiece points as late as 1634, such magic charms are noticeably absent from Thomas Shadwell's radically updated version of Heywood and Brome's play, *Lancashire-Witches* (1682).[40] Magical impotence is fleetingly alluded to, but there is no hint of the actual rituals to bring it about, either in the playtext itself, or even in Shadwell's copious learned references drawn from classical sources, Jacobean drama, and demonological tracts. English witches, it appears, dispensed with magical knots long before their continental counterparts.

Samuel Butler's description of the judiciary astrologer Sidrophel the Rosicrucian, who was consulted by Sir Hudibras concerning his impotence, represents one of the fullest literary accounts of early modern expectations of the professional practice of occult healers, which accorded a prominent role to the diagnosis and treatment of impotence and other infertility problems.[41] In Canto II of the unauthorized Part II, this medical specialism is aggressively marketed by a flamboyant Catholic mountebank from Paris. Mounting his outdoor fairground stage, Monsieur Quack promotes the resurrective powers of his patent cure for impotence in comical broken English, drawing on a venerable literary tradition.[42] Bawdily assisted by his mixed-gender troupe, Quack continues to vaunt his ability to cure—and cause—impotence even after his brutal arrest and capture by the outraged Sir Hudibras and Ralpho:[43]

So on they amble to the place,
Where *Monsieur* spake with a boon grace;
Begar ["by God"] me kill you all, an den
Presan make you alive agen;
Wi dis me do all de gran Cure,
De *Pock,* de *Scab.* de *Calenture;*
Me make de Man strong, pour de Wench.
(Then riseth *Capon* from the Bench)
Look you me now, do you no see
Dead yesterday, now live day be,
Four boon, dey leap, dey dance, dey sing,
May foy, an do de toder ting:
Begar good Medicine do all dis.
Capon makes legs, and Wench doth kiss,
Take hands, and throw their legs about.
[...] Me be de Frenchman, profess Phissick,
Me cure de Pock, de Cough, de Tissick,
De Ish, de Gout, the Ash in bones,
And me begar can cut your Stones [i.e. castrate you].[44]

Rehearsing key themes played out over the poem's three official Parts, the unauthorized Part II anticipates, as well as draws on, Butler's relentless satirical pitting of his Reform protagonists Hudibras and Ralpho against traditional customs such as the skimmington. Performative ceremonies of this type were reviled by hard-line Parliamentarians concerned to repress popular culture with perceived Papist roots.

Butler's Skimmington: Rough Music, Bad Smells and Cuckolds' Horns

In place of the quack troupe of the 1663 unauthorized version, the 1664 authorized edition of *Hudibras* Part II features a colorfully theatrical skimmington that made the poem's title into a byword. A Charing Cross wedding of 1737, for example, was disrupted by what the London press gleefully labelled a "Grand Hudibrastick Skimmington." Involving numerous

"Chairmen [drivers], and others of that Class," it greatly disturbed the mismatched 70-plus-year-old groom and his teenage bride.[45] Literary precedents for the *Hudibras* skimmington can be found in plays such as *The Knave in Graine* (1640, attributed by some to John Day), or Heywood and Brome's *The Late Lancashire Witches* (1634), while it in turn directly inspired writers such as Andrew Marvell, Walter Scott and Edward William Davies, whose detailed fictional skimmington account is previously uncited in this context.[46] The practice was considered stageworthy well into the 18th century, as indicated by works such as *The Country-Wedding and Skimington* (1729), a comic libretto attributed to Essex Hawker.[47]

Like the charivari, the skimmington was habitually accompanied by a terrifying din and heavy-handed allusions to cuckoldry and impotence through the blowing, brandishing, or wearing of horns.[48] The cacophony incorporated mocking laughter, the raucous human voice and "rough music" which, like the demonic music of medieval stage devils, involved martial and rustic instruments such as horns, drums or bagpipes, and noisy makeshift use of women's kitchen implements, such as skimming ladles and pots, pans or griddles. Infernal din contributes materially to the performative impact of stage skimmingtons. In Beaumont and Fletcher's dramatic sequel to Shakespeare's *Taming of the Shrew*, such din is created by a band of noisy women led by the widowed Petruchio's new wife Maria. Rejecting female submission, they "fling main Potlids / like massie rocks, dart ladles, tossing Irons / and tongs like Thunderbolts."[49] Other stage skimmingtons are announced by "a great Hubub and noise, a ringing of basons, a great many Boyes before,"[50] or by an onlooker enquiring: "Whats the matter now, is Hell broke loose?"[51] The arrival of the *Hudibras* skimmington too, is heralded by the fear its commotion instils into Butler's cowardly Sir Hudibras and Ralpho:

When both were parted on the sudden,
With hideous *Clamour,* and a loud one,
As if all sorts of *Noise* had been
Contracted into one loud *Din*:
Or that some Member [of Parliament] to be chosen [i.e. elected],
Had got the *Odds* above a *Thousand;*
And by the Greatness of his Noise,
Prov'd fittest for his *Country's* Choice.
This strange surprisal put the *Knight,*
And wrathful *Squire* into a Fright.[52]

Sir Hudibras and Ralpho's fears were fully justified; but although some charivaris and skimmingtons had been known to lead to serious injury or death, no attempt at regulation had managed to stop this ancient custom. William Prynne's Puritan anti-theatrical treatise of 1633 traces it back to at least 1404, the date of a canon law warning clergy to "be not present at, nor yet play in the play that is called Charevari, in which they use vizards in the shape of divels, and horrible things are there committed: which Play wee prohibit not onely Clergy men, but generally all our subjects under paine of excommunication."[53] Two centuries after this prohibition, Thomas Platter documented unruly French "chalifary" groups of rowdy young bachelors, also disguised in devil masks. They continued to meet nightly to disturb the immediate neighborhood of newlywed couples of unequal age with intolerable smells and unsocial noises, disbanding only on receipt of a handsome bribe from the shamed couple:

each with his own instrument: one has an old kettle, another a pan, the third a drum, the fourth pipes, the fifth a spoon in a salt vat, the sixth a cowhorn and so on … They start playing their instruments at around midnight, and each tries to shout, sing or play more horribly than the rest. This releases such a frightening noise and screaming, that no neighbors within twelve houses' distance are able to get any peace at all.[54]

Platter's description recalls the noisy, smelly, riotous chaos graphically evoked by Butler, as do the historical records relating to a skimmington for the self-proclaimed married couple William and Margaret Cripple. Having set up house together in Burton-on-Trent in 1618, they were soon suspected of being unmarried, even brother and sister. In March 1618, around four hundred locals, many armed or disguised, dragged the newcomers out of their house and through the town to the stocks, "with greate noyce and with ringing of cow bells, basons, candlesticks, fryingpannes and with the sounde of a drumme," shouting "a whore and a knave, a whore, a whore."[55]

William Hogarth's heroic print *Hudibras encounters the skimmington*[56] heightens the rustic riot's burlesque effect by innovatively borrowing the monumental scale traditionally reserved for the most respected category of art: history painting.[57] Directly travestying the musical retinues of classical triumphs, its corpulent central hornblower's[58] massive musical horn draws attention both to the martial din and the motivating cuckoldry of Butler's skimmington, ruled over by the cuckold's horns:

And now the Cause of all their *Fear*,
By slow Degrees approach'd so near,
They might distinguish diff'rent Noise
Of *Horns*, and *Pans*, and *Dogs*, and *Boys*,
And *Kettle-Drums*, whose sullen *Dub*
Sounds like the hooping of a Tub.[59]

Having likened the conventions of his skimmington to some corrupt local political election, Butler goes on to develop satirical parallels to Roman Triumphs:

But when the Sight appear'd in View,
They found it was an Antique Show,
A *Triumph*, that for Pomp and State,
Did proudest *Romans* emulate:
[…] Being mounted in their best Array,

Upon a *Carre*, and who but they?
And follow'd with a World of Tall-*Lads*,
That merry *Ditties* troll'd, and *Ballads*;
Did ride with many a Good-morrow,
Crying, *Hey for our Town*, through the *Burrough*.[60]

These allusions to the important role of the raucous human voice (laughing, shouting, yelling or singing generic doggerel or scurrilous rhymes written for the occasion), are followed by further evocations of rough music:[61]

Next *Pan*, and *Kettles* of all Keys,
From *Trebles* down to *double Base*.
And after them, upon a *Nag*,
That might pass for a forehand Stag,
A *Cornet* rode, and on his Staff,
A Smock display'd, did proudly wave:
Then *Bagpipes* of the lowdest Drones,
With snuffling broken winded tones.[62]

This horned horse alludes to the rundown jade or nag ridden by the theatrical focal point of the skimmington's enactment of the battle of the sexes, the central proxy pair to whom attention is drawn by riotous cacophony.

Within and outside the context of rough music, horns habitually feature in documented skimmingtons. In that held in Quemerford near Calne in 1618, the mob that gathered to shame the local cutler Thomas Mills and his wife Agnes sounded "pipes & hornes ... & rames hornes & buckes hornes carried upon forkes were then and there lifted up and showen." On the morning of May 27, 1618, some dozen rowdy boys and men had been turned away from Quemerford by its womenfolk, who "understanding yt ye drumer & his company came thither for a Skimmington, they made towardes the drumer & cutt a pt of his drum, whereupon he and his company departed towardes Callne." At noon, a group of three or four hundred men from Calne, some armed, arrived with their proxy cuckold, identifiable by his characteristic night-shirt and horns: "a man riding upon a horse, haveing a white night cap upon his head, two shininge hornes hanging by his eares, & counterfayte beard upon his chine made of a deares tayle, a smocke upon the top of his garments."[63] Accusations of cuckoldry and aggressive allusions to horns cut deep. Horning was "an insult that could draw blood."[64] In August 1532, when around 80 rowdy men nightly roamed central Oxford, causing terror by randomly attacking pedestrians with stones or daggers and breaking into houses, but also by threatening them with cuckoldry: "if any one speaks to them out of the windows, they bid him go to bed, cuckold knave, or else come down, and his horns shall be knocked in again."[65]

Butler's Skimmington: Pelting, Riding and the Battle of the Sexes

Another ritual integral to skimmingtons is mutual pelting. Sir Hudibras faces a barrage of eggs wielded by the *Hudibras* mob.[66] Julio, the cheating *Knave in graine*, is pelted with "Pippings, Carrets, or Turneps," while the mashed or spent brewers' grains traditionally used as pig feed or compost referred to in this play's title is confirmed as skimmington ammunition by Marvell.[67] *Hudibras* specifies a less salubrious mixture:

Next, one upon a Pair of *Panniers*,
Full fraught with that, which for good Manners
Shall here be nameless, mixt with *Grains*,
Which he dispenc'd among the *Swains*,
And busily upon the Crowd,
At Random round about bestow'd.[68]

John Locke identifies the unnamed ingredient in an aside directly following a reference to "the bespatterings of Mr *Edward*'s Dunghil," noting that "*Skimmington* Rides in Triumph, driving all before him by the Ordures that he bestows on those that come in his way."[69]

The previously cited skimmington records of 1618 also mention various ritual uses of dung and grain. In Burton-on-Trent, locals cast the "dourte and mier of the streets" on William and Margaret Cripple while dragging them from their own house to the market place and then on to the stocks, where they "did in moste indecent and shamfull mannor cast durte upon [... them] and pissed on their heads," before dragging them back into town "by the feete, their heads lying upon the grownde, throughe the durty channells of the said streets."[70] As in Butler's literary account, the paraded proxy horseman of the 1618 Quemerford skimmington pelted the mob with grain: "he rode upon a red horse wth a paire of potts under him & in them some quantitye of bruinge graines, wch he used to cast upon ye presse of people, rushing over thicke upon him in ye way as he passed.'[71] Specialists, who sometimes view this grain as a malevolent inversion of the benign sprinkling of rice or confetti on newlyweds,[72] rarely comment on a second use of grain in skimmingtons, occurring, for example, after the armed Quemerford crowd forcibly dragged Agnes Mills from the upper floor of her home. They flung her into her "wett hole":[73]

trod upon hir & beried her filthily wth durt, & did beate hir blacke & blewe in many places with an intent ... to have had hir, viz, Agnes, out of their howse to ye horseman & to have sett hir up behind him to carry hir to Callne & there washe hir in the cuckinge stoole, & if she would not be still & sitt quietly, then to stuffe hir mouth wth greines.[74]

The dual role of brewers' grains as both ammunition and force-fed fodder is confirmed in a highly politicized account of a riding allegedly staged at Smithfield Bar (a fortified border then controlling those entering the City of London from the East London district of Smithfield), in January 1650:

Where one that acted Sir *Thomas* a horse-back, with a *Ladle* in his hand, two Baskets of *Prides* Graines before him, and his *Doxie* riding with her face to the horse tayle beihnd; one of them flung a Ladle of Graines in our Commanders face: which he took to be a great affront to a Souldier ... which a Butchers Boy perceiving, presently ... made him swallow his Graines and be thankfull.[75]

At their most typical, skimmingtons unite punishment and festival. Public processional street theatre mocking dominant wives and henpecked or cuckolded husbands enlisted a shamed couple's closest neighbors to reenact their transgressions with a satirical use of transvestite clothing and gendered household items. Some neighbors enthusiastically volunteered to play the role of proxy, with the aim of extracting maximum shame from the couple (and a generous tip or formal payment for their trouble), while others required coercion or refused to participate.[76] *Late Lancashire Witches* describes rowdy street theatre disrupted by the newlywed couple themselves, the bride Parnell and Lawrence, her bewitched and impotent husband. Far from allowing themselves to be drummed out, they unseat the proxy couple and proceed to beat the unfortunate pair with their own mock weapons.[77]

Satirizing the political impotence of English foreign policy, the brief skimmington account in Andrew Marvell's poem "The last instructions to a painter," notes that when a London neighborhood learns of a local husband-beater: "the just Street does the next House invade / Mounting the Neighbour Couple on lean Jade."[78] In a diary entry of 22 February 1563, another Londoner, Henry Machyn, confirms those paraded as the nearest neighbors, not the shamed couple:

The xxij day of Feybruary, was Shroyff-monday, at Charyngcrosse ther was a man cared of iiij men, and a-for hym a bagpype playng, a shame [=shawm] and a drum playhyng, and a xx lynkes bornyng a-bowtt hym, because ys next neybor('s) wyff ded bett [=beat] here hosband; ther-for yt (is) ordered that ys next naybor shall ryd a-bowtt the plase.[79]

Margaret Cavendish argues for abolishing London's "Foolish ... Unjust and Unhandsome Custom" of the skimmington, which shames an "Innocent Person", ... " the next Neighbour " rather than the "Foolish Husband," who should be forced to "Ride in Disgrace, Scorn, and Pain" for allowing his wife to usurp his "Masculine Authority."[80] Knowingly or not, Cavendish betrays no awareness that near neighbors might enjoy heightened opportunities as cuckolders. One such is Julio, the eponymous hero of *The Knave in Graine*. He smugly endures being paraded in a skimmington cart as the proxy of an elderly neighbor who bitterly hints that Julio cuckolded him: "Well he stands heare but for a shew, and I am sure I suffered for it really and indeed."[81]

More often than being paraded in carts, single skimmington proxies were mounted on a horse backwards,[82] or back to back if a couple, as in the Smithfield Bar account of 1650, featuring the couple's two nearest male neighbors raucously enacting the delinquents. One was cross-dressed as a virago, the other wore night clothes and carried domestic items (such as a distaff or spinning wheel), thereby identifying him as an effeminate husband. In *Hudibras*, the proxy playing the henpecked husband is perched backwards, behind his domineering wife:

Then mounted on a Horned *Horse*,
One bore a *Gauntlet* and *Gilt Spurs*,
[…] Next after, on a raw-bon'd Steed,
The Conqueror's *Standard-bearer* rid,
And bore aloft before the *Champion*
A *Petticoat* display'd, and rampant;
Near whom the *Amazon* triumphant,
Bestrid her *Beast*, and on the *Rump* on't
Sat Face to *Tail*, and *Bum* to *Bum*,
The *Warrier* whilom overcome;
Arm'd with a *Spindle* and a *Distaff*,
Which as he rode, she made him twist off.[83]

The backward ride was practiced from the 8th century onwards as a geographically widespread shaming ritual meted out legally as well as informally to those facing sentences for crimes ranging from capital offences to petty social delinquencies.[84] A youthful eye-witness recollection of John Stow (c. 1525–1605) records both carting and backward riding as judicial punishments for cuckolders, in this case the Parish priest of St Michael's Church in Cornhill, London. Having been caught *in flagrante* by John Atwod, the local draper, with his wife:

the Priest being apprehended and committed, I saw his punishment to be thus: He was on three Market dayes conveyed thorow the high street and Markets of the Citie, with a paper on his head, wherein was written his trespasse. The first day hee rode in a Carry; the second, on a horse, his face to the horse taile; the third, led betwixt twaine, and every day rung with Basons, and proclamations made of his fact at every turning of the streets, and also before Iohn Atwods Stall, and the Church doore of his Service, where hee lost his Chauntry of twenty Nobles the yeere, and was banished the Citie for ever.[85]

Hudibras too, alludes to such judicial punishments, as when describing the ignominious journey to the stocks endured by Hudibras and Ralpho "mounted both upon their Horses / But with their *Faces* to the *Arses*," Butler compares backward riders to the spoils of Roman triumphs.[86]

Such triumphs are again evoked when Sir Hudibras labels the skimmington a "prophane … *Show* … a *Paganish* Invention"; only to endure correction by his squire:

Quoth *Ralpho*, You mistake the matter;
For, all th' *Antiquity* you smatter
Is but a *Riding*, us'd of course,
When the *Grey Mare*'s *the better Horse*.
When o'er the Breeches greedy *Women*
Fight, to extend their vast *Dominion*.[87]

Here Butler refers to "the battle for the breeches," waged for household dominance by some marital couples, as depicted in popular prints such as one of 1628 showing a skimmington and a proxy "wife" wearing breeches.[88] Butler continues to subvert well-worn cultural references to the gender power struggle to his own purpose:

And in the Cause Impatient *Grizel*[89]
Has drubb'd her Husband, with *Bull's Pizzle,*
And brought him under *Covert Baron,*
To turn her *Vassal* with a *Murrain;*
When Wives their Sexes shift, like *Hares*
And ride their Husbands, like *Night-Mares,*
And they in mortal *Battle* vanquish'd,
Are of their *Charter* dis-enfranchis'd,
And by the right of War, like *Gills,*
Condemn'd to *Distaff, Horns,* and *Wheels;*
For when Men by their Wives are cow'd,
Their *Horns* of course are understood.[90]

A less rowdy 18th-century stage skimmington features women celebrating their neighbor's victory in a domestic argument over her husband. As they process through the village, they too, sing a ballad referring to "the battle for the breeches":

Good wives, pray learn
Your Husbands Rage to quell:
And follow this Example,
Whenever they rebel.
This man-like buxom Dame,
The Breeches long has worn;
Henceforth no more be tame,
But valiant in your Turn.[91]

The currency of such gender reversals is confirmed by historical accounts. On June 18, 1607, within the framework of other protesting demonstrations, outraged men and women of Wells used the ritual framework of the typical skimmington ritual to ridicule unpopular city leaders. Their procession included the displaying of gendered items of clothing as triumphal trophies, a cross-dressed man with a spinning wheel and distaff, a man with a skimming ladle, and two men mounted on one horse throwing handfuls of grain from a basket.[92]

Recognizing the power of performance and ceremony to build and bind communities and forge perceptions of norms, the early modern Church, the royal court, and city authorities all competed for their control. English religious reform, before and during the Commonwealth, had largely dismantled the Christian festive year that supported the fabric of Catholic European society, although historians such as Underdown caution against interpreting events such as the Wells disorders of 1607 as a straightforward clash between traditionalists and a Puritan minority determined to suppress their May Games.[93] Sir Hudibras and Ralpho's clashes with traditionalist revelers are similarly deserving of nuanced interpretation.

Sir Hudibras roundly condemns the horrors of the traditional English village skimmington as an anti-feminist, Papist, "Dev'l's *Procession*":

'Tis Ethnique and Idolatrous,
From Heathenism deriv'd to us.
Does not the Whore of Babylon ride
Upon her horned Beast astride
[...] It is an Antichristian Opera,
Much us'd in Midnight times of Popery;
[...] To scandalize that Sex, for scolding,
To whom the Saints are so beholding.[94]

His rousing oration in defense of "*Women*, who were our first *Apostles*" is rudely halted in mid-sentence by a volley of eggs and blows. Demonstrating yet again his cowardice and moral impotence, his face and beard "besmear'd with Orange-tawny Slime," and accompanied by Ralpho "smother'd with the Stink" of dung and grain, Hudibras beats "a brave Retreat" from the skimmington mob.[95]

James Stokes identifies the early 17th century as a watershed "moment of great cultural change in which efforts to suppress most festive and performative elements of traditional culture coincided with an end to the acceptance of women in performance."[96] According to Stokes, the skimmington's turning of "punishment of women into a comic performance" parodies the medieval festive elevation of women to central performative roles, as May queens, processional leaders or suchlike. This important insight should not, however, obscure the fact that skimmingtons publicly humiliate weak husbands no less than dominant wives. They reflect gendered anxieties of a transitional period, when radically changing expectations of marriage and its duration (not least due to medical advances in childbed survival rates), increasingly undermined conventional views valuing the public duty of procreation above the private pleasures of companionship.

Conclusion

This essay focuses on Butler's *Hudibras* in the light of evolving cultural reflections of impotence, cuckoldry and the skimmington, with reference to legal and historical records, and literary and factual accounts by diarists and others, both domestic and foreign. The poem's skimmington account unites punitive and festive elements, including rough music, bad smells, cuckolds' horns and pelting with missiles such as eggs, grain and dung, to frame its central performative ritual, the cross-dressed theatrical reenactment of gender conflicts by two back-to-back, mounted proxy actors played by the couple's nearest male neighbors. Through this use of neighbors—innocent or not—as proxies for a transgressing couple, the skimmington lent itself to

Butler's favored themes of individual and collective social responsibility. As literary creation rather than sociological record, his *Hudibras* skimmington contributes to our understanding of the development of persistent cultural conventions and of the opaque relationship between literary texts and historical accounts. Creatively, and with varying degrees of accuracy in reflecting actual practice, Butler draws on and reinforces current cultural conventions. He brings together and illuminates numerous features typical of individual skimmingtons, including the subversion of judicial punishment, and the mockery of political festival, from Roman triumphs to 17th-century election celebrations.

By 1664, when the *Hudibras* skimmington was first published, witchcraft was no longer viewed as the primary cause of impotence, and traditional peasant "wisdoms," encouraging impotent husbands to cuckold themselves by attaining fatherhood through the help of their nearest neighbor, had been largely forgotten. However, such obsolete belief systems indelibly mark the performative practices of the European charivari and related marital shaming rituals. Dramatists and writers viewed magical impotence and skimmingtons as attractive vehicles for introducing into their works erotic energy, combining "the celebratory and the violent"[97] and colorful, exotic elements of occult ritual involving female characters, and systematically utilized them as vehicles for pointed social and political commentary. Although skimmingtons involving marital shaming are rare after 1800, they are historically documented until at least 1930,[98] and feature strikingly in 19th-century novels by Walter Scott, Edward William Davies and Thomas Hardy.

In *Hudibras*, Butler created a vehicle for political satire with much slippery layering of meaning. Although social historians recognize the documentary value of his skimmington account, they have not systematically contextualized it within changing cultural conventions. Suffused with references to the cuckold's horns, it directly develops questions of truth and justice within the context of Butler's sustained social critique.[99] Butler's primary motivation was political rather than domestic; he targeted the private battle between the sexes, but even more the political humiliations of Commonwealth and post-Commonwealth England, and the public hypocrisies of those who imposed them.[100] With numerous knowing nods to popular forms of contemporary print culture such as picaresque fiction, the mountebank's quack bill and the ballad sheet or jest book, *Hudibras* subverts classical texts and chivalric romances. Its skimmington account tellingly combines *Hudibras*'s three mocking strands: style, subject and satire; heroicizing traditional, officially discouraged, "anti-processional" festival practices parodying self-promoting, self-serving Establishment ceremonial culture typified by the Roman triumph. Through his cowardly, hypocritical Hudibras and Ralph, his cheating charlatans, and the shaming rituals of his skimmington mob, Butler satirizes and criticizes Puritans, Catholics, royal and political elites, and the social folly and political impotence of post-Commonwealth England. His bleak pessimism infects all his targets. He satirizes the dishonest dealings of *Hudibras*'s occult protagonists, quacks and central pair, the private cheating of adulterers and their complicit cuckolds,[101] and even more the shameless public cheating of the 17th-century "quacks of government," the political and religious leaders who, in betraying and politically "cuckolding" those on both sides of the Civil War, attracted Butler's sharpest ridicule.[102] *Hudibras* marks a clear watershed in cultural representations of skimmingtons. After 1664, the description and depiction of skimmingtons in art or literature owe as much to Butler as to any folkloric authenticity.

Works Cited

Early Printed Sources (pre-1900)

Anon, *Common Sense or The Englishman's Journal* (London), Saturday, April 16, 1737 (Issue 11).

Anon, *Hudibras the second part*. London, 1663.

Beaumont, Francis and John Fletcher, "The Woman's Prize," *Comedies and Tragedies*. London: Humphrey Robinson and Humphrey Moseley, 1647.

Butler, Samuel, *Hudibras the second part by the Author of the first*. London, 1664.

Butler, Samuel (ed. Zachary Grey), *Hudibras in three parts ... with large annotations and a preface by Zachary Grey*, 2 vols. London: C. Bathurst et al., 1772 (I) and London: Vernor et al., 1806 (II).

Butler, Samuel, *"Dildoides, a Burlesque Poem," with a key explaining several names and characters in Hudibras. Never before printed*. London: J. Nutt, 1706.

Butler, Samuel, *The Posthumous Works of Mr. Samuel Butler (author of "Hudibras") compleat in one volume*. London: R. Reily, 1730.

Cavendish, Margaret (Duchess of Newcastle), *Orations of divers sorts, accommodated to divers places*. London, 1662.

Crouch, John, *The Man in the Moon. Discovering a World of Knavery ... Ianuary 23 to Ian. 31*. London, 1650.

Davies, Edward William, *Frank Raleigh of Watercombe... in three volumes*, III. London: Chapman and Hall, 1877.

D[ay?], J[ohn?], *The Knave in Graine, new Vampt. A witty Comedy, Acted at the Fortune ... written by J. D. Gent*. London: John Nicholson, 1640.

Gayton, Edmund, *Pleasant notes upon Don Quixot*. London: William Hunt, 1654.

Grimm, Jacob (ed.), *Deutsche Rechts Alterthümer*. Göttingen: Dieterische Buchhandlung, 1828.

Grimm, Jacob (ed.), *Weisthümer gesammelt von Jacob Grimm, dritter Theil*. Göttingen: Dieterische Buchhandlung, 1842.

Hawker, Essex, *The Country-Wedding and skimington: a tragic-comi-pastoral-farcical opera*. London: W. Trott, 1729.

Henry VIII, "Henry VIII: August 1532, 16–31," *Letters and Papers, Foreign and Domestic, Henry VIII, Volume 5: 1531–1532* (1880), 536–52, http://www.british-history.ac.uk.libezproxy.open.ac.uk/report.aspx?compid=77491, accessed: December 15, 2012.

Heywood, Thomas and Richard Brome, *The Late Lancashire Witches*. London: Benjamin Fisher, 1634.

Jonson, Ben, *The Workes of Beniamin Jonson*. London: W. Stansby, 1616.

Locke, John, *A second vindication of the reasonableness of Christianity*. London: A. and J. Churchill and Edward Castle, 1697.

Luther, Martin, "Vom ehelichen Leben, 1522." *Der sechste teil der Bücher des Ehrnwirdigen Herrn Doctoris Martini Lutheri*. Wittenberg: Hans Lufft, 1553.

Machyn, Henry, *The Diary of Henry Machyn: Citizen and Merchant-Taylor of London (1550–1563)*, ed. J. G. Nichols. London, 1848, http://www.british-history.ac.uk/report.aspx?compid=45531, accessed: December 3, 2012.

Marten, John, *A Treatise of the Venereal Disease*. London: John Marten, 1711.

Marvell, Andrew, et al., *The third part of the collection of poems on affairs of State*. London, 1689.

Misson, M[onsieur], *M. Misson's Memoirs and Observations in his Travels over England … translated by Mr Ozell*. London: D. Browne et al., 1719.

Pepys, Samuel, *Pepys's Later Diaries*, ed. C. S. Knighton. Thrupp: Sutton Publishing, 2006.

Pepys, Samuel, *The Diary of Samuel Pepys*, 11 vols., ed. William Matthews and Robert Latham. London, 1970–1983.

Platter the Younger, Thomas, *Thomas Platter d. J.: Beschreibung der Reisen durch Frankreich, Spanien, England und die Niederlande 1595–1600*, 2 vols., ed. Rut Keiser. Basel & Stuttgart: Schwabe, 1968.

Prynne, William, *Histrio-Mastix: the Players Scourge, or, Actors Tragædie*. London: Michael Sparke, 1633.

Scott, Walter, *Novels and romances of the author of Waverley, Vol. IV. The Fortunes of Nigel*. Edinburgh: Archibald Constable, 1824.

Shadwell, Thomas, *The Lancashire-Witches and Tegue o Divelly the Irish Priest: a Comedy*. London: John Starkey, 1682.

Stow, John, *The survey of London*. London: Nicholas Bourn, 1633.

Webster, John and William Rowley, *A Cure for a Cuckold. A Pleasant Comedy*. London: Francis Kirkman, 1661.

Secondary Sources and Modern Editions

Alford, Violet, "Rough music or charivari," *Folklore* 70 (1959): 505–18.

Antal, F., "Hogarth and his Borrowings," *Art Bulletin* 29:1 (1947): 36–48.

Barlow, Jeremy, *The Enraged Musician: Hogarth's Musical Imagery*. Aldershot, UK/Burlington, VT: Ashgate, 2005.

Brown, Pamela Allen, *Better a Shrew than a Sheep: Women, Drama and the Culture of Jest in Early Modern England*. Ithaca, NY: Cornell University Press, 2003.

Bruster, Douglas, *Drama and the Market in the Age of Shakespeare*. Cambridge: Cambridge University Press, 1992.

Cunnington, B. Howard, "A Skimmington in 1618," *Folklore* 41.3 (1930): 287–90.

Davis, Natalie Zemon, "The Reasons of Misrule: Youth Groups and Charivaris in Sixteenth-century France," *Past & Present* 50 (1971): 41–75.

Doody, Margaret Anne, *The Daring Muse: Augustan Poetry Reconsidered*. Cambridge: Cambridge University Press, 1985.

Drossbach, Gisela, "Concordia nutrit amorem—Konrad von Megenberg und die Ehe," Edith Feistner, ed. *Konrad von Megenberg (1309–1374): ein spätmittelalterlicher 'Enzyklopädist' im europäischen Kontext*. Wiesbaden: Reichert, 2011. 345–56.

Hardy, Thomas, *The life and death of the Mayor of Casterbridge: a story of a man of character*. New York: Harper, 1920. First published 1886.

Ingram, Martin, "Ridings, Rough Music and the 'Reform of Popular Culture' in Early Modern England," *Past & Present* 105 (1984): 79–113.

Jones, Malcolm, "The English Broadside Print c. 1550–c. 1650," *A New Companion to English Renaissance Literature and Culture, v.1.*, ed. Michael Hattaway. Oxford: Wiley-Blackwell, 2010. 478–526.

Katritzky, M. A., *Healing, Performance and Ceremony in the Writings of Three Early Modern Physicians: Hippolytus Guarinonius and the Brothers Felix and Thomas Platter*. Farnham, UK/Burlington, VT: Ashgate, 2012.

Katritzky, M. A., *Women, Medicine and Theatre, 1500–1750: Literary Mountebanks and Performing Quacks*. Farnham, UK/Burlington, VT: Ashgate, 2007.

Kent, Joan R., "'Folk justice' and royal justice in early seventeenth–century England: a 'Charivari' in the Midlands," *Midland History* 8 (1983): 70–85.

Kümper, Hiram, "'Man greiff manchmallen einer die brüst.' Sexualität und Gewalt in vormodernen Alltagsbeziehungen," *Liebeslust und Ehefrust. Vom Sinn und Unsinn sich zu binden*, ed. Johannes Gießauf, and Andrea Penz. Vienna: Böhlau-Verlag, in press.

Marshall, Ashley, "The Aims of Butler's Satire in 'Hudibras,'" *Modern Philology* 105:4 (2008): 637–65.

Mellinkoff, Ruth, "Riding Backwards: Theme of Humiliation and Symbol of Evil," *Viator* 4 (1973): 153–76.

Middleton, Thomas, *Thomas Middleton the Collected Works*, Gary Taylor and John Lavagnino, eds. Oxford: Oxford University Press, 2010.

O'Connor, Marion, "The witch," *Thomas Middleton the Collected Works*, ed. Thomas Middleton, Gary Taylor and John Lavagnino. Oxford: Oxford University Press, 2010, 1124–8.

Pettitt, Tom, "Customary Drama: Social and Spatial Patterning in Traditional Encounters," *Folk Music Journal* 7:1 (1995): 27–42.

Rösener, Werner, *Bauern im Mittelalter*. München: Beck, 1985.

Schnell, Rüdiger, *Sexualität und Emotionalität in der vormodernen Ehe* (Köln: Böhlau-Verlag, 2002).

Seal, Graham, "A "Hussitting" in Berkshire, 1930," *Folklore* 98.1 (1987): 91–4.

Stokes, James, "Women and Performance in Medieval and Early Modern Suffolk," *Early Theatre* 15:1 (2012): 27–43.

Stokes, James and Robert J. Alexander, *Records of Early English Drama [REED]: Somerset, including Bath*, 2 vols. Toronto: University of Toronto Press, 1996.

Thompson, E. P., "Rough music reconsidered," *Folklore* 103:1 (1992): 3–26.

Underdown, David, "'But the shows of their street': civic pageantry and charivari in a Somerset town, 1607," *Journal of British Studies* 50:1 (2011): 4–23.

Notes

1 My thanks to Sara Matthews-Grieco for inviting me to join her RSA "Cuckolds" panels, to Eric Nicholson for connecting us, and to Pavel Drábek, my co-organizer for "Cuckolds II: Impotence and Cuckoldry in Literary Culture" (RSA 2011, panel 20521), our chair Natasha Korda, co-presenters Hannah Lavery and Joanne Rochester and auditors. Also, for research and conference funding, to The Open University (Arts Faculty FRC Award) and Herzog August Library (Visiting Fellowship, 2011). Except as otherwise noted, translations are mine.

2 Zachary Grey's edition, here referenced throughout as *Hudibras* I and *Hudibras* II, publishes the poem's three authorized parts in two volumes (Butler, Samuel (ed. Zachary Grey), *Hudibras in three parts … with large annotations and a preface by Zachary Grey*, 2 vols. (London: C. Bathurst et al.), 1772 (I) and (London: Vernor et al.), 1806 (II). Both volumes first published in Dublin in 1744. Butler's skimmington account concludes Canto III of Part II.

3 *Hudibras* I, 56–9, 63, 67: "*Ralph* … cou'd foretel what'ever was / By Consequence to come to pass. / … In Men, what gives or cures the Itch, / What makes them Cuckolds, poor or rich."

4 Bruster, Douglas, *Drama and the Market in the Age of Shakespeare* (Cambridge: Cambridge University Press, 1992), 49.

5 Butler, Samuel, *The Posthumous Works of Mr Samuel Butler (author of "Hudibras") compleat in one volume* (London: R. Reily, 1730), 192.

6 *Hudibras* II, 163, 455–6.

7 Webster, John and William Rowley, *A Cure for a Cuckold. A Pleasant Comedy* (London: Francis Kirkman, 1661), II.i , IV.i (sigs. D^v, $E4^v$).

8 Grimm, Jacob (ed.), *Deutsche Rechts Alterthümer* (Göttingen: Dieterische Buchhandlung), 1828, 454. See also below, on divorce of Frances Howard.

9 Grimm, Jacob (ed.), *Weisthümer gesammelt von Jacob Grimm, dritter Theil* (Göttingen: Dieterische Buchhandlung, 1842). For this reference and invaluable information on Grimm's "wisdoms" and their legal context I thank Hiram Kümper.

10 Katritzky, M. A., *Healing, Performance and Ceremony in the Writings of three early modern physicians: Hippolytus Guarinonius and the brothers Felix and Thomas Platter* (Farnham, UK/Burlington, VT: Ashgate, 2012), 108, 302.

11 Grimm, *Alterthümer*, 444–5: "roipen dae sine *naebur* aen, dat sie inne sines wives lives noet helpen weren … sie seinem *nachbar* bringen … der frau an einen schaffen, der ihr ihre pflege thun kann … bitten dar sinen negsten *nabern* dat er siner frauen helfe" (Grimm's italics; minor variants of the first three are republished in Grimm, *Weisthümer*, 48, 70, 311).

12 Rösener, Werner, *Bauern im Mittelalter* (München: Beck, 1985), 168, 190–91.

13 Kümper, Hiram, "'Man greiff manchmallen einer die brüst.' Sexualität und Gewalt in vormodernen Alltagsbeziehungen." Johannes Gießauf, Andrea Penz (eds). *Liebeslust und Ehefrust. Vom Sinn und Unsinn sich zu binden* (Vienna: Böhlau-Verlag, in press).

14 Grimm, *Alterthümer*, 444; Schnell, Rüdiger, *Sexualität und Emotionalität in der vormodernen Ehe* (Köln: Böhlau-Verlag, 2002), 219–20.

15 Gisela Drossbach, "Concordia nutrit amorem – Konrad von Megenberg und die Ehe." Edith Feistner (ed.), *Konrad von Megenberg (1309–1374): ein spätmittelalterlicher 'Enzyklopädist' im europäischen Kontext* (Wiesbaden: Reichert, 2011), 345–56, 345, 351–2.

16 In the broad sense of infertile.

17 Luther, Martin, "Vom ehelichen Leben, 1522." *Der sechste teil der Bücher des Ehrnwirdigen Herrn Doctoris Martini Lutheri* (Wittenberg: Hans Lufft, 1553), sigs. 172r–184r, sigs. 173r–v: "Lieber Man … Vergünne mir /das ich mit deinem bruder oder nehesten freund [literally: "friend" but here almost certainly used in the sense of "blood relative"] ein heimlich Ehe habe."

18 Platter the Younger, Thomas, *Thomas Platter d. J: Beschreibung der Reisen durch Frankreich, Spanien, England und die Niederlande 1595–1600*, 2 vols., ed. Rut Keiser (Basel & Stuttgart: Schwabe, 1968), II, 814: "Unndt haben die weibsbilder … in Engellandt viel mehr freyheit als ettwan an anderen orten, wissen sich auch deßen woll zegebrauchen, dann sie in kleideren überaus prächtig, mehrtheils müeßig spatzieren gehen oder auf gutschen fahren, unndt mießen es die mannen ihnen gar woll lassen gefallen, dörfen ihnen deßwegen nichts arges zufügen, sonder es schlagen woll oft die weiber ihre männer, welches so man es erfahret, setzet man den aller nechsten seinen nachbauren auf einen karren unndt führet ihn dem geschlagenen zu spott durch die gantze statt mitt vermeldung, daß seye sein straff darumb, daß er nicht seinem nachbauren seye zuhülf kommen, als ihn sein frauw geschlagen."

19 Confirmed as the wife ("la pauvre Calomniée") in the original French edition of 1698.

20 Misson, M[onsieur], *M. Misson's Memoirs and observations in his travels over England … translated by Mr Ozell* (London: D. Browne et al., 1719), 129.

21 Alford, Violet, "Rough music or charivari," *Folklore* 70 (1959): 505–18; Davis, Natalie Zemon, "The Reasons of Misrule: Youth Groups and Charivaris in Sixteenth-century France," *Past & Present* 50 (1971): 41–75.

22 Stokes, James and Robert J. Alexander, *Records of Early English Drama [REED]: Somerset, including Bath*, 2 vols. (Toronto: University of Toronto Press, 1996), I, 69.

23 E. P. Thompson discusses this and similar cases ("Rough music reconsidered," *Folklore* 103:1 [1992]: 3–26, 16); Davis indicates a similarly broad role for the French city charivari (66). Butler too refers to the skimmington as a vehicle for social or industrial protest: "So, in this mongrel state of ours, / The rabble are the supreme powers; / That hors'd us on their backs, to show us / A jadish trick at last, and throw us" (*Hudibras* II, 355).

24 Pepys, Samuel, *The Diary of Samuel Pepys*, 11 vols., ed. William Matthews and Robert Latham (London, 1970–1983): December 26, 1662, February 6, 1663.

25 Anon, *Hudibras the second part* (London 1663). This text is known as the "unauthorized" Part II.

26 Probably Butler, Samuel, *Hudibras the second part by the Author of the first* (London 1664). This text, recognized as the "authorized" Part II, was licensed on November 5, 1663.

27 Pepys: November 28, 1663, December 10, 1663, January 27, 1664, October 11, 1665.

28 Pepys: July 19, 1668 (*pace* Marshall, Ashley, "The aims of Butler's satire in 'Hudibras,'" *Modern Philology* 105:4 [2008], 637–65, 638 n. 4).

29 Pepys, Samuel, *Pepys's Later Diaries*, ed. C. S. Knighton (Thrupp: Sutton Publishing, 2006), 142, 188. The copyright of Part III was still separately owned in 1684, when an integrated two-part edition of all three parts was first published. A copy of the three-part 1689 edition is in Pepys's Library.

30 Anon, *Hudibras the second part* (London 1663), 11–13. In the authorized Part II, Sidrophel informs Hudibras that his "Zany" assistant or "under conjurer" Hight Whachum, is the same French quack who robbed him in the unauthorized Part II: "He play'd the Saltinbancho's part, / Transform'd t' a Frenchman by my art; / he stole your cloak, and pick'd your pocket, / Chous'd and Caldes'd ye like a blockhead" (*Hudibras* II, 36–7, 93–4).

31 The authorized Hudibras's deceptive patina of gentle tolerance is borrowed from medieval European traditions of folly literature. Miguel Cervantes, and even more the quirky discursiveness, mild satire and burlesque rhymes of Gayton's commentary to his masterpiece, are major inspirations for Hudibras and its central pair. Gayton, Edmund, *Pleasant notes upon Don Quixot* (London: William Hunt, 1654). "Hudibras at Court" repeatedly refers to Ralph as "Sancho" and his horse as "Rosenante"; Butler's essay "The Assembly-Man" comments "Sometimes, the assembler will venture at the original, and then (with the translator of *Don Quixot*) he mistakes sobs and sighs for eggs and collops" (*Posthumous works*, 7, 9, 232).

32 *Hudibras* I, 340–2, 349–54; *Hudibras* II, 72, 156. On the medical treatment of impotence and sympathetic magical practices such as this one see the essays by Meredith Ray and Laura Giannetti in this volume.

33 See the essay in this volume by Matteo Duni.

34 O'Connor, Marion, "The witch." *Thomas Middleton the Collected Works*, Thomas Middleton, ed. Gary Taylor and John Lavagnino (Oxford: Oxford University Press, 2010), 1124–8, 1124; on this case, see also Katritzky (2012), 181–91.

35 Middleton, 1137: "Knit with these charmèd and retentive knots, / Neither the man begets nor woman breeds, / No, nor performs the least desires of wedlock."

36 Jonson, Ben, *The Workes of Beniamin Jonson* (London: W. Stansby, 1616), 952.

37 Platter I, 274–5; translation: Katritzky (2012), 176–7.

38 Jonson (1616), 947. Butler, too, refers to this classical practice: "Mould 'em as *Witches* do their Clay, / When they make *Pictures* to destroy? / And vex 'em into any Form / That fits their Purpose to do Harm?" (*Hudibras* I, 385–6).

39 Heywood, Thomas and Richard Brome, *The Late Lancashire Witches* (London: Benjamin Fisher, 1634), IV, V (sigs. H3[r], L[r]).

40 Shadwell, Thomas, *The Lancashire-Witches and Tegue o Divelly the Irish Priest: a Comedy* (London: John Starkey, 1682).

41 *Hudibras* II, 11–50. Sidrophel is identified by the anonymous editor of *Dildoides* (Butler, Samuel, *"Dildoides, a Burlesque Poem," with a key explaining several names and characters in Hudibras. Never before printed* (London: J. Nutt, 1706, 13) as Sir Paul Neal FRS; by Zachary Grey as the Commonwealth astrologer William Lilly.

42 Such as Shakespeare's Dr Caius (*Merry Wives of Windsor*), Jonson's Vangoose (*The Masque of Augures*, London, 1622), or Edward Gayton's "French Doctor," 82. This tradition ultimately draws on the "merchant scene" of some European mystery plays, in which holy women, usually the Marys at the Sepulchre, encounter itinerant quacks selling herbs and spices, sometimes also pushing patent medicines, performing cures or claiming to "raise the dead," see Katritzky, M. A., *Women, Medicine and Theatre, 1500–1750: literary mountebanks and performing quacks* (Aldershot, UK/ Burlington, VT: Ashgate, 2007), 33–43.

43 Hudibras's method of dealing with this foreign strolling mountebank was heartily applauded as exemplary by the surgeon John Marten as late as 1711 (*A treatise of the venereal disease* [London: John Marten, 1711], 740–41).

44 Anon, *Hudibras the second part* (London 1663), canto II, 49–50, 78.

45 Anon, *Common Sense or The Englishman's Journal* (London), Saturday, April 16, 1737 (Issue 11).

46 Thompson documents suicides of 1736 and 1853 following rough music, 23 n. 46. Butler is acknowledged in both Walter Scott's and Edward William Davies's literary precedents for Thomas Hardy's skimmington. Davies's main protagonist, Betty Mumford, dies after a brief period of insanity brought on by the shock and shame of a "skymaton"; Hardy's skimmington leads within hours to the death of Lucetta and her unborn child. See: Scott, *Novels and romances of the author of Waverley, vol. IV. The Fortunes of Nigel* (Edinburgh: Archibald Constable, 1824), 294–9. Davies, *Frank Raleigh of Watercombe … in three volumes* (London: Chapman and Hall, 1877), III, chapter 1; Hardy, *The life and death of the Mayor of Casterbridge: a story of a man of character* (New York: Harper, 1920, first published 1886), chapters 36–40.

47 Illustrated with a print based on Hogarth's hugely influential skimmington illustration from his "large" series of *Hudibras* engravings of February 1726 (see below, notes 56 and 57).

48 Ingram, Martin, "Ridings, rough music and the 'Reform of popular culture' in early modern England." *Past & Present* 105 (1984): 79–113, 86–7, 108.

49 Beaumont, Francis and John Fletcher, "The woman's prize," *Comedies and Tragedies* (London: Humphrey Robinson and Humphrey Moseley, 1647), II.v, 106.

50 D[ay?], J[ohn?], *The Knave in Graine, new Vampt. A witty Comedy, Acted at the Fortune ... written by J. D. Gent* (London: John Nicholson, 1640), sig. L4[v].

51 Heywood and Brome, *Late Lancashire witches*, IV (sig. H.3[r]).

52 *Hudibras* I, 402–3.

53 Prynne, William, *Histrio-Mastix: the Players Scourge, or, Actors Tragædie* (London: Michael Sparke, 1633), 600.

54 Platter, *Beschreibung* I, 275–6: "hatt yeder ein besonder instrument, der ein ein alten kessel, der ander ein pfannen, der dritt ein trommen, der viert ein pfeiffen, der fünft ein löfel im saltzfaß, der sechst ein kühhorn u.s.w. … heben ihre instrument ettwan umb mitternacht an zeüben, understehet ye einer heßlicher zu schreyen, singen oder schlahen dann der ander, welches ein solch greülich getümmel unndt geschrey erweket, daß auch kein nachbaur biß in daß zwelfte hauß kein ruhe nitt haben kan." On the closely related Italian public shaming rituals referred to by modern historians as house-scornings, see the essay in this volume by Jacqueline Marie Musacchio.

55 Kent, Joan R, "'Folk justice' and royal justice in early Seventeenth-century England: a 'Charivari' in the Midlands," *Midland History* 8 (1983): 70–85, 73.

56 Plate XII (the "large skimmington") of Hogarth's 12 "large" *Hudibras* engravings of February 1726 (preparatory drawing: Windsor Castle, Royal Library inv. RL 13464). This print's most

distinguished variant is Thomas Rowlandson's *Dr Syntax with the skimmington riders*, published as a colored aquatint by R Ackermann c. 1820 (Huntington Library, 132504, f. 153). An early visual representation of an English skimmington is the original plaster "skymmety" frieze, *in situ* over the fireplace of the Great Hall of Montacute House, Somerset (Ingram, plates 2–3). Finished in 1601, Montacute was inherited in 1614 by Sir Robert Phelips, recipient of a letter of 16 August 1634 by Nathaniel Tomkyns describing the original 1634 production of Heywood and Brome's *The Late Lancashire witches*, and noting its skimmington and magical impotence (Stokes and Alexander, 416).

57 Antal, F., "Hogarth and his Borrowings." *Art Bulletin* 29:1 (1947): 36–48, 38–9; Barlow, Jeremy, *The Enraged Musician: Hogarth's musical imagery* (Aldershot, UK/Burlington, VT: Ashgate, 2005), 60–83. Closely following the anonymously illustrated 1710 edition of *Hudibras*, the skimmington in Plate IX of Hogarth's "small" series of 17 etchings for the May 1726 edition of *Hudibras* observes the low-key conventions of genre composition (preparatory drawing: Windsor Castle, Royal Library inv. RL 13465).

58 Mockingly based on a faun in the Farnese Gallery's monumental *Procession of Bacchus and Ariadne* (Antal, 39). This fresco's artist, Annibale Carracci, had himself not dissimilarly subverted an earlier work (by his master Titian; see the essay by Francesca Alberti in this volume).

59 *Hudibras* I, 403–4.

60 *Hudibras* I, 404.

61 *Hudibras* I, 404–5: "First, He that led the *Cavalcate*, / Wore a Sowgelder's *Flagellate*, / On which he blew as strong a *Levet*, / As well-fee'd *Lawyer* on his *Breviate*; / When over one another's Heads / They charge (three Ranks at once) like *Sweads*." Sowgelders were unqualified veterinary surgeons on the lowest rung of the medical hierarchy, little more than itinerant beggars. As elsewhere in *Hudibras*, they customarily announced their arrival in a new location not with the delicate piping of a flageolet, but with that most unrespectable of instruments, a bellowing rustic horn (*Hudibras* I, 148, 341; *Hudibras* II, 40, 286).

62 *Hudibras* I, 405.

63 Cunnington, B. Howard, "A skimmington in 1618," *Folklore* 41.3 (1930): 287–90, 289. See also Ingram, 82; Brown, Pamela Allen, *Better a Shrew than a Sheep: Women, Drama and the Culture of Jest in Early Modern England* (Ithaca, NY: Cornell University Press, 2003), 119.

64 Brown, 84.

65 "Henry VIII: August 1532, 16–31," *Letters and Papers, Foreign and Domestic, Henry VIII, Volume 5: 1531–1532* (1880), 536–52, http://www.british-history.ac.uk.libezproxy.open.ac.uk/report.aspx?compid=77491, accessed: December 15, 2012.

66 *Hudibras* I, 409–10.

67 D[ay?], sig. Mr; Marvell, Andrew, et al., *The third part of the collection of poems on affairs of State* (London, 1689), 10: "Grains from Kettle fly."

68 *Hudibras* I, 405.

69 Locke, John, "Preface to the Reader," *A second vindication of the reasonableness of Christianity* (London: A. and J. Churchill and Edward Castle, 1697).

70 Kent, 73.

71 Cunnington, 289.

72 Pettitt, Tom, "Customary drama: social and spatial patterning in traditional encounters," *Folk Music Journal* 7:1 (1995): 27–42, 35; Underdown, David, "But the shows of their street: civic pageantry and charivari in a Somerset town, 1607," *Journal of British Studies* 50:1 (2011): 4–23, 15.

73 Variously interpreted as a puddle, pond or outdoor water closet.

74 Cunnington, 290.

75 Crouch, John, *The Man in the Moon. Discovering a World of Knavery … Ianuary 23 to Ian. 31* (Number 40), (London, 1650): 314.

76 In 1586, a participant complained of being short-changed "for his labour for riding" in Cambridge (Ingram, 102 n. 61).

77 Heywood and Brome, IV (sig. H4v): "Enter drum (beating before) a Skimington, and his wife on a horse; Divers country rusticks (as they passe) Par[nell]. pul[l]s Skimington of[f] the horse: and Law[rence]. Skimingtons wife: they beat [th]em. Drum beats alar[m]. horse comes away: The hoydens at first oppose the Gentlemen: who draw [their weapons]: the clownes [rustic peasants] vaile bonnet, make a ring Par. and Skim. fight."

78 In other words, the proxy couple rides a worn out horse. Marvell, 10.

79 Machyn, Henry, *The Diary of Henry Machyn: Citizen and Merchant-Taylor of London (1550–1563)*, ed. J. G. Nichols (London, 1848): "Diary: 1563 (Jan–July)," 298–312. http://www.british-history.ac.uk/report.aspx?compid=45531, accessed: December 3, 2012.

80 Cavendish, Margaret (Duchess of Newcastle), *Orations of divers sorts, accommodated to divers places* (London, 1662), 221–2; directly followed by "an oration against the liberty of women" and "an oration for the liberty of woman." Their passionately opposed arguments recall Sir Hudibras and his beloved widow Tomson's opposing gender perspectives to their concluding debate on marriage (Hudibras II, 419–50); Butler, *Posthumous works*, 311.

81 D[ay?], sigs. M^{r}, M2^{r}.

82 Cavendish, 221: "the next Neighbour Rides through the City Disgracefully … Striding upon a Horse with his Face towards the Tail, or Sitting astride upon a Staff."

83 *Hudibras* I, 406.

84 Mellinkoff, Ruth, "Riding backwards: theme of humiliation and symbol of evil," *Viator* 4 (1973): 153–76, 164–6.

85 Stow, John, *The survey of London* (London: Nicholas Bourn, 1633), 208.

86 *Hudibras* I, 253, 294 ("*Bauds* carted through the Crowd"); *Hudibras* II, 401 ("Cart-loads of bawds to prison sent").

87 Hudibras I, 410.

88 Jones, Malcolm, "The English broadside print c. 1550–c. 1650." *A new companion to English renaissance literature and culture volume 1*, ed. Michael Hattaway (Oxford: Wiley-Blackwell, 2010), 478–526, 482–3, 491.

89 Elsewhere, Butler compares "Patient Grisell" to Job (*Hudibras* I, 167).

90 *Hudibras* I, 410–11.

91 Hawker, Essex, *The Country-wedding and skimington: a tragic-comi-pastoral-farcical opera* (London: W. Trott), 1729, 21–2.

92 Underdown, 14–16.

93 Underdown, 19.

94 *Hudibras* I, 414–15.

95 *Hudibras* I, 419–22.

96 Stokes, James, "Women and performance in medieval and early modern Suffolk," *Early Theatre* 15:1 (2012), 27–43, 28, 35.

97 Doody, Margaret Anne, *The Daring Muse: Augustan Poetry Reconsidered* (Cambridge: Cambridge University Press, 1985), 123.

98 Seal, Graham, "A 'Hussitting' in Berkshire, 1930," *Folklore* 98.1 (1987), 91–4. According to a footnote (referencing *Hudibras*), to the brief allusions to skimmingtons in Walter Scott's historical novel *Fortunes of Nigel* (set in the Jacobean era): "the Skimmington … has been long discontinued in England" (94, 99).

99 *Hudibras* I, 383: "Why should not *Conscience* have *Vacation*, / As well as other Courts o' th' Nation? / Have equal Power to adjourn / Appoint *Appearance* and *Retorn?* / And make as nice Distinction serve / To split a Case; as those that carve / Invoking Cuckolds names, hit joints, / Why should not tricks as slight, do points?"

100 Marshall, 641, 665.

101 *Hudibras* II, 3: "Doubtless the pleasure is as great / Of being cheated as to cheat."

102 *Hudibras* II, 265.

PART II
Impotence, Magic and Medicine

Impotence, Witchcraft and Politics: A Renaissance Case

Matteo Duni

When the 19-year-old Isabella of Aragon arrived in Lombardy in early 1489, she must have been not very optimistic concerning the prospects of her marriage to the 20-year-old duke of Milan, Gian Galeazzo Maria Sforza, who was also her cousin.[1] The first problems had arisen in Naples a few weeks before, just hours after he had married her by proxy, on December 21, 1488: the very next day the Milanese delegation had accused Isabella's grandfather (King Ferrante of Naples) of cheating, alleging that a part of the dowry had been paid in underweight gold ducats. Isabella then undertook an almost three-week journey up the Tyrrhenian Sea through some very rough weather. The bride arrived in Genova so distressed and seasick that she had to rest there for several days. When she finally met her husband for the first time in Tortona under a torrential downpour, Gian Galeazzo tried awkwardly to embrace her in the carriage without dismounting from his horse, but his mount shied and frustrated his intention. This failed first encounter was but a foretaste of the difficulties he was going to have with his new bride, but nonetheless a botched embrace was rather negligible in view of what was still to happen—or rather would not happen—the first night the newlywed couple slept together in the castle of Vigevano on January 28.[2]

A Failed Consummation

Rumors quickly spread that Gian Galeazzo had proved to be extremely cold toward his wife, and thus the marriage had not been consummated. The difficulty was not overcome after the two arrived in Milan on February 1, nor when, a few days later, they moved to their main residence, the castle of Pavia. The Sforza-Aragon marriage was fast becoming the laughing stock of princely courts throughout the Italian peninsula, and everyone seemed to agree that the Duke was to blame: at King Ferrante's court in Naples it was said openly that "the marriage could not be in any way consummated because of the illness of the most Illustrious Duke, who was said to be wholly impotent (*frigidissimo*)."[3]

As far as the diagnosis of Gian Galeazzo's impotence was concerned, two types of explanation were put forth in contemporary court correspondence. Giacomo Trotti, Ferrarese ambassador to the Sforza court and a very well connected gossip monger, had no doubts: "I can attest in all certainty to Your Excellency that he [Gian Galeazzo] is in love and does not dare to look at her," he wrote to Duke Ercole d'Este, ascribing such an attitude to the fact that Gian Galeazzo was still quite immature: "[…] part boy, part simpleton, which proceeds from timidity, as he fears being scoffed at."[4]

Such timidity was willfully strengthened by Gian Galeazzo's uncle, Ludovico il Moro. The *de facto* ruler of Milan and sponsor of the marriage, il Moro actually resorted to lecturing the ducal couple in the presence of the court about "conjugal duty" and its mechanics, and then had the unfortunate newlyweds withdraw to their bedchamber to attempt, once more, the fulfillment of their marital obligation … naturally to no avail.[5] Alternating intimidation with advice, Ludovico would threaten Gian Galeazzo with "Hell if he were not to consummate the marriage, saying that in this case he would be forced to give back not only the dowry he had received … but possibly also his wife."[6] That such tactics could not possibly help a "mortified" Gian Galeazzo improve his performance was clear even to the ambassador Trotti, who commented the situation with a quote from Ovid ("We always strive for what's forbidden [and] want what's denied"). While Ludovico's ambition with regard to Milan was the obvious reason why he would have been happy to have an heirless nephew, the reactions of Isabella's entourage to her husband's indifference could be just as counterproductive as il Moro's "lectures." The duchess of Amalfi, Isabella's lady-in-waiting, joked crudely that if the sexual prowess of Milanese men was to be judged from Gian Galeazzo's, then "Lombard women must have a spider's web on their thing, and need to have someone sweep it away," and concluded, in agreement with Trotti, by urging the new bride to "finally get something done" (*uscire una volta de praticha*).[7]

Poor Isabella also had to endure practical advice in addition to heavy-handed comments. Her grandfather, King Ferrante, had two "expert women" (*matrone*) sent from Naples, with the goal of "encouraging the Duchess help the Duke," hoping that this would finally lead to consummation of the marriage.[8] The intervention of the *matrone* followed a practice recommended by physicians in cases where impotence had to be ascertained for legal reasons (such as the annulment of a marriage). In such situations, while physicians were supposed to examine the couple's genitals to make sure they had no visible deformity or defects which would make sexual intercourse impossible, "expert women" were to assist the spouses by feeding them spicy foods and rubbing their bodies with special ointments, encouraging them to relax and lie together. After having administered such aphrodisiac remedies, these women were supposed to observe what the couple would do, and relate it to the judge.[9] We do not know whether the Neapolitan *matrone* did anything of this sort, nor do we have any information of what they reported back to King Ferrante. We do know that an upset Isabella had later declared that "she'd rather live and stay as she does, than resort to similar expedients."[10]

The husband's mental and physical block—which an inexperienced bride was apparently incapable of dissolving—was not the only explanation invoked for Gian Galeazzo's impediment. Bernardino Corio's *Historia di Milano* (an eyewitness' account of Sforza events, published in 1503) appears to be the first to suggest that the Duke's impotence had non-natural causes: "[...] the Duke was bewitched (*affaturato*) to such degree, that for a long time he was unable to carry out his amorous intentions with his beautiful bride."[11] While Corio was prudently avoiding putting the blame on anyone, the always well-informed Paolo Giovio, in his *Historiae* (first published 1550–1552), relates more extensively that Isabella "was absolutely convinced that, on the very day of the wedding, through Ludovico's intervention, charms and spells had been cast upon herself and her husband by some sorceresses, in order to prevent them from having children."[12] Before Giovio, the official character of this rumor had already been sanctioned by Francesco Guicciardini, who had actually added a new twist to the story: "When Alfonso's daughter Isabella went to Milan to join her husband, Ludovico fell in love with her at first sight and wanted her for his own wife; and in order to obtain his ends (as everyone in Italy believed at that time), Ludovico saw to it by means of sorcery and enchantments that Gian Galeazzo was impotent for many months after his marriage."[13] Guicciardini thus explained the young duke's impotence as a consequence of his uncle's political ambitions and secret designs. While love at first sight was rather improbable, the core of Guicciardini's analysis was well founded: surviving diplomatic correspondence is very explicit on Ludovico's intentions to marry Isabella, which actually predated by at least a year her wedding to Gian Galeazzo.[14] In 1487, il Moro had looked, in fact, at a possible marriage with Isabella as instrumental to secure his hold on the Milanese state with the acquisition of the ducal title, but two years later his plans had changed, and now required Milan to be strongly hostile towards Naples. In this new strategy, the marriage of Gian Galeazzo into the house of Aragon had clearly become problematic, and Ludovico was considering the option of having the match annulled.[15] Failure to consummate a marriage was precisely one of the few accepted motivations for annulment, and this may explain Ludovico's scare tactics towards his nephew as well as the rumors spread about bewitchment.

The details of the supposed *maleficium* remain fuzzy: Giovio writes about women who cast spells (*donne fattucchiare*) but il Moro may even have resorted to much more sophisticated means of intervention. Following in the footsteps of his brother Galeazzo Maria and of his father Francesco, Ludovico relied systematically on astrology and would consult his trusted court astrologer, Ambrogio Varesi da Rosate, before taking any decision of importance. In particular, he believed the choice of the most appropriate moment for lying with one's woman should be guided by astrology in order to maximize the chances of conceiving an heir.[16] However, while astrological talismans or magical formulas and potions based on the influence of the heavenly bodies were believed to be helpful, they could also hinder sexual intercourse and conception. Therefore it would not be too far-fetched to suppose that Ludovico may also have had recourse to Ambrogio's arts, mobilizing the power of the stars (in addition to the power of magic spells) in the hopes of further frustrating Gian Galeazzo's ability to consummate his ill-fated marriage.[17] Whatever the cause of such ducal embarrassment, the story of Isabella's and Gian Galeazzo's sad first year as husband and wife is a good window onto the topic of impotence and magic in the Renaissance as it shows how any sexual failure could be interpreted as the product of several, and often mutually exclusive, factors.

Jurists and Canon Law on Magical Impotence

By the end of the Middle Ages, a long series of authors, both lay and ecclesiastic, had discussed at length the issue of impediments to love, conception and/or sexual intercourse caused by magical means.[18] The matter was described and regulated in the important early medieval text *Si per sortiarias*, which was eventually incorporated into canon law.[19] Ecclesiastical legislation thus gave full credit to the popular belief that sorcery could prevent *copula*, and instructed that couples unable to consummate their marriage should try purification through prayers, fasting and charitable deeds with the assistance of the clergy, and decreed that if the spouses' inability should persist for over three years, they could be separated and eventually remarry. That magically caused impotence gave legitimate grounds for the annulment of a marriage was conclusively confirmed by two of the most authoritative 13th-century canonists, Henry of Susa (Hostiensis) and Raymond of Peñafort, the editor of Pope Gregory IX's *Liber extra* (one of the standard textbooks of canon law).[20] Canonists also importantly distinguished between two possibilities: when a man could not have intercourse with any woman, his impotence (*frigiditas*) was likely due to natural causes. However, as Henry of Susa observed, when the block appeared to be "selective," particularly if it impeded a husband's legitimate conjugal relations but not his sexual activity with other partners, then it was to blame on *sortilegia* and *facturae* (spells and bewitchments).[21] This same point was also made by physicians such as the Florentine Niccolò Falcucci (?–1412) who, in his *Sermones medicinales*, first printed in 1481, stated that when a "learned doctor" (*intelligens medicus*) was unable to diagnose the cause of male impotence, sorcery was likely at work, especially if the man could have sex only with other women but not with his wife.[22] This was perhaps one of the reasons that had led Isabella and other observers to think that the consummation of her marriage had been hindered by magical means: at the same time Gian Galeazzo was shying away from his wife's bed, he was apparently far from being as timid with "other women and men," as Trotti reported.[23]

While 13th- and 14th-century jurists confined discussion of a bewitched couple's problems mostly to the realm of marriage law, from the second half of the 15th century magically caused impotence began being seen as possibly attributable to demons. As Catherine Rider has recently pointed out, the analysis of such an impediment became part of the growing debate on the crime of witchcraft.[24] The German Dominican, Johannes Nider, writing around 1438, discusses the sorcerers' power to provoke excessive love—or violent hate—between a man and a woman. In his *Formicarius*, Nider analyzes five ways in which the Devil, working via the enchantments cast by sorcerers, can interfere with sexual intercourse, and states that a common objective of magic spells was a couple's inability to consummate their marriage. Satan, writes Nider, can assume a material body and physically interpose himself between the spouses; he can excite a man to the sexual act, or on the contrary cool him; he can tamper with a man's imagination, making a certain woman seem repulsive instead of desirable; he can prevent erection and/or the emission of semen, thus making the sexual act a sterile one.[25] While hardly original, and actually largely based on the work of another 14th-century Dominican friar, Pierre de la Palud, Nider's examination of the topic of magical impotence is radically different from that of his predecessor due to a change in cultural context. Spells against the consummation of marriage were now being viewed as part of an unprecedented characterization of the witch as being more threatening: not only as a heretic, but also as a member of the Devil's sect and thus part of a conspiracy against Christianity.[26] Nider's influential tract clearly left a mark. In the 1450s, another Dominican, the inquisitor Nicolas Jacquier, dwelled at length on the ways in which demons, with or without the intervention of magicians and sorceresses, were able to harm men's health and more specifically prevent the "union of the flesh" (*copula carnalis*).[27] Jacquier was struck especially by the violent repulsion between spouses which could be provoked by enchantments, and reported having personally witnessed numerous cases in which, as soon as a bewitched person would get close to his/her spouse, he or she would suddenly begin "being tortured by the spell, and so tormented in the whole body, as to be forced to flee, sometimes even screaming loudly."[28] Jacquier's colorful account should not be discounted as an exaggeration, since near-contemporary archival records confirm that a "love" charm could be suspected any time husband and wife seemed to be forced to stay away from each other by unnatural, violent physical reactions. A 1520 case examined by the Modenese inquisition relates how a certain Baila, a woman from Campogalliano widely believed to be a sorceress, had bewitched a couple by feeding first the husband, then his wife, a charmed *placenta* (a type of cake). The effects had been quite spectacular: the husband, Jacopo Cantini, had started to hate his wife and children while loving and following Baila, "although she was a most disgusting and stinking woman;" most remarkably and symmetrically, Jacopo's wife "began loathing him, to the point that, when she approached her husband, or he approached her, they seemed to each other to stink unbearably."[29]

The Church's growing concerns about magically caused impotence were also apparent in the famous bull *Summis Desiderantes*, issued by Pope Innocent VIII in 1484. The bull denounces in apocalyptical tones the diabolical plan of sorcerers and witches, who are currently attacking fertility and fecundity by destroying the reproductive capabilities of humans, animals and plants. The Pope's alarm reaches its climax when it denounces witches who "keep the men from fathering children and the women from conceiving by impeding their ability to render the conjugal act to each other."[30] The 1484 bull was addressed to two German inquisitors, Jacob Sprenger and Heinrich Institoris (Kramer), and was eventually included as a sort of foreword in the book published by the latter in 1486, the notorious *Malleus Maleficarum*.[31] In tune with the Pope's concerns, Kramer devoted three lengthy *quaestiones* and no fewer than four chapters to the subject of witches' and demons' threat to fertility and sexual potency.[32] Some of Kramer's discussions follow rather traditional lines, such as examining "Whether sorceresses can impede the faculty to procreate or the sexual act" (Part One, Question 8), but other passages introduce additional types of bewitchment.[33] Thus in the first part of the *Malleus Maleficarum* (Question 9), Kramer debates "Whether sorceresses work on male members through a magical illusion as if these limbs were completely pulled out of the body."[34] The cases he reports, such as that of a young man from Ravensburg, who after breaking up with his fiancée found himself deprived of his member "with the result that he could not see or feel his body as anything but smooth" in the relevant area, show to what extent the inquisitor believed in the power of witches over human—and especially male—sexuality.[35] Having castrated men, even though only through an illusion, witches appear in the *Malleus Maleficarum* as always eager to consort with unfailingly potent *incubi* demons who, in their shape as *succubi*, had previously received the semen of (preferably) criminal men.[36] Satan could thus bring about the impregnation of a witch, in a perfectly asymmetrical triangle (man, demon, witch). Such "un-natural" copulations could then be crowned by the conception of progeny which could be considered demonic, if not in a strict sense, then doubtless due to the satanic inclinations of its witch–mother and the diabolic nature of its vicarious father.

Skepticism with Regard to Impotence Magic

Several authoritative voices dissented from Kramer's nightmarish vision. Lawyers and jurists such as Ulrich Molitor (1442–1507) and Ambrogio Vignati (?–c. 1480), both early witchcraft skeptics, argued that sexual relations between humans and demons, if at all possible, could never be fertile.[37] However, even Molitor in his *De lamiis et pythonicis mulieribus* (1489)—in many respects a sort of anti-*Malleus*—does not have very much to say about magically caused male impotence, aside from confirming that it was very frequent, and that in such cases the best course of action was for the bewitched couple to keep trying for three years, after having performed devout practices.[38] Somewhat surprisingly, we have to turn to a theologian and demonologist, Pierre Mamoris, to find a more original, detailed analysis.[39] In his *Flagellum maleficorum*, written between 1460 and 1462 and first published around 1486, Mamoris addresses, over and above the bewitchment of the *vis coeundi* (erectile function), the fact that strong reciprocal dislike or outright hate between spouses could be the main cause of a couple's inability to consummate the marriage. He relates at length the case of a young woman from his hometown (Poitiers), who had been "bewitched" (*maleficiata*).[40] Indeed, having been married for ten years, she was still a virgin because she felt an extraordinary, insurmountable loathing towards her husband—who, by the way, was impotent. Through a rather clever strategy, Mamoris led the woman to define and measure the level of her aversion:

> 'If you were alone at night in a wood, having on one side a wolf just waiting to devour you, and on the other side your husband ready to defend you, which one would you go to?' She answered that she would rather go to the wolf, or even to a lion ... I asked her whether she would go with her husband or rather with the Devil. She answered that she would not go with the Devil, but would rather go with her husband. Finally the spell was broken, and love followed between the spouses as well as the begetting of children.[41]

By having the woman take a stance against the Devil, Mamoris managed to make her take a position in favor of her husband, and the evil charm was dispelled.

Mamoris was clearly more interested in a pastoral approach to such problems than in the simple repression of witchcraft. His suggestions on how to overcome marital problems indeed go beyond the usual series of devotional practices wife and husband should perform, and include advice for the moral and spiritual support a confessor should offer to the afflicted couple. The priest should try to have the spouses react against the Devil's intention, which was to dishonor the sacrament of marriage. At the same time he should instill into them love for the children they will beget if they overcome their mutual aversion. "You would drink a very bitter medicine [the confessor should tell them] if you were gravely ill and you hoped to be cured by it. Although it would have a repulsive taste, you would force yourself to drink it in order to recover your good health."[42] But immediately after providing the text of a special prayer that husband and wife should recite together to proclaim their contempt for the Devil and their willingness to perform the "conjugal act," Mamoris shifts to a tone of doubt. Magically caused impotence, he warns, is often falsely claimed by men or women so that they may have their marriage annulled and thus be free to enjoy the carnal favors of their lovers or mistresses. In truth, this is *incerta materia* (uncertain ground). Therefore, judges examining such cases should always be "discerning ... cautious, and shrewd," for Mamoris evidently considered the wiles of men to be as subtle as those of the Evil one.[43]

Both latent and explicit skepticism with regard to magically induced impotence was probably more widespread than such a cursory examination of writings on the subject would seem to imply. Physicians, for example, were often unwilling to admit that sorcery was to blame for a couple's inability to copulate: Giovanni Michele Savonarola (1384–1468) wrote around the middle of the 15th century that as far as impotence magic went, he had "heard many things, but seen few"; nevertheless, he would not rule out entirely the possibility of demonic agency in such matters.[44]

Resistance to the supernatural explanation of marriage problems turns up in unexpected circles. Around 1505, another Isabella of royal blood and Iberian ancestry, Isabella of Castile, came across magically caused impotence, although only indirectly. The niece of one of her ladies-in-waiting, the countess of Haro, had been *ligata* (bewitched) and could not satisfy the conjugal debt. In a discussion with the Inquisitor General Diego de Deza, Isabella explicitly challenged the idea that the Devil could tamper with the sacrament of matrimony, arguing that "in such a holy thing the illusions of the Devil or the operations of a demon cannot achieve any effect."[45] Deza was clearly embarrassed, and while standing by the current demonological view that such things did indeed happen, he was cornered by the Queen into admitting that this was not an article of faith. Isabella could therefore conclude the conversation by insisting that, if it was not against the faith, "I will certainly not believe that the Devil can exert any power over those conjoined in matrimony and 'bind' them (*ligare*), as they say. For these divisions (*divisiones*) are more due to discord among humans (*hominum discordantium*) than to interference by powerful demons."

The Castle (Finally) Conquered

Judging conjugal troubles to be a wholly human affair, the Queen of Castile would probably have agreed with Trotti, the Ferrarese ambassador, that the best course of action for Isabella of Aragon was to "make up for the Duke's failings and to tame or sooth him (*domesticarlo*); for women must and will do anything in bed with their husbands."[46] We don't know if Isabella followed such advice, or if she tried any other of the remedies we have mentioned. What we do know is that her marital problems came to an end about a year after the wedding celebration, and that everyone found out almost immediately. On April 27, 1490, the papal nuncio in Milan, Giacomo Gherardi, announced to Pope Innocent VIII in minimally allusive language that the previous night "the door that, so to speak, had remained tenaciously closed, has been finally opened, and even she, whose castle is said to have been conquered, seems to confirm it with virginal modesty."[47] Il Moro's court poet, Bernardo Bellincioni, hurried to celebrate the happy event:

And now, what will the critics say?
She is; she's not; she can't; yes, she can; yes, she wants.
The thorns have become roses and violets
And all the bad humors will be purged.
[...]
O mischievous and envious lot, what will you say
Seeing the loyalty and the deeds of my dear Moro,
Who only thirsts for his nephew's good?
[...]
While the Duke has consummated his marriage,
Il Moro is preserving his patrimony.[48]

Bellincioni's reference to "the critics" is a direct allusion to rumors putting the blame on il Moro for the couple's plight, and suggests that such speculations must have been widespread. At the same time, his mention of "humors" puts the problem soundly in the area of medical ailments, and provides a clever way to dismiss suspicions of foul play: the Duke's impotence would have been due to a pathology which the purgation of "bad humors" had resolved. The court poet is thus adding yet another explanation for the impotence of Gian Galeazzo, one that the other sources examined here do not take under consideration. This explanation was what physicians called *impotentia naturalis* (natural impotence),[49] which was diagnosed as stemming from either an anatomical problem (such as deformity of the genitals), or an alteration in the *complexio*, that is, in "the balance of the qualities of hot, wet, cold and dry resulting from the mixture of the elements in the human body."[50]

"Natural" *Versus* "Magical" Impotence

Since classical antiquity, medical authors had discussed and proposed a range of remedies meant to heal the imbalance in the bodily humors that caused impotence,[51] but it was not easy to make a clear distinction between natural impotence and *maleficium*. Indeed, a number of physicians agreed with theologians that demons could afflict both women and men in the sexual arena by acting upon their bodies: either directly, as a succubus/incubus, or indirectly, through spells cast by human agents.[52] Some authoritative medical treatises described in detail how to nullify the magic spell and restore the spouses' ability to perform the sexual act. Constantine the African's *Pantegni* (XI century) was the earliest and most influential discussion of the bewitchment of sexual activity.[53] A work derived from a much earlier, Hellenic–Arab medical encyclopedia, the *Pantegni* suggested remedies that were as based on magical principles as much as the spells supposedly cast on the couple. For example, "If the bride and groom keep with them the bile of some fish, and especially *zangarinus,* in a box of juniper wood and if, when they go to bed, they put it on hot coals so that they are fumigated by it, all of the above-mentioned spells will vanish."[54] Another, simpler cure was destined to several centuries of success: "Similarly, if mercury (*argentum vivum*) is taken and put into a reed sealed with wax without the bride and groom's knowledge, no spell will harm them in the place where it is put."[55] This particular remedy, based on the widespread belief in the magical properties of mercury, was to be included by Petrus Hispanus (later Pope John XXI) in his greatly popular collection of recipes, *Thesaurus pauperum* (c. 1250). In a chapter titled "Against bewitchments and demons: that is, spells," the Portuguese scholar suggested: "[...] take mercury and pour it into a hollow reed or in an emptied hazelnut, and put it under the pillow of the bewitched, or else under the threshold of his home: it will unmake the spell."[56] The success of the *Thesaurus pauperum*, and the prestige of its author, guaranteed wide currency to this recipe, and thus lent renewed credibility to the belief that impotence could be caused by spells. Three centuries after its composition, even the established author Pietro Bairo, court physician to Duke Carlo II of Savoy, would still offer, as a cure for "those who are so tied (*legati*) and bewitched, that they cannot have sex with women" a recipe in his *Secreti medicinali* (1561) clearly drawn from the *Thesaurus* (but probably based also on a direct reading of the *Pantegni*): "Take mercury and pour it into a hollow reed or in a pierced walnut, seal it with wax, and put it under the pillow of the bewitched, or else under the threshold of his bedroom or home: it will unmake the spell."[57]

Despite the currency of such remedies, there was, however, no consensus among Renaissance physicians regarding the idea that bewitchments worked through demonic intervention. On the contrary, certain medical authorities, such as Antonio Guaineri or Jacques Despars, both active in the first half of the 15th century, suggested that the efficacy of spells was due either to the natural virtues of their component parts or to the power of human imagination.[58] Nevertheless, the equally authoritative Giovanni Michele Savonarola warned that the Devil was behind the incantations concocted by witches and sorcerers, and even Guaineri had to admit that "although I put no faith in these [magical remedies], nonetheless I hear unbelievable things every day in those parts, where in that year many women were burned on account of it [their acts of sorcery]."[59] Guaineri is possibly talking about Piedmont, where some of the earliest trials for witchcraft took place in the 1420s.[60] Be that as it may, this reference clearly indicates that the witch-hunt was already taking hold also amongst medical authorities, who were increasingly drawn to concede the diabolical character of love spells. Over one hundred years later the Dutch physician Johann Wier (or Weyer), the most prominent among the Renaissance defenders of the witches, defined "selective" male impotence as being the Devil's work while denying emphatically that a sorceress' intervention was necessary for this kind of bewitchment to be effective.[61] In terms of the more general, ambitious plan of his major book, *De praestigiis daemonum* (1563), Wier was here trying to prove that witches could not be held responsible for certain types of crimes that could be directly attributable to Satan. Once more, we see that sexual impotence was a condition which different observers could ascribe to a variety of causes depending on each observer's outlook and agenda: timidity due to youth, incapacity due to bad humors, marital discord, magic spells, the Devil or witchcraft.

In the story of Isabella of Aragon's unhappy marriage, no one had a clearer agenda than Ludovico il Moro. Fearing that Gian Galeazzo, pressured by his wife and father-in-law, could finally claim his full authority over the duchy, il Moro had him poisoned gradually over the course of several months in 1494.[62] He died a very painful death on October 21, at age 25. Ironically, the official version—reported by Guicciardini—credited his decease to "immoderate coitus" (*coito immoderato*).[63] In the minutes of the letters prepared by the Sforza chancery to inform the crowns and governments of Italy and Europe, a blank space significantly shows where the cause of Gian Galeazzo's death should have been indicated. Like his impotence, his long and ultimately fatal illness seemed to elude any definitive diagnosis.[64]

Works Cited

Early Printed Sources (pre-1900)

Corio, Bernardino, *L'historia di Milano volgarmente scritta dall'eccellentissimo oratore m. Bernardino Corio gentil'huomo milanese.* Venezia, Giovanni Maria Bonelli, 1554.

Bairo, Pietro, *Secreti medicinali di m. Pietro Bairo da Turino, già medico di Carlo secondo duca di Savoia.* Venezia, Giacomo Cornetti, 1592.

Giovio, Paolo, *Delle istorie del suo tempo di mons. Paolo Giouio da Como, vescouo di Nocera, tradotte da m. Lodouico Domenichi.* Venezia: Altobello Salicato, 1572.

Ioannes <papa; 21>, *Thesaurus pauperum di Messer Pietro Hispano,* Venetia, Benedetto di Bendoni, 1531.

Jacquier, Nicolas, *Flagellum haereticorum fascinariorum. autore F. Nicolao Jacquerio,* Francofurti ad Moenum, apud Nicolaum Bassaeum, 1581.

Mamoris, Pierre, *Flagellum maleficorum,* in Institoris, Henricus, *Malleus maleficarum, maleficas et earum haeresim framea conterens,* Lugdunii, apud Claudium Bourgeat, 1669, vol. II, tome 3.

Molitor, Ulrich, *De lamiis et pyhonicis mulieribus,* in Institoris, Henricus, *Malleus maleficarum, maleficas et earum haeresim framea conterens,* Lugdunii, apud Claudium Bourgeat, 1669, vol. I, tome 1, part I.

Nider, Johannes, *Formicarius,* Augustae, per Anthonium Sorg, c. 1484.

Secondary Sources and Modern Editions

Azzolini, Monica, *The Duke and the Stars: Astrology and Politics in Renaissance Milan.* Cambridge, MA: Harvard University Press, 2013.

Bailey, Michael, *Battling Demons: Witchcraft, Heresy and Reform in the Late Middle Ages.* University Park, PA: Pennsylvania State University Press, 2003.

Behringer, Wolfgang, "Malleus Maleficarum," in *Encyclopedia of Witchcraft. The Western Tradition,* ed. Richard M. Golden. Santa Barbara, CA: ABC–CLIO, 2006, vol. III, 717–23.

Bever, Edward, "Molitor, Ulrich," in *Encyclopedia of Witchcraft. The Western Tradition*, ed. Richard M. Golden, Santa Barbara, CA: ABC–CLIO, 2006, vol. III, 776–7.

Broedel, Hans Peter, *The Malleus Maleficarum and the Construction of Witchcraft*. Manchester, UK: Manchester University Press, 2003.

Carusi, Enrico (ed.), *Dispacci e lettere di Giacomo Gherardi nunzio pontificio a Firenze e Milano*. Roma: Tipografia Poliglotta Vaticana, 1909.

Céard, Jean, "The Devil and Lovesickness: Views of 16th Century Physicians and Demonologists," in *Eros and Anteros: The Medical Traditions of Love in the Renaissance*, ed. Donald A. Beecher and Massimo Ciavolella. Toronto: University of Toronto—Dovehouse Editions, 1992, 33–47.

Corio, Bernardino, *Storia di Milano*, ed. Anna Morisi Guerra. Torino, UTET, 1978.

Danielle Jacquart, "Le regard d'un médecin sur son temps: Jacques Despars," in Ead., *La science médicale occidentale entre deux renaissances (XIIe s.–XVe s.)*. Aldershot, UK: Variorum, 1997.

Darmon, Pierre, *Le tribunal de l'impuissance: virilité et défaillances conjugales dans l'ancienne France*, Paris: Éditions du Seuil, 1979.

Dina, Achille, *Isabella d'Aragona Duchessa di Milano e di Bari, 1470–1524*. Milano: Tip. San Giuseppe, 1921.

Duni, Matteo, "Molitor, Ulrich," in *Dizionario storico dell'Inquisizione*, ed. Adriano Prosperi, Vincenzo Lavenia and John Tedeschi. Pisa: Edizioni della Normale, 2010, vol. II, 1061–2.

Duni, Matteo, *Tra religione e magia: storia del prete modenese Guglielmo Campana (1460?–1541)*. Firenze: Olschki, 1999.

Duni, Matteo, "Vignati, Ambrogio," in *Dizionario storico dell'Inquisizione*, ed. Adriano Prosperi, Vincenzo Lavenia and John Tedeschi. Pisa: Edizioni della Normale, 2010, vol. III, 1690–91.

Guicciardini, Francesco, *History of Italy*, ed. and trans. Sidney Alexander. New York/London: Macmillan, 1969.

Guicciardini, Francesco, *Storia d'Italia*, ed. Silvana Seidel Menchi. Torino: Einaudi, 1971.

Hansen, Joseph, *Quellen und Untersuchungen zur Geschichte des Hexenwahns und der Hexenverfolgung im Mittelalter*. Bonn: Carl Georgi, 1901.

Herzig, Tamar, *Christ Transformed into a Virgin Woman: Lucia Brocadelli, Heinrich Institoris, and the Defense of the Faith*. Roma: Edizioni di storia e letteratura, 2013.

Institoris (Kramer), and Jacobus Sprenger Henricus, *Malleus maleficarum*, ed. and trans. Christopher S. Mackay. Cambridge: Cambridge University Press, 2006.

Jacquart, Danielle and Claude Thomasset, *Sexualité et savoir médical au Moyen Age*. Paris: Presses Universitaires de France, 1985.

L'imaginaire du sabbat: édition critique des textes les plus anciens (1430 c.–1440 c.), ed. Martine Ostorero, Agostino Paravicini Bagliani, Katrin Utz Tremp et al. Lausanne: Université de Lausanne, 1999.

Lopez, Guido, *Moro! Moro! Storie del Ducato sforzesco*. Milano: Camunia, 1992.

Muccillo, Maria, "Falcucci, Niccolò," in *Dizionario biografico degli Italiani*. Roma: Istituto dell'Enciclopedia italiana, 1994, vol. 44, 403.

Mugnai Carrara, Daniela, "Guaineri, Antonio," in *Dizionario biografico degli Italiani*. Roma: Istituto dell'Enciclopedia italiana, 2003, vol. 60, 111–15.

Ostorero, Martine, *Le diable au sabbat: littérature démonologique et sorcellerie (1440–1460)*. Firenze: Sismel-Edizioni del Galluzzo, 2011.

Pellegrini, Marco, *Ascanio Maria Sforza: la parabola politica di un cardinale-principe del Rinascimento*. Roma: Istituto Storico Italiano per il Medio Evo, 2002.

Rider, Catherine, *Magic and Impotence in the Middle Ages*. Oxford: Oxford University Press, 2006.

Scrivano, Riccardo, "Bellincioni, Bernardo," in *Dizionario biografico degli Italiani*. Roma: Istituto dell'Enciclopedia italiana, 1970, vol. 7, 687–9.

Siraisi, Nancy G., *Medieval and Early Renaissance Medicine: an Introduction to Knowledge and Practice*. Chicago: University of Chicago Press, 1990.

Stephens, Walter, *Demon Lovers: Witchcraft, Sex, and the Crisis of Belief*. Chicago: University of Chicago Press, 2002.

Vaglienti, Francesca M., "Gian Galeazzo Maria Sforza," in *Dizionario biografico degli Italiani*. Roma: Istituto dell'Enciclopedia italiana, 2000, vol. 54, 391–17.

Vaglienti, Francesca M., "Isabella d'Aragona," in *Dizionario biografico degli Italiani*. Roma: Istituto dell'Enciclopedia italiana, 2004, vol. 62, 609–15.

Weyer, Johann, *Witches, Devils, and Doctors in the Renaissance: Johann Weyer, De Praestigiis Daemonum*, ed. George Mora and Benjamin Kohl, trans. John Shea. Binghamton, NY: Medieval and Renaissance Texts and Studies, 1991.

Notes

1 Isabella was the daughter of Alfonso, duke of Calabria, and of Ippolita Maria Sforza, sister of Galeazzo Maria, father of the bridegroom. Francesca M. Vaglienti, "Gian Galeazzo Maria Sforza," in *Dizionario biografico degli Italiani* (henceforth *DBI*) (Roma: Istituto dell'Enciclopedia italiana, 2000), vol. 54, 391–17, and Eadem, "Isabella d'Aragona," *DBI*, 2004, vol. 62, 609–15, provide the basic information on the two protagonists. Achille Dina, *Isabella d'Aragona Duchessa di Milano e di Bari, 1470–1524* (Milano: Tip. San Giuseppe, 1921) (offprint from *Archivio Storico Lombardo*, 48, 1921, 269–457), provides rich information on Isabella's life from various primary sources (some of them unpublished). Guido Lopez, *Moro! Moro! Storie del Ducato sforzesco* (Milano: Camunia, 1992), also provides useful information (although often without quoting sources properly). But see now Monica Azzolini, *The Duke and the Stars: Astrology and Politics in Renaissance Milan* (Cambridge, MA: Harvard University Press, 2013), which discusses the case of Gian Galeazzo's marriage, quoting additional sources on his impotence. It unfortunately came to my attention too late to be taken fully into account in the present article.

2 Cf. Dina, *Isabella d'Aragona*, 20–21.

3 "… era fatto intendere a la Maestà Sua [i.e. *Ferrante*] che non poteva, per modo alchuno, sortire effetto la consumazione del matrimonio fra Sue Eccellenze, per l'indisposizione dell'Illustrissimo Duca di Milano, quale intendeva essere frigidissimo." These were the words of Camillo Cruciati, envoy of the king of Naples to Milan, gathered by the papal nuncio Giacomo Gherardi (cf. *Dispacci e lettere di Giacomo Gherardi nunzio pontificio a Firenze e Milano*, ed. Enrico Carusi [Roma: Tipografia Poliglotta Vaticana, 1909], 436, n. 4). This and all following translations from the Italian or Latin are mine, unless otherwise indicated.

4 "Certifico Vostra Signoria chel gli è innamorato e non ardisse guardarla … habe del puto e del scempio, che procede da vergogna, dubitando essere dilegiato" (Dina, *Isabella d'Aragona*, 34, quoting Trotti's letter from March 4, 1489. Trotti's unpublished correspondence is in the Archivio di Stato of Modena, Archivio Segreto Estense, Cancelleria sezione Estero, Carteggio ambasciatori. I have not been able to compare Dina's transcriptions with the originals).

5 Ibid.

6 Dina, *Isabella d'Aragona*, 39, quoting Trotti's letter from December 31: "... li dipinse lo inferno per chel non consumava el matrimonio ... dicendoli che non solamente se restituiria la dota hauta, ma che forse anche se bisognaria restituire la dona, del che il povero sire tuto stete mortificato, ma non ne sarà più de quello che sia stato per il passato, secondo il juditio mio, perché *Nitimur in vetitum semper, cupimus negata*" (the Latin quote is from Ovid's *Amores*, 3, 4, 17). The reason for this brutal treatment of Gian Galeazzo lay obviously in Ludovico's political plans: see below, notes 12, 13.

7 "... le donne lombarde debbono havere la telarina a la lor faccenda, et haver bisogno che gliela spaccino via," in Lopez, *Moro! Moro!*, 106, quoting from Trotti's letter of February 14.

8 Azzolini, *The Duke and the Stars*, 151, note 75.

9 On this practice see Danielle Jacquart, Claude Thomasset, *Sexualité et savoir médical au Moyen Age*, Paris, Presses Universitaires de France, 1985, 230–36; a broader overview of its legal application in later periods in Pierre Darmon, *Le tribunal de l'impuissance: virilité et défaillances conjugales dans l'ancienne France* (Paris: Éditions du Seuil, 1979).

10 "... che piuttosto vole vivere et star come la sta, che usar simili termini," in Dina, *Isabella d'Aragona*, 35 (quoting from Trotti's letters of February 14).

11 Bernardino Corio, *Historia di Milano*, Venezia, Giovanni M. Bonelli, 1554, parte VI, ff. 447r–v: "... il duca in tal forma restò affaturato, che gran tempo stette che non poté con la bella sposa compiere gli amorosi intenti" (in the modern edition of the original 1503 publication, *Storia di Milano*, ed. Anna Morisi Guerra (Torino: UTET, 1978), this passage is in vol. II, 1475). According to Corio the supposed bewitchment had happened when the couple returned to the Castello sforzesco after having participated in the repeat of the wedding ceremony at the Duomo on February 2.

12 Paolo Giovio, *Delle istorie del suo tempo*, Venezia, Altobello Salicato, 1572, lib. I, 11–12: "... ella teneva certo, che per opera di Ludovico nel giorno istesso delle nozze al marito et a lei fossero stati fatti incanti, et malie da donne fattucchiare, perché non potessero haver figliuoli ...."

13 Guicciardini's *Storia d'Italia* was completed in 1540: Francesco Guicciardini, *History of Italy*, ed. and trans. Sidney Alexander (New York/London: Macmillan, 1969), 33. "Quando Isabella figliuola d'Alfonso andò a congiungersi col marito, Lodovico, come la vide, innamorato di lei, desiderò di ottenerla per moglie dal padre; e a questo effetto operò, così allora fu creduto per tutta Italia, con incantamenti e con malie, che Giovan Galeazzo fu per molti mesi impotente alla consumazione del matrimonio." *Storia d'Italia*, ed. Silvana Seidel Menchi (Torino: Einaudi, 1971), vol. I (bk. I, ch. 6), 51.

14 Cf. Marco Pellegrini, *Ascanio Maria Sforza: la parabola politica di un cardinale-principe del Rinascimento*, Roma, Istituto Storico Italiano per il Medio Evo, 2002, vol. I, 218, 228. Many thanks to Pellegrini for having kindly and promptly answered my queries about il Moro's political designs in those years.

15 Ibid., 254, 256.

16 Cf. Azzolini, *The Duke and the Stars*, 170–75.

17 Ibid., 148–51.

18 My discussion of the relevant literature relies largely on Catherine Rider, *Magic and Impotence in the Middle Ages* (Oxford/New York: Oxford University Press, 2006).

19 The text was written by Hincmar, archbishop of Rheims in the IX century, the first author to distinguish impotence magic from other forms of love magic, according to Rider, *Magic and Impotence*, 31 (see Rider's English translation of *Si per sortiarias*, ibid., 40).

20 Rider, *Magic and Impotence*, 119–21.

21 Ibid., 126.

22 Ibid., 197 and n. 40 (but the title of Falcucci's book is misspelled, see Maria Muccillo, "Falcucci, Niccolò," in *DBI*, vol. 44, 403).

23 Dina, *Isabella d'Aragona*, 35, quoting from Trotti's letter of February 22.

24 Rider, *Magic and Impotence*, ch. 10, *passim*.

25 Johannes Nider, *Formicarius*, Augustae, Anthonius Sorg, c. 1484, bk. V, ch. 5, ff. 262r. (frequency of spells against marriage and fertility), 263 r. (ways in which the Devil can prevent the union). I have utilized the digitized version of this edition, available online from the Bayerische Staatsbibliothek at Munich.

26 On *Formicarius* see *L'imaginaire du sabbat: édition critique des textes les plus anciens (1430 c.–1440 c.)*, eds. Martine Ostorero, Agostino Paravicini Bagliani and Katrin Utz Tremp et al., Lausanne, Université de Lausanne, 1999, 101–265 (which anyway does not analyze the question of magic and impotence). On Nider's life and works see Michael Bailey, *Battling Demons: Witchcraft, Heresy*

and Reform in the Late Middle Ages (University Park: Pennsylvania State University Press, 2003). On Pierre de la Palud (Petrus a Palude) and his influence on the discussion of love magic in later authors such as Gabriel Biel (but not in Nider) see Rider, *Magic and Impotence*, ch. 8 and 10.

27 On Jacquier see Martine Ostorero, *Le diable au sabbat: littérature démonologique et sorcellerie (1440–1460)* (Firenze, Sismel-Edizioni del Galluzzo, 2011), 451–502 and *passim*.

28 "... maleficium statim tamen torquetur, et toto corpore interius vexatur et cogitur ex vehementia vexationis fugere, quandoque cum validis clamoribus" (Nicolas Jacquier, *Flagellum haereticorum fascinariorum*, Francofurti ad Moenum, apud Nicolaum Bassaeum, 1581, 89–90).

29 "[Jacopo] uxorem et filios abhominatus fuerit et dictam Bailam, tametsi turpem et fetidam, super modum dilexerit et sequutus fuerit. Insuper dicunt quod a dicto Jacobo cognoverunt qualiter uxor illius per idem tempus comedit de quadam alia placenta facta ex pasta eis data ab illa Baila, et ex tunc illa quoque abhominata est virum suum, ita quod cum viro appropinquat, vel ille sibi, appareant sibi invicem intollerabiliter fetentes" (Archivio di Stato di Modena, Inquisizione, Busta 2, Processi 1489–1549, 11 April 1520, deposition of Niccolò Borgola and several other witnesses).

30 "... eosdem hominesque ne gignere et mulieres ne concipere, virosque ne uxoribus, et mulieres ne viris actus coniugales reddere valeant, impedire," in Henricus Institoris (Kramer), Jacobus Sprenger, *Malleus maleficarum*, ed. and trans. Christopher S. Mackay, 2 vols. (Cambridge: Cambridge University Press, 2006), vol. I, 199 (translation in vol. II, 19).

31 Although the attribution to both Kramer and Sprenger has been long accepted, recent scholarship tends mostly to conclude that Kramer was the sole author of the book (see Wolfgang Behringer, "Malleus Maleficarum," in *Encyclopedia of Witchcraft. The Western Tradition*, ed. Richard M. Golden, Santa Barbara, CA, ABC–CLIO, 2006, vol. 3, 717–23; but see also a more tentative perspective in *Malleus Maleficarum*, 103–21). On Kramer and his view of female sexuality and witchcraft as being inextricably linked see Hans Peter Broedel, *The Malleus Maleficarum and the Construction of Witchcraft* (Manchester, UK: Manchester University Press, 2003). The best extensive treatment of Kramer's life (and especially of his lesser known works), is Tamar Herzig, *Christ Transformed into a Virgin Woman: Lucia Brocadelli, Heinrich Institoris, and the Defense of the Faith*, Roma, Edizioni di storia e letteratura, 2013.

32 These are Question 8, 9 and 11 of Part One, and chapters 5, 6, 7 and 13 in Question 1 of Part Two.

33 "An generativam potentiam seu actum venereum malefice impedire possunt [*sic*], quod maleficium in bulla continetur" (*Malleus Maleficarum*, vol. I, 307). This *quaestio* is mostly based on the discussion of the same issue in *Formicarius*, one of Kramer's key sources (large sections of the *Malleus* are a word-by-word copy of the *Formicarius*).

34 "An malefice prestigiosa illusione operantur circa membra virilia quasi illa omnino sint a corporibus evulsa" (*Malleus maleficarum*, vol. 1, 314).

35 "... ut nihil videre aut tangere preter planum corpus posset": Part Two, *Quaestio* 1, ch. 7, "The way in which they regularly take away male members" ("De modo quo membra virilia auferre solent," ibid., vol. 1, 428).

36 *Malleus maleficarum*, Part Two, Quaestio I, ch. 4 (vol. I, 411–ff.): "De modo quo se incubis demonibus subiiciunt" ("The method by which they subordinate themselves to incubi demons").

37 On Vignati see Matteo Duni, "Vignati, Ambrogio," in *Dizionario storico dell'Inquisizione*, eds. Adriano Prosperi, Vincenzo Lavenia and John Tedeschi (Pisa: Edizioni della Normale, 2010), vol. III, 1690–91; on Molitor, Id.,"Molitor, Ulrich," ibid., II, 1061–62; Edward Bever, "Molitor, Ulrich," in *Encyclopedia of Witchcraft*, vol. 3, 776–7.

38 Ulrich Molitor, *De lamiis et pyhonicis mulieribus*, in *Malleus maleficarum, maleficas et earum haeresim framea conterens* (Lugdunii: Claudius Bourgeat, 1669), vol. I, tome 1, part I, 22.

39 On Mamoris see Ostorero, *Le diable au sabbat*, 165–98, and *passim*.

40 Pierre Mamoris, *Flagellum maleficorum*, in *Malleus maleficarum, maleficas et earum haeresim*, vol. II, tome 3, 153 (quoted at length and analyzed in Ostorero, *Le diable au sabbat*, 546–7).

41 Ostorero, *Le diable au sabbat*, 547 (translation from the Latin is mine).

42 Mamoris, *Flagellum*, 157–8 (Ostorero, *Le diable au sabbat*, 548 n. 127).

43 "discretos ..., circumspectos atque sagaces," Mamoris, *Flagellum*, 158 (Ostorero, *Le diable au sabbat*, 546, n. 125).

44 Rider, *Magic and Impotence*, 199–200.

45 Walter Stephens, *Demon Lovers: Witchcraft, Sex, and the Crisis of Belief* (Chicago/London: University of Chicago Press, 2002), 313–15 (the Spanish source is in Joseph Hansen, *Quellen und Untersuchungen zur Geschichte des Hexenwahns und der Hexenverfolgung im Mittelalter*, Bonn, Carl Georgi, 1901, 262).

46 "... supplire a li manchamenti del duca et domesticarlo; perché le donne volgiono et debbono fare ogni cosa in lecto cum li mariti" (quoted in Lopez, *Moro! Moro!*, 106).

47 "Portam enim quae (ut dicitur) usque ad extremum clausa fuerat, apertam tandem affirmant omnes, atque illa ipsa cuius castra expugnata dicuntur, ingenua quadam verecundia virginali id ipsum quodammodo fateri videtur" (*Dispacci e lettere di Giacomo Gherardi*, 463).

48 "Orsù, che diranno ora e' detrattori? / Ell'è; non è; non può; sì può; sì vuole / Le spine fatte son rose e viole / E purgati saran tutti gli umori. ... / Dispettosi e invidiosi or che direte / Alla fede e agli effetti del mio Moro, / che sol del ben di suo nipote ha sete? ... / S'el duca ha consumato el matrimonio, / el Moro gli conserva il patrimonio" (Dina, *Isabella d'Aragona*, 44). On Bellincioni and his role at the Sforza court see Riccardo Scrivano, "Bellincioni, Bernardo," in *DBI*, 1965, vol. 7, 687–9.

49 Rider, *Magic and Impotence*, 8–9.

50 Nancy G. Siraisi, *Medieval and Early Renaissance Medicine: an Introduction to Knowledge and Practice* (Chicago: University of Chicago Press, 1990), 101.

51 See Jacquart, Thomasset, *Sexualité et savoir médical au Moyen Age*, 230–36; Rider, *Magic and Impotence*, 162–3, discussing 13th century physician Gilbertus Anglicus and his analysis of impotence as the result of natural causes.

52 Cf. Jean Céard, "The Devil and Lovesickness: Views of 16th Century Physicians and Demonologists," in *Eros and Anteros: The Medical Traditions of Love in the Renaissance*, eds. Donald A. Beecher and Massimo Ciavolella (Toronto: University of Toronto—Dovehouse Editions, 1992), 33–47.

53 Rider, *Magic and Impotence*, 45–51.

54 Ibid., 47.

55 Ibid., 68–9.

56 *Thesaurus pauperum di Messer Pietro Hispano*, Venetia, Benedetto di Bendoni, 1531, f. 49v: "Contra le malie et demoni: cioè fature"; "... metti argento vivo in una penna [evidently a wrong translation of the original Latin *calamo*] o nuocella vuota, et poni sotto lo capezale del letto del amaliato over sotto la soglia del uscio donde entra: disfa le malie." Petrus Hispanus, born in Lisbon around 1210, author of works of logic and medicine, was elected pope in 1276, dying the following year. The *Thesaurus pauperum* (whose attribution to the Portuguese thinker is not entirely certain), dating from the middle of the XIII century, enjoyed a remarkable and long-lasting fortune: the book survives in circa one hundred manuscripts, and it was published in no less than eighty editions (in several languages), from the late 15th to the early 18th century.

57 "Metti argento vivo in calamo, o in nose straforata stroppando con cera, et metti sotto el capezzale de maleficiati, overo sotto il sogliaro della porta, per la qual s'entra in camera o in casa, et si disfarà l'incanto": *Secreti medicinali di M. Pietro Bairo da Turino* (Venezia: Giacomo Cornetti, 1592), f. 217r. I have discussed more fully this recipe, its complex tradition, and its application by non-academic medical practitioners in my *Tra religione e magia: storia del prete modenese Guglielmo Campana (1460?–1541)* (Firenze: Olschki, 1999), 258–61.

58 Rider, *Magic and Impotence*, 202–4; on Despars (c. 1380–1458), see also Danielle Jacquart, "Le regard d'un médecin sur son temps: Jacques Despars," *Bibliothèque de l'École des Chartes*, 138, 1980, 35–86 (now in Ead., *La science médicale occidentale entre deux renaissances (XIIe s.–XVe s.)* (Aldershot, UK: Variorum, 1997). On Guaineri (c. 1390–c. 1455) see also Daniela Mugnai Carrara, "Guaineri, Antonio," in *DBI*, 2003, vol. 60, 111–15 (on the power of the imagination in particular cf. 114).

59 "Verum etsi his fidem nullam adhibeam, non credenda tamen quotidie istis in partibus audio, ubi anno isto ob hoc cremate sunt plurime," quoted in Rider, *Magic and Impotence*, 203.

60 Rider, *Magic and Impotence*, 198 (Guaineri was employed by the Duke of Savoy, and elsewhere in his work mentions a case of bewitchments he had treated in Pinerolo, the site of trials for magic and heresy in 1427).

61 *Witches, Devils, and Doctors in the Renaissance: Johann Weyer, De Praestigiis Daemonum*, eds. George Mora and Benjamin Kohl, trans. John Shea (Binghamton, NY: Medieval and Renaissance Texts and Studies, 1991), 334 (Bk. IV, ch. 20).

62 Poisoning is indicated as a near-certain cause of the death of Giangaleazzo by Guicciardini, *Storia d'Italia*, bk. I, ch. 13, and this indication is accepted by Vaglienti, "Gian Galeazzo Maria Sforza," 396. Azzolini, *The Duke and the Stars*, analyzes at length the duke's sickness and its treatment by Milanese astrologers and physicians (see esp. 153–66). However, while admitting that Ludovico had a vested interest in getting rid of his nephew and all opportunities for having him poisoned, Azzolini stresses that available documentation does not provide conclusive evidence that Gian Galeazzo was actually poisoned.

63 Guicciardini, *History of Italy*, 54 (*Storia d'Italia*, vol. I, 92).

64 Vaglienti, "Gian Galeazzo Maria Sforza," 396.

5

The Satyr in the Kitchen Pantry[1]

Laura Giannetti

In the fourth act of Machiavelli's *Clizia* (1525) old Nicomaco tells his servant Pirro how he intends to prepare for a night of love with the beautiful young Clizia: before dinner he plans to take a sexually reinvigorating concoction, the *satirión*, followed by a serving of cooked onions, a mixture of spiced broad beans and a half-cooked pigeon.[2] Nicomaco's planned dinner sums up the general advice of food literature at the time on how to ensure sexual potency. Traditionally "windy" and "warm" foods such as onions and *fave* (broad beans) were thought to be excellent for "exciting Venus," while the meat of a still bloody pigeon would give an old lover the necessary strength.[3] But the most potent ingredient in Nicomaco's plan went beyond dietary aids: it was a medicinal potion regularly sold by Italian apothecaries at this time. The *satirión* was a concoction made with the bulbous root of a special orchid, the *Satyrion*, or with the similar *testiculus vulpis* ("fox testicles") cooked and dressed with spices and seeds noted for their aphrodisiacal virtues.[4]

Renaissance Viagra

Machiavelli's Messer Nicomaco exemplified a character common to many comedies of the period: the old man in love with a young woman, usually ridiculed and sometimes punished (at the end of the play) for his erotic desires and amorous schemes. The search for the right medicinal concoction and special foods to revive and sustain virility was often part of the comic plot and served to point out how infatuated old men had lost their reason, and no longer conformed to the current social ideal of dependable and sober patriarchal behavior. The attention paid to aphrodisiacs in many comedies, along with the description of the erotic properties of food and other supposedly aphrodisiacal substances, effectively constitutes a discourse on the sexual impotence of elderly patriarchs and the problems they have in satisfying their unflagging sexual desires, a discourse that humanistic literature of the time often shunned or found inappropriate. In contrast, however, the permanence of erotic urges in the aged and the difficulty they had in satisfying them were fully recognized by both medical and the commonplace culture of the time, and reworked by imaginative literature.[5] Authors drew extensively upon dietary, herbal, pharmaceutical and medicinal tracts, adapting their specialized language and instructions to humorous effect. Renaissance comedy was the genre that most delighted in the description of libidinous old men, their sexual desires, their performance anxiety and their sentimental expectations. In the exploration of characters of old fools in love and their search for the right erotic aid, dramatists had an opportunity to address some of the deepest social and sexual tensions of Renaissance society.

Following a repeated script, probably first inspired by Machiavelli's *Clizia*, enamored old men ask their servants to go to an apothecary shop and procure a potion often referred to as a *lattovaro/lettovaro*, a tonic drink made with several ingredients whose name derived from the common medicinal term *elettuario*.[6] If it is not a servant it is a friend (usually of an equally advanced age) who buys the proper foods and spices for the infatuated elderly swain. Particularly popular in comedies are *pinochiati*, a type of cake made from flour, egg whites, pine nuts and sugar, pistachios and marzipan.[7] In the Florentine comedy *Il vecchio amoroso* (written c. 1533–1536), for example, Teodoro's friend Arrigo went to the apothecary shop, not to the food market, to buy four marzipan confections, many *pinochiati* and some vaguely described *confezioni* for his friend.[8] But as these foods were widely recognized as having an amorous effect, the eating of the aphrodisiacal ingredients and remedies is often carried out in secret. In *Il vecchio amoroso* old Teodoro tells the audience: "I shut myself up in my bedroom where I drank two glasses of *malvagia* [*malvasia*] wine and had a little candied orange, two pieces of ginger root and I do not know what type of *confezioni*."[9] Usually specific vegetables, roots and nuts made up the lion's share of the most popular foods consumed by old characters in love, notably truffles, artichokes, ginger thistles and garden celery.[10] Servants sent to the market will also be told to buy fowl such as partridges, pheasants and sparrows, considered in Renaissance perception and imagination as "hot" foods able to stimulate the senses, and thus an essential ingredient of a preparatory dinner for libidinous old men.[11] The clever servant Tracanna in *Fortunio* (1593) reminded his master that he would need an entire series of aphrodisiacal birds, in addition to the mysterious *confettioni* and sweet/potent wines.[12]

A crucial source for many 16th-century recipe books was the most successful food treatise of the 15th century, *De honesta voluptate and valetudine* (first Italian edition 1487) written by Bartolommeo Sacchi, known as Platina (1421–1481). Platina lists an impressive number of foods and recipes with aphrodisiacal properties, among them onions and tubers, broad beans, rocket, pine nuts, turnips, marzipan and pies in a special broth,[13] while truffles, oysters and partridges are considered particularly powerful in exciting even "flagging' or "deadened' passion.[14] In the 16th century, many of Platina's recipes were repeated or slightly revised and recycled in the highly successful *La singolar dottrina di Domenico Romoli sopranominato Panunto* (1560), where highly reputed aphrodisiacs were vegetables such as onions, carrots, chick peas, artichokes, rocket, marjoram, pine nuts and leeks.[15] Similar dietary notions are to be found in Baldassare Pisanelli's *Trattato della natura de' cibi et del bere* (1583), one of the best examples of a new, popular genre that fell between the culinary and the nutritional.[16] Among authors of food treatises there was in fact a general agreement that foods promoting sexual performance included meat, oysters, wine, bread and eggs, which were considered to be particularly nourishing (strengthening) foods, while capers, chickpeas, pine nuts, artichokes, asparagus, turnips, truffles, arugula and parsley were "hot" foods (inciting lust), and leeks, carrots, parsnips and tubers in general were deemed "windy" (inflating) foods.[17] Dietary lore was still basically informed by classical authorities, but authors of cook books and health treatises in the 16th century often added pragmatic advice related to their own experience. In many cases the aphrodisiacal properties of food for the young and the aged were presented as if they were common knowledge accessible to everybody. In fact, cook books and food treatises explored the medicinal properties of food in a process of mutual exchange, imitation and simple copying, to the extent that there was seldom a clear-cut distinction between food treatises and health manuals, especially in the 15th and 16th centuries. Works such as the *Libreto de tutte le cosse che se manzano* (c. 1450–1452) dedicated to Borso d'Este by the physician Michele Savonarola (c. 1385–1466), or the *Libro de homine* (first ed. 1474) by Girolamo Manfredi (1430–1493), were at the same time culinary and medical works. In the volume dedicated to Borso d'Este, the entry on truffles first illustrates the properties of the plant according to classic Galenic theory, includes several preparation and cooking suggestions in the last paragraph, and at the very end adds, almost as an afterthought, that truffles were a meal perfect for "old men with beautiful wives."[18]

Renaissance comedies refer to other remedies for impotence beyond foods and potions. Besides the mysterious *confetioni/confetti*[19] there are occasional mentions of expensive rubs, such as in Cornelio Lanci's *Ruchetta Comedia* (1584), where Beco asks old Averardo about the purpose of the pricey lotion he has bought. Averardo responds: "To rub myself. It has so much power that it is able to resurrect the dead."[20] In *La Cortigiana.* written in 1526 by Pietro Aretino, the expert *ruffiana* (procuress) Alvigia also speaks about a lotion that is purportedly able to "resurrect the flesh of the codpiece."[21] To return to Machiavelli, the fertility potion of the mandrake root had a central place in his famous comedy *Mandragola* (written 1518), but the potion Lucrezia was given to drink in effect was "hypocras," a mulled wine mixed with spices, considered to be both aphrodisiacal and digestive.[22] The issue of the impotence of the elderly husband was also broached in the *Mandragola* when Messer Nicia, anxious to defend himself from doctor Callimaco's doubts, asserts: "Impotent me? Are you joking? I doubt there is another man in Florence as rugged and hard as I am."[23] In Machiavelli's *Clizia,* Messer Nicomaco more modestly recognized that he needed some help and decides to have recourse to the *satirión,* possibly the most famous remedy of the time, to enhance his virility.[24]

The Satyrion Potion

The notion that certain plants or herbs could stimulate or restore sexual potency in the elderly existed well before Renaissance comedy exploited this *topos*. Already in the Greco–Roman period, from Dioscorides to Pliny the Elder, there were repeated mentions in medical and naturalist treatises of the quasi-legendary plant of the orchid family called satyrion [in Latin, *Satÿrion*] whose well-known aphrodisiacal properties also played a literary role in the famous *Satyrica* [in English, *The Satyricon*] by Petronius Arbiter.[25] Why was the bulbous root a particularly strong sexual symbol across the centuries? The root's similarity to human testicles and the flower's often striking resemblance to a human phallus were possibly the most important factors. Phallic images of this plant circulated in medieval *herbaria,* in early modern medical and dietary treatises, and in early modern botanical texts, such as the particularly explicit representation found in Giambattista Della Porta's work *Phytognomonica* (1588). The plant's properties, as described by such treatises, were invariably described as aphrodisiacal: eaten alone, mixed with other ingredients or simply held in one's hand, the root was effective in provoking lust.[26] Underlying this conception was the belief in the doctrine of "signatures," already known in ancient times but clearly defined by Paracelsus (Philippus Aureolus Theophrastus Bombastus von Hohenheim, 1493–1541) in the 16th century. According to the Swiss-born physician and alchemist, all plants and animals had a purpose or virtue precisely inscribed in their shape, color or appearance, which is why the orchid's roots had medicinal properties that could be beneficial for male genitals.[27] Although Paracelsus may have systemized the notion of "signatures" from a theoretical point of view, it was a widely held piece of common wisdom and as such it was included in many *Books of Secrets* published in the 16th century or earlier. According to the *Medicinal Secrets* (1561) by the doctor Pietro Bairo, simply keeping in the mouth a little piece of *verga di lupo seccata* (dried wolf penis) was believed to have an immediately stimulating effect for performing the sexual act.[28] Similarly, quail testicles are used as the main ingredient for an ointment "to erect the member' in *I Segreti de la Signora Isabella Cortese* (1561), a popular recipe book.[29]

Medieval herbaria contained drawings of the *testiculus vulpis* plant and dedicated similar entries to the *satureja hortensis* (summer savory), a plant also considered to have aphrodisiacal powers.[30] The original recipe for the satyrion potion, sometimes called simply *confetto,* was reportedly invented by the famous doctor Yūwas r ibn Māsawaih (known in Europe as Mesué) who lived in Baghdad in the IX century. It continued to enjoy great popularity for centuries in medical, pharmaceutical and dietary literature up to the 17th century. The recipe for the "original" Arab electuary was provided, for example, in the entry for "*Diasatyrion*" attributed to Mesué that appears in the *Nuovo Receptario*, a collection of medical recipes approved by the College of Doctors in Florence that was first published in 1498 and often reprinted in the following century.[31] The Florentine apothecary Stephano Rosselli includes no less than two recipes for biscuits containing satyrion root in a manuscript book of instructions for his sons (1593) and affirms that they had been sold in his shop "for a long time' with "great effects" and also "sent many times to Rome," which assertion was meant to demonstrate that these aphrodisiacal biscuits were in demand even outside of Tuscany.[32] Rosselli also left a *Zibaldone di segreti diversi* (now in the Biblioteca Marucelliana in Florence), in which appears a recipe titled *"morselletti da eccitar Venere"* (little biscuits to excite Venus),[33] while an ointment defined as being useful *"a eretione"* (to provoke erection) was made with the satyrion root and 18 other ingredients, some hard to identify due to bizarre names such as *carpobalsamo* and *astrologia*, while other ingredients were more familiar, such as ginger, pepper and pine nuts, well known also to our characters in comedies.[34] In that many medicinal treatises of the first half of the 16th century included the satyrion root amongst the ingredients for their recipes, it comes as no surprise that Machiavelli and other playwrights were well aware of the various Viagra recipes of their time, and used them to humorous effect in their comedies.

On the whole, the satyrion potion enjoyed a solid reputation in medical, pharmaceutical and dietary manuals, as well as in the literary production of early modern Italy. A host of different factors, as we have seen, contributed to its fame. The circular exchange of ideas regarding the natural world, medical and scientific theories, word metaphors and shape similarities helped form the legend of the potent satyrion potion in a wide range of disciplines and genres. An apt example of how many factors interacted in this mythical remedy can be seen in the explication a satyrion recipe found in a 17th-century treatise, the *Theatro farmaceutico dogmatico e stagirico* a pharmaceutical *summa* by Tomaso Donzelli (1596–1670). While providing one stock recipe for the "Diasatyrion by Mesué," Donzelli adds an explanation regarding the plant called *testicoli di volpe* that humorously summarizes the cultural spectrum of the discourse on the plant. He begins by relating its mythical origins: the roots of that plant were called "Satirij," because they were discovered and used by satyrs to boost their libido while chasing nymphs who fled into the woods. Immediately, however, he added a judicious qualification noting that some more discretely argued that the name came from the root's power "to provoke an erection, called Satyriasis, by the Greeks."[35] The full range of medical, botanical, etymological, and literary knowledge was thus accounted for in one short entry.

From the plant name *satyrion* came the subsequent etymological cluster—and confusion in meanings—of words such as *sàtiro* (satyr), *satìrio*/*satìrij* (satyrion root/roots), *sàtira* (satire), *satirióne*/*satiriónne* (potion) and *satirión* (both a potion and a poisonous mushroom).[36] The Machiavellian reference to the remedy *satirión* in its loose derivation from the word satyrion calls to mind the ithyphallic satyr, the half man, half animal creature that pagan mythology, followed by medieval and early modern culture, saw as the "embodiment of lust."[37] It is fascinating to note that at the same time that the satyrion root and satyrion potions became popular in the early modern period in medical, herbal and pharmaceutical treatises, lascivious images of satyrs with an erect phallus began to circulate broadly in visual media, sculpture and painting, while satyr scenes were even to become a favorite staple of late 16th-century pastoral literature.[38]

The bulbs of the exotic orchid were often substituted with the roots of a more commonly available domestic plant called *testiculus vulpis* or *testiculus canis* as Pietro Matthioli explains in his medical *Discorsi on Dioscorides* (first edn. 1544).[39] According to Prospero Borgarucci, a 16th-century doctor and apothecary working in Venice, several *spezieri* in his city regularly prepared the *satirión* with the *testiculus canis* root instead of the satyrion as it was more difficult to obtain.[40] However, he warned that for problems related to sexual impotence, it was best to use only the bigger roots because the smallest would have a contrary effect.[41] One of these recipes called for boiling the roots in a chickpea broth and adding, among other things, rocket seeds, asparagus, cinnamon, long pepper [the dried fruit of the Indian plant *piper longum*] pine nuts, pistachios and two ounces of sparrow brain. Given the ingredients, Borgarucci promised, the recipe would produce "marvelous effects."[42] The Venetian doctor Giovanni Marinello in his *Le medicine pertinenti alle infermità delle donne* (1574), listed 16 pages of *elettuari, satiriónni* and foods for restoring lost virility.[43] While his preoccupation with a functional sexuality in marriage is understandable—impotence could be the legal ground for annulment of a marriage—the attention he devoted to old men and their problems is particularly noteworthy.[44] Following humoral theory, Marinello suggested substances that were believed to increase the flow of blood and warm the cold body of the elderly, such rocket seeds, various kinds of pepper, mustard, saffron, cinnamon and cardamom.[45] His inventive formulas often added satyrion to the mix and, in one case, an especially potent prescription called for thirty sparrow brains (the sparrow was notoriously libidinous) to make a *nociuola* or pill to be eaten before going to bed with a woman.[46] Marinello followed medical tradition and popular lore, but he did add some savvy and practical advice. He suggested that having a satisfying sexual relation involved more than potions or lotions, it also required the right environment, the absence of preoccupations, the role of imagination and general moderation in eating and drinking.[47]

The purported properties of the satyrion potion continue to appear in medical lore well into the 17th century, although even specialized literature becomes a bit vague about what it is exactly. For example, the *Antidotario Romano Latino e Volgare* (1668), a *summa* of medical remedies, gives several recipes for *Diasatyrion* made with the *testiculus canis* root, but guiltily admits that there is uncertainty about what root it is and suggests that one might make do with any bulbous root regularly consumed in everyday cooking such as onions, leeks and scallions.[48] It would seem that the popular medical lore circulating in the 16th-century *Book of Secrets* with its exotic ingredients has been abandoned in favor of more commonplace items from the larder, but with equally guaranteed effect.

Lustful Senescence: Literary Humor *Versus* Humanist Denial

To return to Renaissance comedy, the enormous popularity of Platina's work with its multiple editions and translations, along with the proliferation of food treatises and health manuals in the 15th and 16th centuries, can certainly account for the repeated mentions of specific foods and cures for impotence that appear in many plays.[49] But did dramatists believe in the power of *lattovari* and special foods as did (apparently) doctors and the authors of health and dietary treatises? Should playwrights be seen as being more skeptical than not, considering that the "miraculous" properties of many remedies were usually playfully discussed or even mocked in comedies? The gullibility of the amorous old fools who believed in such popular aids and remedies for impotence was often underscored in scenes specifically dedicated to them, while clever servants usually reveled in revealing the foolish credulity of their masters. In the comedy *Calandra* (1513) by the future Cardinal Bernardo Dovizi da Bibbiena there is a famous line by the servant Fessenio where he laughingly comments on the power of love, saying it was "Just like truffles! They both make young men's affairs come to a head and old men fart."[50] This scathing comment was typical of a series of mocking tropes on contemporary medical and dietary literature that were to appear in Renaissance plays. For example, in the comedy *Fortunio* by Vicenzo Giusti (published 1593), Messer Anselmo conferred with his servant Tracanna about what to eat to prepare for a night of love. Tracanna responded using a parody of a "scientific" explanation to dissuade his master from eating oysters, arguing that they were a "cold" food, useful to excite young people but with unpleasant effects on the aged.[51] In Loredano's *Li vani amori* (1588), Garbino waits in line an hour at the apothecary shop for a preparation of a *lattovaro* for his master Crispo. When the servant returned with the fresh potion, Crispo feared it would not suffice to overcome his problems and urged him to return to the market to buy garden celery and thistles. Garbino tried to dissuade his master, warning him humorously about the properties of garden celery by pointing out that he would not be able to do anything beyond a windy serenade from the "lower regions" of his body, as this particular remedy would make him full of wind.[52] Later, Garbino speaks openly to the audience about the foolishness of his master, mockingly describing him about to gulp down "recipes" believed to be able to resurrect the dead.[53] In another comedy by Francesco Mercati da Bibbiena, *Il Lanzi* (1566), servants decide to have fun at the expense of their foolish master Ruberto and teach him that his sexual appetites were not appropriate for one of his age. To this end they made Ruberto meet with a (false) doctor who would supposedly provide him with a miraculous *lattovaro,* made with the "youth apple from Calicut" to make him young again.[54] In Giovan Battista della Porta's *La Furiosa* (1609), the strategy is told from a feminine perspective: the protagonist is a young wife married to an old doctor who is desperate for a cure for her husband's impotence. She laments to a servant that her husband's cures and attempts to "revive dead bodies" were of no use to her because he could not revive his own member "more dead than death itself" neither with ointments nor with caresses.[55]

Besides plays, other literary texts express doubts on the power of aphrodisiacal foods, while admitting that they had a recognized role in the popular imagination as cures for impotence. In Pietro Aretino's *Ragionamenti* (1534–1536), for example, Nanna instructs her daughter Pippa on the supposed power of certain foods for would-be libidinous old men, such as oysters, hot *lattovari* from France, truffles, thistles and pepper. She also noted mockingly that Pippa, during such meals, could eat without restraint since the old men were too busy, anxiously stuffing themselves with fortifying foods in preparation for what they hoped was to follow.[56] Unfortunately for these elderly swains, in another section of the dialogue Nanna admits to her friend Antonia that the most popular aphrodisiacal foods, such as truffles, artichokes and *lattovari*, did not actually seem to have much effect.[57] Similarly, in a short 16th-century novella by Anton Francesco Doni an old man, Lombardo, marries a beautiful young woman and "after taking many *lattovari* and using several unguents" tries to make love to her, but to no avail.[58] Desperate, he tried standing naked on the balcony, singing the *Magnificat* in the hopes that as in church everything would stand up at the sound of that sacred song.[59]

At the same time as Renaissance comedy was encountering widespread success, along with its humorous treatment of erotic topics, 15th- and 16th-century humanist writing about old age, love and desire offered a decidedly less humorous and less hopeful perspective on elderly men and cures for their impotence.[60] It is interesting to note that humanist writing often makes reference to the same sexual themes treated in comedies, but adopted an entirely different approach to the problem, relying strictly on ancient texts and the theory of the four humors in their assessment of geriatric impotence. The main explanation found in humanist treatises regarding old men's sexual dysfunction is based on Galenic theory and the astrological claim that a different planet and humor dominate the body at different ages. Thus old men were under the control of Saturn, they were cold and dry, lacking in strength and unable to function sexually. Following this line of thought, Marsilio Ficino, in his *De vita libri tres* (published in 1489), recommended that saturnine people "avoid the Venereal act, which takes away most of the life even of people who are young."[61] Since elderly men already lacked inner warmth and moisture, they should certainly not engage in sexual intercourse as they would risk losing their entire remaining vital humors. Ludovico Guicciardini in *L'ore di recreazione* (1565) and Cardinal Gabriele Paleotto (1524–1597) in his highly moralistic *Libro del bene della vecchiezza* (1597), also supported the Galenic notion that the diminution of excess heat in old age finally freed men from the tyranny of the senses and "all unrestrained impulses."[62] Despite this respectable pedigree, such conclusions were certainly not attributed by dramatists to characters of old lovers. In direct opposition to Ficino and contemporary conduct literature, Messer Ambrogio in Giovan Maria Cecchi's *Assiuolo* (written and staged in 1549) described himself as someone who had "fire inside" while old Filippo in *La stiava* (also by Cecchi, 1550) both echoed Petrarchan concepts and contradicted humoral theory by affirming that he fell in love because he possessed the two crucial elements: "kindness of heart and warmth of blood."[63] In *Olivetta* by Cornelio Lanci (1587), a dialogue between two patriarchs, Lippo and Lando, centered on the hot–cold dichotomy between young women and old men. Lando warned his friend that old men, similar to old wood, cannot make a good fire, while women catch fire immediately.[64] Teodoro, in Donato Giannotti's *Il vecchio amoroso* (written c. 1533–1536) also contradicted Ficinian theory by boasting that he was sixty and happily enamored of the young slave Diamante.[65] Similarly, the 70-year-old Messer Ricciardo in *Il commodo* by Antonio Landi (1566) patently ignored all medical dictates regarding sex in old age when he proclaimed: "[...] regarding this other thing I always did what I wanted to do."[66] In *Il Saltuzza* by Andrea Calmo (1551), old Melindo undertakes a long monologue that playfully mixes Venetian dialect and macaronic Latin to explain that doctors were wrong when they affirmed that old men like himself lacked the virtues of "*diritiva, premitiva, sustentativa*" [becoming erect, penetrating and enduring].[67] In sharp contrast to humanistic literature based on Galenic theory, comedies reveal that old patriarchs, even though they were supposed to be cold and dry, had "fire inside" and might fall in love, even if they were unable to live up to the desires that they still strongly felt.

The humanist image of old age as a period of life almost free of carnal desires was also contradicted by a significant body of medical knowledge of the time that recognized the existence of sexual desire in the elderly and the troubles it caused. The Veronese physician Gabriele Zerbi, in his *Gerontocomia* (1484), acknowledged the power of sex "because of the great delight it produces," and admitted how difficult it was for old men to "curb the use of it."[68] Alessandro Trajano Petronio, doctor of Pope Gregorio XIII in his treatise *Del viver delli Romani et del conservar la sanità* (1592), advised men over 63 years of age that sex should be avoided because semen emission would weaken the body. But if one was "forced by nature" or by the desire to have children to engage in intercourse, he recommended at first a surprisingly humble soup of bread and raw egg whites, and then went on to suggest a series of more elaborate traditional remedies, including pigeon cooked in red wine, sparrow meat, aphrodisiacal mushrooms and the "*confetto* called diasatyrion."[69] In his introduction on the causes of impotence, Giovanni Marinelli, author of *Le medicine pertinenti alle infermità delle donne* (1574), expressed a certain compassion with regard to age-induced impotence suffered by "those who cannot exercise sex with women and know very well what it means."[70] Yet even authors such as the *speziale* [pharmacist] Matteo Palmieri, in his *De vita civile* (written 1438–1439, published 1529), who condemned lust in general but denounced the desires of old men as being particularly "abominable and ugly," nonetheless had to admit that it could pose no small problem for the elderly.[71]

Conclusion

Dramatists and authors of *novelle* and other literary forms took full advantage of the comic possibility offered by the character of the amorous old fool, and often used such figures to explore contemporary views about sexuality in general and geriatric sexuality in particular. What was then the "social and cultural script"[72] to be found in comedies that mocked but at the same time empathized with the elderly characters in love? As I have argued elsewhere in more detail, comedies were an imaginative terrain where traditional age stereotypes and gender definitions were playfully discussed. The characters of old lovers were certainly an important part of that imaginative arena. Comedies elaborated on at least three competing sets of problems concerning old men and sex in 16th-century society: the age disparity in arranged upper-class marriages that often saw old men married to much younger wives;[73] the necessity of proving virility and manhood in such marriages by producing offspring; and lastly the difficult relationship between the old and the young, especially in gerontocratic societies such as Venice and Florence.[74]

This contrast was often dramatized in Italian comedies that ended with the final triumph of the young, allowing at least in the imaginary world of the comedy the overturning of "the more normal subordination of young males to older male patriarchs."[75] A significant number of plays portray young male characters temporarily dressed as women and successfully passing as such, a ploy that openly alluded to life offstage where youths were regularly kept in a submissive and thus "feminine" social position. Significantly, however, the shedding of the female dress at the end of the comedy was invariably preceded by a scene of phallic revelation that served to reassure the audience that the cross-dressed character had evolved into an adult male. In several comedies, phallic revelations even spill over into phallic celebrations where young, well-equipped men reverse (at least at the sexual level) the normally dominant position of their elders. Certainly the young phallus celebrated in these comedies served primarily to exclude any residual femininity in cross-dressed characters and provided an eloquent theatrical metaphor for the contrast between young and old men, and for their respective sexual prowess and sexual weakness.[76]

While, in some cases, the shaming and ritual humiliation of lustful old men bring them back to a more socially appropriate role (as in Machiavelli's *Clizia*), in others the lovelorn patriarchs remain blissfully unaware that they have been made a fool, but no matter what the end result may have been, the scripting of old fools in love was quite distant from the image that prescriptive humanist literature depicted and society demanded. In comedies most of the characters never managed to carry out their erotic plans, being thwarted by an alliance against them that included servants, young men and women, all of whom were usually subjugated to patriarchal power. Often old men were punished with charivari-like pranks until they regained both their senses and their *virtù*, whereby traditional patriarchal reason and sexual order were reassuringly restored. To soften the bitter medicine of their failure in love, old fools are occasionally redeemed by the sentimental discovery that the object of their affection is actually a long-lost daughter. At other times an elderly swain finally sees the light and graciously steps aside in favor of his son, virtually always a sympathetic character who finds himself in amorous competition with not just the older generation, but his own father. Such is the genre of comedy, where almost every character is given a role in the final happy end, with the return of harmony and the triumph of youth and love. In comedy's complex rendering of amorous old men it is thus possible to read a critique of the contemporary humanistic view of senescence as a period of self-control and *saviezza* (wisdom) that certainly did not correspond with reality. In contrast to the normative humanist ideal of the savvy patriarch who has relinquished erotic desires, both comedy and medical lore recognize that masculine old age was hardly chaste. Not only was this stage of life portrayed as being subject to passions and desires, but it was also seen as attempting (somewhat pathetically) to recover the pleasures of youth with invigorating foods, stimulating lotions, and the most potent remedy of all: the legendary *satirión*.

Works Cited

Manuscripts and Early Printed Sources (pre-1900)

Antidotario Romano Latino e Volgare, tradotto da Ippolito Ceccarelli. Li Ragionamenti, e le aggiunte dell'Elettione de' Semplici, e Prattica delle Compositioni. Con le annotazioni del Signore Pietro Castelli Romano e trattati della Teriaca romana e della teriaca Egittia. Rome: per il successore al Mascardi, 1668.

Bairo, Pietro, *Secreti medicinali di M. Pietro Bairo da Turin, già medico di Carlo Secondo Duca di Savoia.* Venice: Appresso F. Sansovino, 1561.

Boerio, Giuseppe, *Dizionario del dialetto veneziano.* Venice: Reale Tipografia di Giovanni Cecchini, 1867.

Borgarucci, Prospero, *La fabrica de gli spetiali, partita in xii distintioni. Nuovamente composta dall'Eccellente Medico e Filosofo Prospero Borgarucci.* Venice: Vincenzo Valgrisio, 1566.

Cecchi, Giovanni Maria, *La stiava comedia di Gio. Maria Cecchi Fiorentino.* Venice: Gabriel Giolito de Ferrari, 1550.

Cortese, Isabella, *I Secreti della Sign. Isabella Cortese. Ne' quali si contengono cose minerali, medicinali, arteficiose, e alchimistiche. Et molte de l' arte Profumatoria, appartenenti a ogni gran Signora. Con altri bellissimi segreti aggiunti.* Venice: Appresso gli heredi di Iacomo Simbeni, 1588.

Dolce, Lodovico, *Fabritia Comedia di M. Lodovico Dolce.* Venice: Aldi Filii, 1549.

Doni, Antonfrancesco, *Tutte le Novelle, Lo Stufaiolo Commedia e La Mula e La Chiave Dicerie di Antonfrancesco Doni.* Milan: G. Daelli e Comp. Editori, 1863.

Donzelli, Giuseppe, *Teatro farmaceutico dogmatico e spagirico del dottor Giuseppe Donzelli, Napoletano, Barone di Dogliola.* Naples: A Spese degli Socii, 1726.

Falloppia, Gabriel, *Secreti diversi, e miracolosi raccolti dal Faloppia e approbati da altri medici di gran fama. Nuovamente ristampati e a commun beneficio di ciascuno, distinti in tre libri.* Venice: Pietro Miloco, 1620.

Giusti, Vicenzo, *Fortunio Comedia Nuova di M. Vicenzo Giusti da Udine.* Venice: Nicolò Moretti, 1593.

Lanci, Cornelio, *Olivetta Commedia. Del Sig. Cavaliere Cornelio Lanci.* Florence: Sermartelli, 1587.

Lanci, Cornelio, *Ruchetta Comedia del Signor Cavaliere Cornelio Lanci.* Florence: Sermartelli, 1584.

Landi, Antonio, *Il commodo* (Florence: Appresso i Giunti, 1566).

Loredan, Giovan Francesco, *Li vani amori del Signor Gio. Francesco Loredano.* Venice: All'insegna della speranza a San Giuliano, 1588.

Marinello, Giovanni, *Le Medicine Partenenti alle infermità delle Donne. Scritte per M. Giovanni Marinello. Divise in Tre Libri.* Venice: Appresso Giovanni Valgrisio, 1574.

Matthioli, Pietro, *I Discorsi di M. Pietro Matthioli Sanese, Medico Cesareo, et del Serenissimo Principe Ferdinando Archiduca D'Austria & c. Nelli sei libri di Pedacio Dioscoride Anazarbeo della materia Medicinale. Hora di Nuovo dal suo istesso autore ricorretti, & in più di mille luoghi aumentati. Con le figure grandi tutte di nuovo rifatte, & tirate dalle naturali & vive piante, & animali, & in numero molto maggiore che le altre per avanti stampate,* 5 vols. Venice: Vincenzo Valgrisi, 1568.

Nuovo Receptario composto dal Famosissimo Chollegio degli Eximii Doctori Della Arte et Medicina Della Inclita Ciptà di Firenze (1498) in http://www.pluteus.it ed. Olimpia Fittipaldi.

Paleotto, Gabriele, *Libro del bene della vecchiezza,* trans. M. F. Pietro da Piombino Agostinaio. Rome: Appresso Luigi Zannetti, 1597.

Palmieri, Matteo, *Della vita civile Trattato di Matteo Palmieri cittadino fiorentino.* Milan: Giovanni Silvestri, 1825.

Petronio, Alessandro, *Del viver delli Romani et di conservar la sanità. Libri cinque. Tradotti dalla lingua latina nella volgare, dall'eccellente medico M. Basilio Paravicino de Como.* Rome: Appresso Domenico Basa, 1592.

Pisanelli, Baldassare, *Trattato della natura de' cibi et del bere del Sig. Baldassare Pisanelli, Medico Bolognese. Nel quale non solo tutte le virtù, & i vitij di quelli minutamente si palesano; ma anco i rimedij per correggere i loro difetti ….* Carmagnola: Bellone, 1589.

Romoli, Domenico, *La singolar dottrina di M. Domenico Romoli sopranominato Panonto, dell'ufficio dello scalco, de i condimenti di tutte le vivande, le stagioni che si convengono a tutti gli animali, uccelli, e pesci, banchetti di ogni tempo ….* Venice: Giov. Battista Bonfadino, 1593.

Rosselli, Stephano, *Zibaldone di diversi segreti,* Biblioteca Marucelliana MS C.145, "Morselletti da eccitar Venere cap. LXXV."

Targioni Tozzetti, *Ottaviano, Dizionario Botanico Italiano che comprende i nomi volgari italiani specialmente toscani e vernacoli delle piante raccolti da diversi autori e dalla gente di campagna col corrispondente latino botanico compilato dal dottore Ottaviano Targioni Tozzetti.* Florence: a spese dell'editore, 1858.

Secondary Sources and Modern Editions

Albala, Ken, *Beans: A History*. Oxford/New York: Berg, 2007.

Albala, Ken, *Eating Right in Renaissance Italy*. Berkeley/Los Angeles: University of California Press, 2002.

Aretino, Pietro, "La Cortigiana," in Pietro Aretino, *Tutte le Commedie*, ed. G. B. De Sanctis. Milan: Mursia, 1994.

Aretino, Pietro, *Ragionamento-Dialogo*, ed. Carla Forno. Milan: Biblioteca Universale Rizzoli, 1988.

Battaglia, Salvatore, *Grande Dizionario della lingua italiana*. Turin: UTET, 1961–.

Battisti, Carlo, and Giovanni Alessio, *Dizionario Etimologico Italiano*. Florence: G. Barbèra 1968.

Bennett, Jane, *The Enchantment of Modern Life: Attachments, Crossings, and Ethics*. Princeton, NJ: Princeton University Press, 2001.

Bourne, Molly, "Vincenzo Gonzaga and the Body Politic: Impotence and Virility at Court."

Calmo, Andrea, *Il Saltuzza*, ed. Luca D'Onghia. Padua: Esedra, 2006.

Calmo, Andrea, *Il Travaglia. Comedia di Messer Andrea Calmo, nuovamente venuta in luce, molto piacevole e d varie lingue adornata, sotto bellissima invenzione. Al modo che la fo presentata dal detto autore nella città di Vinegia*, ed. Piermario Vescovo. Padua: Editrice Antenore, 1994.

Campbell, Julie D., "Introduction," in *Isabella Andreini La Mirtilla: A Pastoral*, translated with an Introduction by Julie D. Campbell. Tempe: Arizona, 2002.

Camporesi, Piero, *I balsami di Venere*. Milan: Garzanti, 1989.

Carroll, Linda, "Money, Age, and Marriage in Venice: A Brief Biocultural History," in *Politics and Culture*, Issue 1 (2010). http://www.politicsandculture.org/2010/04/29/money-age-and-marriage-in venice-a-brief-biocultural-history/.

Carroll, Linda, "Who's on top? Gender as Societal Power Configuration in Italian Renaissance Painting and Drama," *The Sixteenth Century Journal* 20 (1989): 531–58.

Castiglioni, Luigi, *Storia delle piante forastiere. Le più importanti nell'uso medico, od economico*, ed. Luigi Saibene. Milan: Jaca Book, 2008.

Cecchi, Giovanni Maria, "Assiuolo" in *Commedie del Cinquecento*, ed. Nino Borsellino, 2 vols. Milan: Feltrinelli, 1962.

Cox, Virginia, *The Prodigious Muse: Women's Writing in Counter-Reformation Italy*. Baltimore, MD: Johns Hopkins University Press, 2011.

Del Turco, Giovanni, *Epulario e segreti vari. Trattati di cucina toscana nella Firenze Seicentesca 1602–1636*, ed. Anna Evangelista. Bologna: Forni, 1992.

Della Porta, Giovan Battista, "La Furiosa," in Giovan Battista della Porta, *Teatro Quarto tomo-Commedie*, ed. Raffaele Sirri, 4 vols. Naples: Edizioni Scientifiche Italiane, 2003.

Dovizi da Bibbiena, Bernardo, "The Comedy of Calandro," in *Five Comedies from the Italian Renaissance*, ed. and trans. Laura Giannetti and Guido Ruggiero. Baltimore, MD: Johns Hopkins University Press, 2003.

Ellis, Anthony, *Old Age, Masculinity, and Early Modern Drama. Comic Elders on the Italian and Shakespearean Stage.* Farnham, UK/Burlington, VT: Ashgate, 2009.

Faraone, Christopher A., *Ancient Greek Love Magic.* Cambridge, MA: Harvard University Press, 1999.

Faraone, Christopher, "Encolpius' Impotence and the Double Dose of Satyrion," in *The Ancient Novel: Classical Paradigms and Modern Perspectives,* ed. J. Tatum and Gail M. Vernazza. Hanover, NH: Dartmouth College, 1990.

Ferraro, Joanne M., *Marriage Wars in Late Renaissance Venice.* Oxford/New York: Oxford University Press, 2001.

Finucci, Valeria, "There's the Rub: Searching for Sexual Remedies in the New World," *Journal of Medieval and Early Modern Studies,* 38.3 (Fall 2008): 523–57.

Finucci, Valeria, *The Manly Masquerade. Masculinity, Paternity and Castration in the Italian Renaissance.* Durham, NC: Duke University Press, 2003.

Galli Stampino, Maria, "Pastoral Constraints, Textual and Dramatic Strategies: Isabella Andreini's *La Mirtilla* and Torquato Tasso's *Aminta,*" in *Italian Culture* 22 (2004): 1–20.

Giannotti, Donato, "Il vecchio amoroso," in *Commedie del Cinquecento,* ed. Nino Borsellino, 2 vols. Milan: Feltrinelli, 1962.

Grazzini, Anton Francesco, "Le Cene" in *Opere di Anton Francesco Grazzini,* ed. Guido Davico Bonino (Turin: UTET, 1977, 2nd ed.).

Grieco, Allen, J., "From Roosters to Cocks: Italian Renaissance Fowl and Sexuality," in, *Erotic Cultures of Renaissance Italy,* ed. Sara Matthews-Grieco. Farnham, UK/ Burlington, VT: Ashgate, 2010. 89–140.

Kaske, Carol V., and John R. Clark, eds., *Marsilio Ficino Three Books on Life. A Critical Edition and Translation with Introduction and Notes.* Tempe: AZ, 1998, 1st ed., 1989.

Kaufmann, Lynn Frier, *The Noble Savage: Satyrs and Satyr Families in Renaissance Art.* Ann Arbor, MI: UMI Research Press, 1984.

Machiavelli, Niccolò, "Clizia," in *Niccolò Machiavelli Teatro Andria Mandragola Clizia,* ed. Guido Davico Bonino. Turin: Einaudi, 1979.

Machiavelli, Niccolò, "The Mandrake Root," *Five Comedies from the Italian Renaissance,* ed. and trans. Laura Giannetti and Guido Ruggiero. Baltimore, MD: Johns Hopkins University Press, 2003.

Matthews-Grieco, Sara, "Satyr and Sausages: Erotic Strategies and the Print Market in Cinquecento Italy," in *Erotic Cultures of Renaissance Italy,* ed. Sara Matthews-Grieco. Farnham, UK/Burlington, VT: Ashgate, 2010.

McLaren, Angus, *Impotence: A Cultural History.* Chicago: University of Chicago Press, 2007.

Mercati, Francesco da Bibbiena, *Il Lanzi* in Erica Lynn Westhoff, "Il Sensale," "Il Lanzi," "L'Imbroglia: *Reconsidering Renaissance Comedy through the Plays of Francesco Mercati.* PhD Diss.: UCLA, 2010.

Mintz, Sidney W., *Sweetness and Power: The Place of Sugar in Modern History.* New York: Penguin Books, 1986.

Montanari, Massimo, *Nuovo Convivio: Storia e Cultura dei piaceri della tavola nell'età moderna.* Rome: Laterza, 1991.

Pezzella, Salvatore, *Gli erbari. I primi libri di medicina (le virtù curative delle piante)* (Perugia: Grifo, 1993).

Piccolomini, Alessandro, *Alessandro*, ed. Florindo Cerreta. Siena: Accademia Senese degli Intronati, 1966.

Platina, Bartolomeo (Sacchi), *On Right Pleasure and Good Health* [*De honesta voluptate et valetudine*], ed. and trans. Mary Ella Milham. Tempe, AZ: Medieval and Renaissance Texts and Studies, 1998.

Ray, Meredith, "*La castità conquistata*: The Function of the Satyr in Pastoral Drama," in *Romance Languages Annual* 9 (1998): 312–21.

Rees, Katie, "Female-Authored Drama in Early Modern Padua," *Italian Studies* 63.1 (Spring 2008): 41–61.

Rosselli, Stefano Francesco Di Romolo, *Mes secrets: à Florence au temps des Médicis, 1593: pâtisserie, parfumerie, médecine*, ed. Rodrigo de Zayas. Paris, 1996.

Ruzante (Angelo Beolco) *L'Anconitana*, in *Ruzante Teatro*, ed. Ludovico Zorzi. Turin: Einaudi, 1967.

Savonarola, Michele, *Libreto de tutte le cosse che se magnano: un'opera di dietetica del sec. xv*, ed. Jane Nystedt. Stockholm: Almquist & Wiksell, 1988.

Shaw, James and Evelyn Welch, eds., *Making and Marketing Medicine in Renaissance Florence.* Amsterdam: Rodopi, 2011.

Simons, Patricia, *The Sex of Men in Premodern Europe: A Cultural History.* Cambridge: Cambridge University Press, 2011.

Szirmai, Julia, *La syrinx au bucher. Pan et les satyres a la renaissance et a l'age baroque.* Geneva: Droz, 2005.

Van Passen, Anne Marie and Lodovico Guicciardini, eds., *L'ore di ricreazione.* Rome: Bulzoni, 1990.

Vitullo, Juliann, "Taste and Temptation in Early Modern Italy," The *Senses and Society* 5.1 (March 2010): 106–18.

Waddington, Raymond, *Aretino's Satyr. Sexuality, Satire, and Self-Projection in Sixteenth-Century Literature and Art.* Toronto: University of Toronto Press, 2004.

Warren, Jeremy, "Bronzes," in *At Home in Renaissance Italy*, ed. Marta Ajmar-Wollheim and Flora Dennis. London: Victoria & Albert Museum Publications, 2006.

Wheeler, Jo with the assistance of Katy Temple, *Renaissance Secrets: Recipes & Formulas.* London: Victoria & Albert Museum Publications, 2009.

Zerbi, Gabriele, *Gerontocomia: On the Care of the Aged and Maximianus, Elegies on Old Age and Love*, trans. L. R. Lind. Philadelphia, PA: American Philosophical Society, 1988.

Notes

1 I am deeply grateful to Sara Matthews-Grieco for inviting me to collaborate on the volume and for providing invaluable comments and suggestions on earlier drafts of this essay.

2 "Nicomaco: "... ed ho ordinato una cena a mio modo: io piglierò prima una presa d'uno lattovaro, che si chiama satirión." Pirro: "Che nome bizzarro è cotesto!" Nicomaco: "E' gl'ha più bizzarri e fatti, perché e' gli è un lattovaro che farebbe, quanto a quella faccenda, ringiovanire uno uomo di novanta anni, non che di settanta, come ne ho io. Preso questo lattovaro, io cenerò poche cose, ma tutte sustanzievole: in prima, una insalata di cipolle cotte, di poi una mistura di fave e spezierie ..." Pirro: "Che fa cotesto?" Nicomaco: "Che fa? Queste cipolle, fave e spezierie, perché sono calde e ventose, farebbono far vela ad una caracca genovese! Sopra queste cose, si vuole uno pippione grosso arrosto, così verdemezzo, che sanguini un poco ... " See Niccolò Machiavelli, "Clizia," IV, ii, in Guido Davico Bonino (ed.) *Niccolò Machiavelli Teatro Andria Mandragola Clizia* (Turin, 1979), 139–201 at 179–80.

3 In early modern Europe the idea persisted (based on Greek medicine) that erection was due to warm air or spirits. Regarding the circulation and diffusion in Europe of this notion see Angus Mc Laren, *Impotence: A Cultural History* (Chicago, 2007), 39. Ken Albala explains the vision of *fava* beans as windy and therefore an aphrodisiacal food: "Yet, more surprisingly, beans inflate not just the stomach but the whole body. This creates a kind of artificial aid to sex, an early modern Viagra, if you will." Ken Albala, *Beans: A History* (Oxford/New York, 2007), 58.

4 Because of its shape the root was called in ancient Greek *òrchis-eos* (from which orchid) which means "testicle."

5 Besides comedies, in the *novella* genre it is common to find the character of the old impotent husband who is jealous of his young wife. See for instance "ebbe per ventura una fanciulla, giovane, nobile, e bella: la quale era da lui, *in fuora che nel letto* (my emphasis), contentata di tutte quante le cose che ella sapeva chiedere." Anton Francesco Grazzini, "Le Cene" in Guido Davico Bonino (ed.), *Opere di Anton Francesco Grazzini* (Turin, 1977, 2nd ed.), "Prima Cena," no. X, 525–33 at 525.

6 See *Li vani amori del Signor Gio. Francesco Loredano* (Venice, 1588), IV, ii, c. 91r.; *Fortunio Comedia Nuova di M. Vicenzo Giusti da Udine* (Venice, 1593), I, ix, c.19r. and *Fabritia Comedia di M. Lodovico Dolce* (Venice, 1549), where the servant Turchetto buys "pignocate" and "marzapani" for his master (II, viii, c. 22r.). A *lattovaro/lettovaro* (and/or *lactovaro*) may contain different components and usually honey is one of the main ingredients. The medicinal term *lattovaro* is common in literature well before the 16th century. For instance see Giovanni Boccaccio, *Decameron* , VII, 3.

7 *Pinochiati* are defined as "small individual cakes made from pine-nuts and sugar" in James Shaw and Evelyn Welch (eds.) *Making and Marketing Medicine in Renaissance Florence* (Amsterdam, 2011), 202. See Giovan Maria Cecchi, "Assiuolo" in Nino Borsellino (ed.), *Commedie del Cinquecento*, vol. I (Milan, 1962), III, iv, 161, for mentions of *pinochiati* and a *lattovaro*. *Assiuolo* was first published in 1550. For two examples of *pinochiato* and *pinochiato alla veneziana* recipes see: Giovanni Del Turco, *Epulario e segreti vari. Trattati di cucina toscana nella Firenze Seicentesca 1602–1636*, ed. Anna Evangelista (Bologna, 1992), 86, 97. In a well-known Lenten sermon delivered in Florence by St. Bernardino in 1424, Florentine apothecaries are "damned" for selling *pinochiati* and marzipans along with other foods responsible for the sins of sodomy and lust. Quoted in Juliann Vitullo, "Taste and Temptation in Early Modern Italy," The *Senses and Society* 5.1 (March 2010): 106–18 at 106. Pistachios were particularly recommended for old men in *La fabrica de gli spetiali, partita in xii distintioni. Nuovamente composta dall'Eccellente Medico e Filosofo Prospero Borgarucci* (Venice, 1566), c. 41: "molto son commendati da Medici à vecchi, non solamente per mangiare così alla giornata, ma anche nelle medicine, che si fanno per Madonna Venere ... di maniera che i vecchi di questo frutto ne ritranno diverse utilità prima per mantenersi grassi, e freschi, overo per divenire tali e poi per mantenersi ne fatti d'Amore gagliardamente."

8 Arrigo: "Io ho tolto quattro marzapani, parecchi pinochiati, ed altre confezioni, delle quali io penso che abbi ad avere bisogno, perché tu sai come sono fatte le giostre amorose." Donato Giannotti, "Il vecchio amoroso," in Nino Borsellino (ed.), *Commedie del Cinquecento*, III, v, 46.

9 "mi serrai in camera; e da me, bevvi due bicchieri di malvagia, e mangiai un poco di ranciata e due barbe di gengiovo e non so che confezioni." Donato Giannotti, *Il vecchio amoroso*, IV, i, 53. The term *confezione/confettione/confetione* in general refers to a medicinal preserve. Old Collofonio in *Il travaglia* takes note of the money he spent after he fell in love and includes in his list "soldi 3 e piccoli 2" for *moscardini* [a sweet pastry] and hair-washing session: Andrea Calmo, *Il Travaglia. Comedia di Messer Andrea Calmo, nuovamente venuta in luce, molto piacevole e d varie lingue adornata, sotto bellissima invenzione. Al modo che la fo presentata dal detto autore nella città di Vinegia*, ed. Piermario Vescovo (Padua, 1994), II, 16, 139. *Il travaglia* was first published in 1556.

10 "Sèleno" is the word used for garden celery. See the entry "sèleno" in Giuseppe Boerio, *Dizionario del dialetto veneziano* (Venice, 1867), 642. Many thanks to Karen Reed and William Eamon who helped me to identify the name of the plant. Garden celery and thistles in *Li vani amori*, IV, iv,

c. 91r.; pine nuts and pistachios in *Ruchetta Comedia del Signor Cavaliere Cornelio Lanci* (Florence, 1584), III, i, c. 46r. Truffles and artichokes are the choice for old Gostanzo in Alessandro Piccolomini's *Alessandro*, ed. Florindo Cerreta (Siena, 1966), II, iii, 162. Gostanzo is also planning to eat "macaroni" an aromatic plant with a taste similar to the asparagus not to be confused with "maccheroni." *Alessandro* was written in 1544.

11 Allen J. Grieco, "From Roosters to Cocks: Italian Renaissance Fowl and Sexuality," in Sara Matthews-Grieco (ed.), *Erotic Cultures of Renaissance Italy* (Farnham, UK/Burlington, VT, 2010), 89–140.

12 Tracanna: "Ci vole altro a pari vostri. Buone confettioni, buoni Caponi, starne, Fagiani, Moscati, Vini … . See *Fortunio*, I, ix, c. 19r. Wines are considered good for different reasons, but sweet/potent wines convey strength.

13 See Platina, *On Right Pleasure and Good Health*, ed. and trans. Mary Ella Milham (Tempe, AZ: 1998). Onions and tubers (Book III, 187) rocket (B. III, 199) turnips (B. VII, 319) pine nuts (B. III, 177) pie in broth (B. VIII, 377) pie which they call marzipan (B. VIII, 379). Many recipes were adapted and translated into Latin from Maestro Martino da Como, the most noted cook of the 15th century.

14 Platina, *On Right Pleasures*: see [Partridges] *partridges* (B. V, 255–7), [Truffles] *truffles* (B. IX, 411), and [Oysters] *oysters* (B. X, 437).

15 *La singolar dottrina di M. Domenico Romoli sopranominato Panunto, dell'ufficio dello scalco, de i condimenti di tutte le vivande, le stagioni che si convengono a tutti gli animali, uccelli, e pesci, banchetti di ogni tempo* … (Venice, 1593). The fourth book, dedicated to exemplary menus, opens with advice for the first day of Lent (March 10, 1546) when the goal was to suppress the senses and lust: the antipasto includes figs, walnuts, a lettuce salad and different types of fish. Lettuce was considered by all food treatises and health manuals as the anti-lust food *par excellence*.

16 Baldassar Pisanelli, *Trattato della natura de' cibi et del bere del Sig. Baldassare Pisanelli, Medico Bolognese. Nel quale non solo tutte le virtù, & i vitij di quelli minutamente si palesano; ma anco i rimedij per correggere i loro difetti* … . (Carmagnola, 1589).

17 As Ken Albala explains, "In Renaissance physiology, sexual appetite is directly linked to nutrition. Production of sperm is merely the last step of the entire digestive process, and it is generated directly from an[d] excess of nutritive material remaining after the body has been nourished." Ken Albala, *Eating Right in Renaissance Italy* (California, 2002), 144. See the entire discussion at 143–54.

18 "E pur finalmente qui dirò che sè pasto da veghij che hanno belle moglie." Michele Savonarola, *Libreto de tutte le cosse che se magnano: un'opera di dietetica del sec. xv*, ed. Jane Nystedt (Stockholm, 1988), 105.

19 The term *confetti* usually refers to sweets made with fruit, spices and cane sugar. See Sidney W. Mintz, *Sweetness and Power: The Place of Sugar in Modern History* (New York, 1986), 28–9 and Massimo Montanari, *Nuovo Convivio: Storia e Cultura dei piaceri della tavola nell'età moderna* (Rome, 1991), 107. In comedies it usually refers to a nut-shaped concoction with aphrodisiac properties.

20 "Per ungermi. Che l'ha tanta virtù, che farebbe rizzare un morto." Cornelio Lanci, *Ruchetta*, III, i, c. 46r. Rubs to help in impotence were already known in medieval medicine. See for example the recipe contained in the *herbarium* manuscript Aushburn 731 in the Biblioteca Medicea-Laurenziana in Florence (c. 1450): "Prendi un luccio ed estraigli la mascella inferiore: pestala bene e passala al setaccio. Con la composizione così ottenuta ungiti il pene, dopo averlo prima lavato con vino bianco in cui siano state bollite delle rose." Quoted in Salvatore Pezzella, *Gli erbari. I primi libri di medicina (le virtù curative delle piante)* (Perugia, 1993), 150.

21 "Per resuscitar la carne della brachetta." "La Cortigiana," in Pietro Aretino, *Tutte le Commedie*, ed. G.B. De Sanctis (Milan, 1994), II, vii, 147.

22 Valeria Finucci, *The Manly Masquerade. Masculinity, Paternity and Castration in the Italian Renaissance* (Durham, NC: 2003), 88.

23 "Impotente io? Oh voi mi farete ridere! Io non credo che sia el più ferrigno ed il più rubizzo uomo, in Firenze, di me." Translation from: Niccolò Machiavelli, "The Mandrake Root," *Five Comedies from the Italian Renaissance*, trans. and eds. Laura Giannetti and Guido Ruggiero (Baltimore, 2003), II, ii, 83.

24 For an informative and entertaining treatment of what early modern European and New World pharmacopoeia had to promote sexual vigor in aging men, see Valeria Finucci "There's the Rub: Searching for Sexual Remedies in the New World," *Journal of Medieval and Early Modern Studies* 38.3 (Fall 2008), 523–57. For a cultural history of masculinity and the male physical body that "historicizes and redefines" the pre-modern phallus, see the groundbreaking book by Patricia Simons, *The Sex of Men in Premodern Europe: A Cultural History* (Cambridge: Cambridge University Press, 2011).

25 Christopher Faraone, "Encolpius' Impotence and the Double Dose of Satyrion," in *The Ancient Novel: Classical Paradigms and Modern Perspectives*, J. Tatum and Gail M. Vernazza (eds.) (Hanover, NH, 1990), 114–16.

26 *Del Satirio erithronio. Cap. CXXXVIII*: "Tenuta la sua radice in mano provoca (secondo che dicono) al coito: ma molto piu bevendosi nel vino." *I Discorsi di M. Pietro Matthioli Sanese, Medico Cesareo, et del Serenissimo Principe Ferdinando Archiduca D'Austria & c. Nelli sei libri di Pedacio Dioscoride Anazarbeo della materia Medicinale. Hora di Nuovo dal suo istesso autore ricorretti, & in più di mille luoghi aumentati. Con le figure grandi tutte di nuovo rifatte, & tirate dalle naturali & vive piante, & animali, & in numero molto maggiore che le altre per avanti stampate*, vol. 3 (5 vols., Venice, 1568), 931.

27 "Nature endows everything with the form which is also the essence, and thus the form reveals the essence." Jane Bennett, *The Enchantment of Modern Life: Attachments, Crossings, and Ethics* (Princeton, NJ, 2001), 34–5.

28 "Taglia in pezzetti verga di lupo seccata al fumo et tiene in bocca un pezzetto e farà opera." *Secreti medicinali di M. Pietro Bairo da Turin, già medico di Carlo Secondo Duca di Savoia* (Venice, 1561).

29 Isabella Cortese, *I Secreti della Sign. Isabella Cortese. Ne' quali si contengono cose minerali, medicinali, arteficiose, e alchimistiche. Et molte de l' arte Profumatoria, appartenenti a ogni gran Signora. Con altri bellissimi segreti aggiunti* (Venice, 1588). See "A far drizzare il membro," 89.

30 A beautiful image of the *testiculus vulpis* plant is held in the Biblioteca Mediceo-Laurenziana in Florence: Ms. Cod. Aushb. 731 at c. 78r. The image is reproduced in Salvatore Pezzella, *Gli Erbari*.137. See also the entry "Santoreggia' in Pezzella, *Gli Erbari*, 58: "La Sanctoreggia è calda et seccha. Questa herba mangiata con pepe et con mele, meravigliosamente conmuove la luxuria." Florence, Biblioteca Marucelliana, MS. C/168: della virtù della sanctoreggia," f. 23 r.

31 *The Nuovo Receptario composto dal Famosissimo Chollegio degli Eximii Doctori Della Arte et Medicina Della Inclita Ciptà di Firenze* (1498) in http://www.pluteus.it (site accessed on 2.17.2012) ed. Olimpia Fittipaldi. See p. 69 (II.I. 2 Diasatyrion). The recipe appears in the group of "Lactovari Dolci."

32 The recipe is reproduced in: Jo Wheeler with the assistance of Katy Temple, *Renaissance Secrets: Recipes & Formulas* (London, 2009), 90–91. The manuscript "Questo libro e' di Stephano di maestro Romolo Rosselli, speziali all'insegnia di S.to Francesco in sul canto del gilio et di Franc.o et Vinc.io suo figlioli ... cominciato con il nome di Dio alli X di Agosto, il di' di S.to Lorenzo 1593 a Firenze," is held in Biblioteca Zayas, Seville, MS C-IV-15 [Private collection of Rodrigo de Zayas in Seville] and published in Stefano Francesco Di Romolo Rosselli, *Mes secrets: à Florence au temps des Médicis, 1593: pâtisserie, parfumerie, médecine*, ed. Rodrigo de Zayas (Paris, 1996). The two manuscripts in Florence precede this one. Thanks are due here to Jo Wheeler who provided me with the correct source for the recipe and information about Rosselli's manuscripts. On Stefano Rosselli and his apothecary shop in Florence see also *Making and Marketing Medicine*, eds. James Shaw and Evelyn Welch, 304–7.

33 For an example of the use of *morselletti*, see the essay by Molly Bourne in this volume, "Vincenzo Gonzaga and the Body Politic: Impotence and Virility at Court," chapter 2.

34 Rosselli Stephano, *Zibaldone di diversi segreti*, Biblioteca Marucelliana MS C.145, "Morselletti da eccitar Venere cap. LXXV." The term "astrologia' probably was a corruption of "aristolochia' an herb with curative properties. See the voice "aristolochia" in *Dizionario Botanico Italiano che comprende i nomi volgari italiani specialmente toscani e vernacoli delle piante raccolti da diversi autori e dalla gente di campgna col corrispondente latino botanico compilato dal dottore Ottaviano Targioni Tozzetti* (Florence, 1858, 2nd ed.), 24. The term "carpobalsamo" indicates the fruit/semen of the plant called "Balsamo." See the voice "Opobalsamo ossia balsamo della Mecka," in Luigi Castiglioni, *Storia delle piante forastiere. Le più importanti nell'uso medico, od economico*, ed. Luigi Saibene (Milan, 2008), 359–66.

35 "I Testicoli delle Volpi sono quelle radici bulbose, chiamate volgarmente Satirij, detti così, perche credono alcuni, che fussero state ritrovate, e poi usate dai Satiri, acciò se gl'accendesse più la libidine, mentre seguitavano le Ninfe per la selva. Alcuni poi più sensatamente dicono, chiamarsi queste radici Satirij, perche fanno erigere la verga virile, e tale erezzione da Greci è chiamata *Satyriasis*." *Teatro farmaceutico dogmatico e spagirico del dottor Giuseppe Donzelli, Napoletano, Barone di Dogliola* (Naples, 1726), 20 r. The work was first published in Venice in 1681.

36 Raymond Waddington explains that in the sixteenth century there was "a false etymology deriving *satire* from *satyr*." Thus it was commonly held that the literary genre of *satire* came from the satyr plays, while the word *satire* derives from the Latin adjective *sàtura* [full]. The wrong identification was corrected in the 17th century in the work of Isaac Casaubon, *De Satyrica Graecorum Poesi & Romanorum Satira* (1605); see Raymond Waddington, Aretino's *Satyr. Sexuality, Satire, and Self-Projection in Sixteenth-Century Literature and Art* (Toronto, 2004), 94–9. According to Carlo Battisti and Giovanni Alessio, *Dizionario Etimologico Italiano* (Florence, 1968) the words "satìrio," "satirióne" and "sàtiro" indicate respectively: 1) a tonic drink based on the root of

satìrio, 2) the plant "testiculus vulpis" (*himantoglossum hircinum*) whose root is good to excite libido, which is also a kind of orchid called *giglio di prato* 3) a lascivious person. Salvatore Battaglia, *Grande Dizionario della lingua italiana* (Turin, 1961–) indicates for *satirióne* 1) an orchid plant with attributed aphrodisiacal properties, 2) a poisonous mushroom (*phallus impudicus* today called *Satirione*). A beautiful image of the *phallus impudicus* mushroom—also called *fungus priapeius*—appears in the *acquerello* series by Ulisse Aldovrandi housed at the University of Bologna, AMS Historica, *Collezione digitale di opere storiche*.

37 Quoted in Sara Matthews-Grieco, "Satyr and Sausages: Erotic Strategies and the Print Market in Cinquecento Italy," in *Erotic Cultures*, ed. Sara Matthews-Grieco, 19–60 at 28. On the uses of the satyrion root in the Greco-Roman period see Christopher A. Faraone, *Ancient Greek Love Magic* (Cambridge, 1999), 19–21. Dioscorides and Pliny both cite the plant satyrion.

38 Particularly fashionable were artistic engravings representing episodes of pagan mythology in morality prints and emblem books, such as Andrea Alciato's *Diverse Imprese* (1551) where *Lussuria* is symbolized by the goat-legged satyr. See Sara Matthews-Grieco, "Satyr and Sausages," p. 31. Small bronze satyrs were kept in private spaces such as a scholar's study: especially famous were the couple of *Satyr and Satyress* made by Padua bronze artist Andrea Briosco (c. 1470–1532). See Jeremy Warren, "Bronzes," in *At Home in Renaissance Italy*, eds. Marta Ajmar-Wollheim and Flora Dennis (London, 2006), 294–306 at 303–4. Pietro Aretino even commissioned a number of portrait medals of himself tellingly with a satyr image on the reverse "announcing his intertwined sexuality and identity as a satirist." Raymond Waddington, *Aretino's Satyr*, "Introduction," xix. The satyr scenes became a classic in Italian and English pastoral plays towards the end of the 16th century. See Meredith Kennedy Ray, "*La castità conquistata*: The Function of the Satyr in Pastoral Drama," in *Romance Languages Annual* 9 (1998): 312–21, on the role of the satyr in the most important pastoral plays of the period. The satyrs' episodes are particularly interesting in two works by female writers: Isabella Andreini's *Mirtilla* (1588) and Valeria Miani's *Amorosa speranza* (1604). Julie D. Campbell explains how "Andreini takes liberties with the traditional theatergram" (i.e. of the satyr); see Julie D. Campbell, "Introduction," in *Isabella Andreini La Mirtilla: A Pastoral*, translated with an Introduction by Julie D. Campbell (Tempe, AZ, 2002), xix. See also Maria Galli Stampino, "Pastoral Constraints, Textual and Dramatic Strategies: Isabella Andreini's *La Mirtilla* and Torquato Tasso's *Aminta*," in *Italian Culture* 22 (2004): 1–20. In the later *Amorosa speranza* by Miani the nymph takes revenge on the satyr: see Katie Rees, "Female-Authored Drama in Early Modern Padua," *Italian Studies* 63.1 (Spring 2008): 41–61, especially 50–51. Virginia Cox notes that "Miani's emphasis on the satyr's advanced age brings her version close, as well, to the classic comedic stereotype of the humiliation of the *senex* who presumes to fall in love." Virginia Cox, *The Prodigious Muse*: *Women's Writing in Counter-Reformation Italy* (Baltimore, 2011), 113. On the satyr *topos* in Renaissance art and culture, see also: Lynn Frier Kaufmann, *The Noble Savage: Satyrs and Satyr Families in Renaissance Art* (Ann Arbor, MI, 1984); Julia Szirmai, *La syrinx au bucher. Pan et les satyres a la renaissance et a l'age baroque* (Geneva, 2005).

39 See *Satirioni, & Testicoli di cane, & loro essame*. "Errore di molti: errano veramente à i tempi nostri la maggior parte de i medici, & degli spetiali, togliendo communemente per il Satirione amendue i testicoli di cane. Imperoche le spetie de i Satirioni scritti da Dioscoride sono assai diverse nelle fattezze loro da i Testicoli di cane" in *I Discorsi di M. Pietro Matthioli Sanese*, vol. 3, 932.

40 "Questa presente conserva, ò condito che ne vogliam dire, ho io molte volte veduto preparare in Venetia in diverse spetiarie; ma in luogo di questo Satirione ho veduto che sempre pigliano le radici amendue di quell'herba chiamata testicolo di cane." *La fabrica de gli spetiali, partita in xii distintioni. Nuovamente composta dall'Eccellente Medico e Filosofo Prospero Borgarucci* (Venice, 1566), c. 16.

41 "Usasi per le cose veneree la radice piu alta, e piena, perche la piu bassa, la quale è grinza, dicono che fa contrario effetto." *La fabrica de gli spetiali*, c. 17.

42 "Chi ben considera tutte le cose che entrano in questa presente compositione, di necessità potrà conoscere ella dover operare tutto quello che dice Mesué. Et quantunque alcuna cosa vi sia, che con fattica si possa ritrovare, e conservare: non di meno è da credere per fermo che componendola si possa vedere di mirabili effetti." "Discorso del Borgarucci nel secondo Diasatirione' in *La fabrica de gli spetiali*, c. 28.

43 Giovanni Marinello, *Le Medicine Partenenti alle infermità delle Donne. Scritte per M. Giovanni Marinello. Divise in Tre Libri* (Venice, 1574), vol. I, cap. X.

44 For examples of such arguments in legal cases in 16th-century Venice see: Joanne M. Ferraro, *Marriage Wars in Late Renaissance Venice* (New York: 2001), ch. 3, "Bedtime Stories."

45 Ken Albala summarizes the types of food that were commonly held to be aphrodisiacs in medical and culinary treatises of the time: heating foods "which helps the circulation of blood and eventually the production and delivery of sperm" (examples: leeks, garlic, oysters, chickpeas, turnips, truffles, cloves, almonds, partridges), anything salty, "windy foods that cause flatulence" (carrots, parsnips, arugula), etc. Ken Albala, *Eating Right*, 146–50.

46 "Ai vecchi debili si vede giovare sommamente il seguente, ove si ripongono quattro oncie di seme di ruchetta, e una di pepe in polvere, e con melle (honey) spumato l'accompagnano meschiando bene. Si fanno etiandio alcune nociuole artificialmente: le quali hanno grandissima virtù di accendere ad amore carnale. E il modo è questo. Togliensi ben trenta cervelli di passeri, e anche più, e meno secondo il piacere di colui, che ne vorrà, et dimeninsigli con diligenza in alcuna scutella capace. Appresso prendesi altrotanta quantità di quello sevo di becco subito ammazzato, che sta d'intorno alle reni, et ben netto meschiasi co' cervelli, e poi amendue frigansi insieme in alcuna patella. Quindi tratti con melle spumato facciasi cuocere tanto, che s'induriscano come uno elettuario, di che facciansene piccole palle, quali sono le nociuole, di queste avanti che l'huomo vada in letto, ne mastichi una: e conoscerà quanto beneficio recano a chi le usa." See Giovanni Marinello, *Le Medicine*, c. 31r–v. Often Marinello feels the need in his work to reassure his readers especially women (to whom the book is dedicated), that his recipes had marvelous effects on old men even if in some cases they tasted bad (c. 33r.). In a book of secrets that claims to be a compilation of Falloppio's medicinal recipes, after giving a list of remedies "a far lussuriare oltra modo" the author [probably Borgaruccio who wrote the "Introduction'] affirms: "che vederai veramente miracolo tu buon vecchietto o giovane galante innamorato." *Secreti diversi, e miracolosi raccolti dal Faloppia e approbati da altri medici di gran fama. Nuovamente ristampati e a commun beneficio di ciascuno, distinti in tre libri* (Venice, 1620), 120–21.

47 "Se il non poter usare con donna, viene da poco desiderio e da non sentire stimolo della carne, egli è di bisogno confortare il corpo e l'animo con allegrezza, diletto, esercitio temperato e simili cose di poi mangiare vivande, che facciano grasso, e che sono facili ad essere digerite brodi di gallina." Giovanni Marinello, *Le Medicine*, at c. 23r.

48 "Circa il seme del bulbo vi è grande lite perche non essendo stata descritta dalli Antichi la sua effigie, non si può affermare niente di certo, tanto più che ora non usiamo mangiare altri bulbi, che le cipolle, li porri, le scalogne." A *lettovaro* based on these bulbs is warm and windy, increases the strength for coitum and it is good to old men who are married. See *Antidotario Romano Latino e Volgare, tradotto da Ippolito Ceccarelli. Li Ragionamenti, e le aggiunte dell'Elettione de' Semplici, e Prattica delle Compositioni. Con le annotazioni del Signore Pietro Castelli Romano e trattati della Teriaca romana e della teriaca Egittia* (Rome, 1668), c. 44r.

49 In the comedy *Fabritia* by Lodovico Dolce, the parasite Melindo, thanking a friend for an excellent lunch, quotes Platina: "Io non credo che Carlo Magno né il Soldano facesse mai convito così bravo e così stupendo, come è stato il desinare che m'havete dato oggi in casa vostra e se la cena di questa sera si conformerà seco, infino ad hora io la frego a Platina e a Cinciglione." III, i, c. 25v.

50 Bernardo Dovizi da Bibbiena, "La Calandra," in *Five Comedies*, eds. Laura Giannetti and Guido Ruggiero, I, ii, 10.

51 Tracanna: "Voi vi siete mal informato, perdonatemi, elle non conferiscono al vostro stomaco: perche sono troppo fredde e di troppo tarda digestione. [...] L'ostreghe fanno a i giovani muovere l'appetito e a i vecchi tirar coreze." *Fortunio Comedia Nuova*, I, x, c. 19r. In *Anconitana* by Ruzante there is a marked class difference between what the old master and the young servant will eat to prepare for their amorous adventures in Arquà. Messer Tomao recurs to a *confetto*, pine nuts and expensive spices whose names are twisted to comic effect (such as "mostachi, morlachi" not a food in itself, but a name recalling that of a eastern population—Morlacchi—presumably like an exotic spice, and whose sound was similar to the word "pistacchi"). The servant Ruzante more modestly had cheese crusts, bread and wine. "Oh, sea laldò Dio! Andarón pur stasera tuti a Arquà. El vegio no arà magnò indarno el confeto e i pignuoli arpigiè, né de qui che ven d'oltra mare, mostachi, morlachi, che fa bona forza. Gniam mi a' n'arè magnò indarno le croste de formaio salò, né qui tri pan tanto fati, né bevú indarno de quel vin, che ha una vena de reçento, che Mare Biata!" Ruzante (Angelo Beolco) *L'Anconitana*, in *Ruzante Teatro*, ed. Ludovico Zorzi (Turin, 1967), V, iv, 773–881 at 875.

52 Garbino responds with a technical explanation to Crispo: "Dalla ventositate che havete in corpo: essendo la proprietà del seleno di farla à vecchi, essalare par di sotto." *Li vani amori*, IV, iv, c. 91r.

53 "Voglio dopo fatta la spesa entrare in casa per la porta del giardino e stare in aguato per vederlo trangugiare i recipe creduti da lui poter resuscitare i morti." Ibid.

54 Spinello: "All'hora fui io per ridere: e fu bella inventione darli innanzi pasto quel lattovaro, con dirli ch'era composto del pomo della gioventù venuto di Calicut." Francesco Mercati da Bibbiena, *Il Lanzi* , III, iv. The comedy is studied and entirely reproduced in Erica Lynn Westhoff, *"Il Sensale," "Il Lanzi," "L'Imbroglia": Reconsidering Renaissance Comedy through the Plays of Francesco Mercati* (PhD Diss., UCLA, 2010). See 327.

55 "Che giovano a me le sue medecine e che resusciti i morti, se non fa risuscitar le sue membra che son più morte della morte stessa? Che né per losinghe, onzioni e carezze che gli si faccino, ponno resuscitare." Giovan Battista della Porta, "La Furiosa," in Giovan Battista della Porta, *Teatro Quarto tomo-Commedie*, ed. Raffaele Sirri. (Naples, 2003), I, iii, 115 [101–70].

56 "I boriosi e volenterosi, sperando nel pevere, nei tratufi, nei cardi e in certi lattovari calidi che vengono di Francia, ne fanno maggiori scorpacciate che i contadini de l'uva; e inghiottendo l'ostrighe senza masticarle, vorrebber pur far miracoli. A così fatte cene puoi tu manicare quasi senza cerimonie." Pietro Aretino, *Ragionamento-Dialogo*, ed. Carla Forno (Milan, 1988), 319.

57 "né per tartufi, né per carcioffi, né per lattovari potè mai drizzare il palo, e se pur l'alzava un poco, tosto ricadeva giuso." Ibid., 261.

58 "Un vecchio Lombardo per disperazione intuona il Magnificat, giudicandolo buon rimedio per la sua impotenza." Novella viii in *Tutte le Novelle, Lo Stufaiolo Commedia e La Mula e La Chiave Dicerie di Antonfrancesco Doni* (Milan, 1863), 22–3.

59 "... Voi dovete sapere' disse il vecchio 'ch'io ho provato tutt'i modi e usato tutte le vie ché costui si levi in piedi (accennando dove bisognava) e si cavi la berretta, facendo honore a me e alla sua sposa; e non v'è stato ordine. Ho ultimamente veduto a' vespri della mia parrocchia, quando si tocca i tasti dell'organo, e che si canta il *Magnificat* che ognuno si rizza; onde io voleva provar questo rimedio ancora (poiché non m'erano giovati gli altri) per vedere se costui si voleva rizzare con questo mezzo." Ibid.

60 This topic has been studied in details by Anthony Ellis, *Old Age, Masculinity, and Early Modern Drama. Comic Elders on the Italian and Shakespearean Stage* (Burlington, VT, 2009), especially at 70–72 and 133–5.

61 Carol V. Kaske and John R. Clark, eds. *Marsilio Ficino Three Books on Life. A Critical Edition and Translation with Introduction and Notes* (Tempe: AZ, 1998, 1st ed. 1989). See II, viii, "The Diet, Mode of Life, and Medicine of the Elderly": "Those who have already completed their forty-ninth year and are nearing their fiftieth, should reflect that young people are signified by Venus, while old people are signified by Saturn, and that according to astronomers these stars are the most hostile of all to each other. Therefore those saturnine people should avoid the Venereal act, which takes away most of the life even of people who are young. For she takes no thought for things already born, but for those about to be born, and even dries up the green plants as soon as they have produced seed" (189). The idea was that sex in the aged was dangerous because it used up their (declining) heat and moisture, and damaged moist organs such as the brain and the eyes; see Ken Albala, *Eating Right*, 144–5.

62 See "Venere nuocere a' vecchi e non giovare a giovani," in *Lodovico Guicciardini, L'ore di ricreazione*, ed. Anne-Marie Van Passen (Rome, 1990), 283. Quoted in Anthony Ellis, *Old Age*, 71. Gabriele Paleotto, *Libro del bene della vecchiezza*, trans. M. F. Pietro da Piombino Agostinaio (Rome, 1597), 107–8.

63 Ambrogio: "In fatti chi ha "l fuoco dentro, bisogna che ne mandi fuori il fumo." "Assiuolo," in *Commedie del Cinquecento*, ed. Nino Borsellino, II, I, 141. Filippo: "Lo innamorarsi viene da gentilezza di cuore e da caldezza di sangue." *La stiava comedia di Gio. Maria Cecchi Fiorentino* (Venice, 1550), I, v, c. 8v.

64 Lippo: "A noi vecchi interviene el medesimo che succede delle legne di quercia vecchia che si logorano, e si consumano a poco, a poco, facendo un fuoco tanto stentato, che non ne gode persona; e le giovani s'accendono subito, e fanno un fuoco che tutta la brigata se ne rallegra e se ne riscalda." *Olivetta Commedia. Del Sig. Cavaliere Cornelio Lanci* (Florence: 1587), I, iii, c. 24–5.

65 Teodoro: "Oh questa è bene la più nuova cosa che si sentisse mai! Chi sarebbe mai quello che la credesse, che uno vecchio di sessant'anni s'innamorasse? E pure è vera; ed io sono quel desso che ne veggo l'esperienza." Donato Giannotti, "Il vecchio amoroso," II, ii, 24.

66 Ricciardo: "Horamai io ho presso che i miei settanta, e sempre mi son fatto beffe di riguardarmi e mangio d'ogni cosa, e anche di quell'altra faccenda ho fatto sempre quello che mi è venuto voglia." Antonio Landi, *Il commodo* (Florence, 1566), IV, no scene, c. 66.

67 "Altri me dise può che me dieba destiore, e che oramai el sol va al monte, e che'el me manca la vertue diritiva, premitiva e sustentativa," in Andrea Calmo *Il Saltuzza*, ed. Luca D'Onghia (Padua, 2006), I, iii, 57. As the editor explains in n. 34, the Latinate adjectives are derived from verbs such as "drizzare, premere e sostenere" that suggest the sexual act. Obviously Calmo is poking fun at Melindo who claims to be sexually potent but a little later admits openly his impotence: "Poh! Che so-io mi? E' son vegnuo de pallazzo e intra una cosa e l'altra e' son tanto storno, che no posso tegnir la testa su." I, iii, 62.

68 "Nevertheless, it is difficult for old men as it is for those at the other stages of life to curb the use of sex since, as they say, sobriety vanishes when the check rein is removed. So it is with this act because of the great delight it produces." See Ch. XVIII, "Permission and Prohibition of Sex in the Resumptive Regimen," in Gabriele Zerbi, *Gerontocomia: On the Care of the Aged and Maximianus, Elegies on Old Age and Love*, trans. L. R. Lind (Philadelphia, PA,1988), 274–5.

69 "... si farà una minestra di pan fresco e di chiari d'ovi mal cotti, la qual sia ridotta a forma di latte e la pigliarà per tre o quattro giorni ogni mattina e sera inanzi pasto, né credo che si possa trovar cosa più al proposito in questo caso, se bene alcuni lodano gli piccioni co'l vino rosso e con specie, alcuni il latte di pignoli, alcuni gli stinchi, altri le passere, altri quella specie di fonghi che si chiama

Bulbo, e altri il confetto chiamato diasatirion." Alessandro Petronio, *Del viver delli Romani et di conservar la sanità. Libri cinque. Tradotti dalla lingua latina nella volgare, dall'eccellente medico M. Basilio Paravicino de Como* (Rome, 1592), 340–41. Originally published in latin as *Mensa Romana* (1581). Quoted in Piero Camporesi, *I balsami di Venere* (Milan, 1989), 27–8.

70 "Che cosa sia il non poter usare carnalmente con donna, coloro il sanno troppo bene, che il provano, ò ne lo hanno provato." "Le cagioni, i segni e la cura di quegli che sono debili, e impotenti al generare" in Giovanni Marinello, *Le medicine*, c. 19v.

71 "La lussuria in ogni età è brutta ma ne' vecchi quanto più può è scellerata, abominevole e bruttissima," in *Della vita civile Trattato di Matteo Palmieri cittadino fiorentino* (Milan, 1825), II, 127.

72 Introduction in Laura Giannetti, *Lelia's Kiss: Imagining Gender, Sex and Marriage in Italian Renaissance Comedy* (Toronto, 2009), 10.

73 The most famous example is perhaps the young Lucretia married to Messer Nicia in *Mandragola*; see also Oretta married to old Messer Ambrogio in *Assiuolo* by Giovan Maria Cecchi. Examples of unsuccessful attempts to marry young daughters to old men are present in comedies such as *Ingannati, Il ragazzo, La sporta*: see Laura Giannetti, *Lelia's Kiss*, 217.

74 The theme is developed by Anthony Ellis in *Old Age, Masculinity and Early Modern Drama* chapters 3 and 4, with the study of a group of comedies (written and staged in Florence and Venice) where the generational and political conflict between the foolish old men in love and their young sons or other young males is particularly relevant. Linda Carroll, in a series of fundamental studies dedicated to gender and drama in Venice at the beginning of the 16th century, has shown how masculine and patriarchal power at that time was in a position of weakness and difficulty [Linda Carroll, "Who's on top? Gender as Societal Power Configuration in Italian Renaissance Painting and Drama," *The Sixteenth Century Journal* 20 (1989): 531–58.] In a more recent study on the social identity of Venetians she uses the figure of the mask Pantaloon to signify the decline of Venice in this period. "Pantaloon is comical, even farcical, an image of the lecherous old age given over to its still-youthful appetites. That image of age is very different from an image of the wise elder judiciously husbanding the resources of his state. Buttock-baring youths flirting with dominant foreign powers, libidinous old men who never quite grew up. These are the icons of Venice in its decline." See Linda Carroll, "Money, Age, and Marriage in Venice: A Brief Biocultural History," in *Politics and Culture*, Issue 1 (2010). http://www.politicsandculture.org/2010/04/29/money-age-and-marriage-in venice-a-brief-biocultural-history/.

75 Laura Giannetti, *Lelia's Kiss*, 144.

76 Laura Giannetti, *Lelia's Kiss*, 142–52.

6

Impotence and Corruption: Sexual Function and Dysfunction in Early Modern Italian Books of Secrets

Meredith K. Ray

The early modern compilations of recipes concerning alchemy, medicine, cosmetics, perfumery and household management known as *libri di segreti*, or books of secrets, flourished amid the culture of empiricism that took root in 16th-century Italy. Despite the claims to privileged knowledge put forth by their titles, these vernacular works—unlike their more arcane Latin predecessors—were accessible and pragmatic manuals, spilling "secrets" to a wider, non-specialist audience of early modern men and women even as they promoted the exclusivity of their contents. Whether offering recipes for conducting true alchemical experiments (such as producing alchemical gold) or proposing formulas for skin creams and medicines, books of secrets emphasized practice over theory, extolled the virtues of trial and error, and prized efficacy above all else.[1]

With their expansive catalogues of remedies for ailments ranging from rashes, worms and rotting teeth to sciatica, epilepsy and cancer, books of secrets offer rich territory for exploring a variety of early modern concerns about the body, including a myriad of problems related to reproductive health and sexual function. Their contents reflect the vast array of medical conditions for which the early modern public sought advice, the kinds of approaches that were proposed as preventive or curative therapies, and many of the underlying tensions around the body and its functions that pervaded Renaissance culture.[2] Scholarship by William Eamon, Elaine Leong, Alisha Rankin and others has been instrumental in investigating many facets of these texts.[3] However, the specific place and role of sexual health and behavior, which figure prominently in books of secrets, remains to be fully examined. This essay draws from a selection of early modern books of secrets, focusing particularly on a manuscript attributed to Caterina Sforza (1463–1509), the charismatic ruler of Imola and Forlì, to examine the physiological aspects of sexual function described in such works as well as the attendant cultural concerns raised by questions of sexual performance. The primary focus of this essay will be to address the problems that are most frequently dealt with in relation to each of the sexes: specifically, female virginity and its opposite, "corruption," and male virility and impotency. What do book of secrets suggest about early modern notions of gender and sexuality? How do the mechanics of sexuality—male and female—intersect with fears about issues such as adultery and, especially, cuckoldry? Finally, how are medical approaches to sexual function influenced by the alchemical practices that pervade the pages of early modern books of secrets?

Books of Secrets and Matters of Sex

Sexual activity, as Patricia Simons notes, was a "medicalized topic" in the early modern period, with coitus belonging to the list of "non-naturals," or external elements (such as air, exercise, food and sleep) that could have potentially harmful or beneficial effects on bodily health.[4] A rich history of both learned and popular medical writing—ranging from medieval adaptations of ancient works such as the Arabic *Tacuinum Sanitatis* to the Pseudo-Albertus Magnus's *De Secretis Mulierum*—laid the groundwork for early modern approaches to sexuality and reproduction.[5] Some works, such as the 12th-century compendium known as the *Trotula*, took a more clinical tack toward matters of sex, while others—including the influential *De secretis*—were infused with a censorious approach to sexuality, particularly in regard to women.[6] The question of biological sexual function and its role in the marital union would continue to develop well into the seventeenth century in marriage manuals such as Nicolas Venette's popular *Tableau de l'amour conjugal* (1686) and *Aristotele's Masterpiece* (1684).[7] As Giuseppe Palmero points out, an enormous variety of works dealing with medical matters, including problems relating to sexual and reproductive health, circulated in the late medieval and early Renaissance periods in both manuscript and print.[8] From this "cultural crucible" emerged widely-circulated works such as the *Secreti di don Alessio Piemontese* (*Secrets of Alexis of Piedmont*, 1555), which inaugurated the "golden age" of the *libri di segreti* in print, and Pietro Bairo's *Secreti medicinali (Medicinal Secrets*, 1561), both of which devoted entire sections to male and female sexual biology and practice.[9] Similarly, manuscript collections of recipes compiled for private use, including Sforza's collection of *Experimenti* (*Experiments*), also paid careful attention to questions of sex.[10] Chief among the concerns that emerge in such texts are, for women, problems related to virginity (especially ascertaining its presence or absence), issues pertaining to conception and fertility and sexual pleasure and sexual attractiveness. For men, sexual potency (or lack thereof) takes primary stage, along with sexual health complications such as venereal disease, both of which constituted sources of deep and widespread anxiety in early modern Europe.[11] Underlying the discussion of male and female sexual matters was a continual tension between the practical (and sometimes not so practical) therapeutic advice offered to the reader and an implicit cultural anxiety relative to the social regulation of sexuality, especially in the case of women. This anxiety is directed above all toward the specter of cuckoldry. Considered to be an almost inevitable consequence of sexual (dys)function on the part of husbands, the automatic association between impotence and cuckoldry appears at all levels of society, and is explored in depth by the other studies in this volume.

In framing instructions for rectifying sexual and reproductive problems, books of secrets turn to the pervasive language and imagery of alchemy, both in their assessment of the intertwined nature of all things and in their assumption that substances (and bodies) may, as a result, be manipulated and transformed through practical experiment. As Jonathan Hughes notes, the broader "flowering of alchemical medicine" in the early modern period centered on sexual and reproductive functions "in a specific, medical, biological way."[12] The preparation of ingredients for recipes related to coitus and procreation thus relies heavily on alchemical techniques such as distillation and multiplication, while the twinned alchemical principles of simulation and transformation subtend the goals of treatment.[13] Such alchemical notions were central to both learned and popular medical advice literature in the early modern period. Books of secrets capitalized on their familiarity and on their promise of efficacy, enticing readers with formulas for transformation (of lead into gold, or flagging virility into performative potency) and providing instructions for simulation (an imitation of gold, or of virginity). Recipes treating matters of sex—from proving female purity to managing male performance—are thus dependent, like all alchemical recipes, on the notion of simulating a natural state that is not present or transforming the body through the use of natural ingredients (such as foods, herbs, minerals) and alchemical operations. Such recipes promise not simply to demonstrate virginity, but to feign it where it is lacking, in order both to guarantee the market value of a promised bride and secure a conjugal contract predicated on female virtue. The "secret" formulas promise not merely to enhance male sexual potency, but to counterfeit an increased degree of physical endowment that will ensure a female partner's devotion and transform an unstable intimate bond into a stable and faithful union. The 16th-century fascination with practical (as opposed to philosophical) alchemical principles thus spills over into the physical territory of the body and of sexual function, as well as into the cultural conventions and social arena of marriage.[14]

Recipes for ameliorating problems related to sexual health and facilitating conception and childbirth were by no means confined to the pages of books of secrets. Advice about such matters proliferated in a variety of medical self-help literature, from the *De Secretis Mulierum* to vernacular publications including Giovanni Marinello's *Le medicine pertinenti alle infermità delle donne* (1574), [Giovanni] Michele Savonarola's *Libro della natura e virtù delle cose* (1575), Nicholas Culpepper's *Directory for Midwives* (1661) and Venette's *Tableau de l'amour conjugale* (1686). Like all manuals in this period that deal with sexuality and procreation, books of secrets similarly promoted and reinforced the heterosexual (and marital) partnership,[15] while the socially sanctioned goal of sexual intercourse remained, predictably, that of generation.[16] As Castor Durante cautioned in his *Tesoro della sanità* (1588), a reference manual of foods and herbs and their various salutiferous effects: "The object of lovemaking must be the generation of children with the wife who is joined to you in holy matrimony."[17] Echoing a commonly voiced opinion, Durante added that even marital sex must be "practiced in moderation."[18] While limited sexual activity could be considered necessary for health, intercourse should be regulated and practiced within the marital bond, not outside of it.

In offering remedies for forms of sexual dysfunction ranging from a lack or excess of libido—male and female—to problems of infertility and impotence, books of secrets sought to create healthy bodies and enhance salubrious sexual practice, but also to ensure that the heterosexual union would produce children. These practical medical handbooks thus faithfully reflect the cultural norms and gender constructs of their era. At the same time, when addressing the physiology of the gendered body and questions of sexual performance, the *libri di segreti* medicalize rather than moralize sexual behavior. Problematic scenarios such as infidelity, impotence and cuckoldry constitute a specific type of "medical" problem to be treated through the recipes provided.

Female Virginity

Determining the state of a woman's reproductive status occupies a central place in books of secrets, both private and published. Recipes found in printed works as well as in manuscript collections center on determining when a woman is fertile and, if she cannot conceive, discovering whether the problem lies with her or her partner. As Katharine Park has noted, the interior, hidden nature of the female reproductive system conferred upon it a status of particular mystery among medieval and early modern physicians and medical writers, complicating and frustrating attempts to understand and explain its workings.[19] Accordingly, recipes relating to female reproductive biology seek to establish techniques for an external verification of an internal condition, for the uterus's concealed position inside the body meant that "its state and contents could be inferred only indirectly, through the woman's testimony or through external signs."[20] A common method to determine whether or not a woman is fertile instructs her to urinate over a mallow plant. If the mallow deteriorates over a period of three days, she can conceive. Such information could be useful to either achieve or avoid pregnancy, depending on the circumstance.[21] Similarly, the integrity of a woman's virginity could be ascertained by external signs. Many recipes suggest that the woman drink sal ammoniac [ammonium chloride] with water, a mixture often used as a mild diuretic. Since the urinary and reproductive systems were considered to be one, a compromised hymen would cause fluid to move more quickly through the body,[22] whereas, according to more than one 16th-century manuscript: "if she is a virgin [the mixture] will have no effect."[23]

This recipe to determine virginity, which has numerous antecedents in medieval medical treatises,[24] also appears in the manuscript compiled by Caterina Sforza (1463–1509). Best known for her regency of Imola and Forlí after the assassination of her first husband, Girolamo Riario, Caterina Sforza was also keenly interested in collecting alchemical, medical and cosmetic secrets.[25] Her *Experimenti,* a collection of over three hundred such recipes and formulas, has been characterized as "the most complete and important document" of its kind for the early sixteenth century.[26] It offers a valuable opportunity to examine connections between the kinds of remedies that circulated in printed books of secrets and those that were collected privately; and, especially, to consider the kinds of recipes that women compiled for personal use or interest. In fact, Sforza's *Experimenti* bears close resemblance to many of its manuscript and published counterparts, suggesting that *libri di segreti* indeed acted as vehicles for a shared culture of popular medical practice, variously transmitted by word of mouth, by manuscript collations and by printed works that responded to a market demand for this type of self-help literature. In the *Experimenti,* Caterina Sforza, like the authors of many such compendiums, also suggests the use of sal ammoniac to assess virginity:

> How to tell if a woman is a virgin, or rather corrupt. Take sal ammoniac and dissolve in water and give it to drink to whoever you wish. If she is a virgin, it will have no effect; if she has been corrupted, she will urinate immediately.[27]

The action of the mineral salts upon the body, once ingested, serves to create an external demonstration of what cannot otherwise be easily observed or proven without a physical examination.

The language of such entries on virginity seems at first to reflect prevailing early modern moral prescriptives regarding female sexuality. Women's bodies are either virginal (intact and pure) or corrupt (penetrated and despoiled), and it is essential to have a noninvasive means by which to confirm their state. In addition to its regular appearance in medical treatises, the virginity test for women is a common literary motif, and usually centered upon the same basic ingredients and processes.[28] The rationale for a virginity test, however, could be pragmatic as well as moral. As Kathleen Coyne Kelly points out in a study of medieval practices, such examinations could constitute proof not just of a woman's virginity, but of a partner's impotence, thereby providing grounds for divorce.[29] An unconsummated union could also have a significant impact on issues such as inheritance and paternity. Perhaps not surprisingly, given the high stakes attendant on the results of such "tests," Sforza and the compilers of other similar collections often seem to be as interested in demonstrating how to simulate virginity as in how to ascertain its actual presence.

Indeed, Sforza's collection includes several recipes that detail methods for counterfeiting virginity. Because her collection, like most books of secrets, lacks a clear narrative framework and voice, there is no explicit explanation as to the purpose of these recipes. It is the result that counts, and the instructions include assurances as to the degree of their effectiveness. Recipes for simulating virginity rely closely, as noted earlier, on the ingredients and procedures common to alchemical experiment and are steeped in the notion of simulation and transformation. The simplest of Sforza's recipes, for example, calls for distilling sage and water in an alembic, a basic transformative stage of the alchemical process. Applying the resulting mixture to the vagina over a period of time will return the woman's organ to its virginal state: a "true and marvelous" recipe (*verissima a maraviglia*).[30] Another, more complicated, recipe includes more than 10 ingredients and calls for a preparation (again based on heating and distilling) that requires more than two weeks to complete; it promises results that the user herself cannot fail to realize: "[…] you will see that thing become so narrow [tight] that you yourself will be in admiration" (*tu vederai quella cosa cusí stretta devenir che tu medesima ne admiraraj*).[31] A pessary of pulverized carnations in wine promises to achieve the same results for women or girls, of any age, who have been "corrupted," so they can return to the state of "the most natural and perfect virgin" (*A fare che una donna o putta de che età se voglia essendo conrupta demonstrarà naturalissima vergine expertum*).[32]

Attention to simulating or "restoring" virginity is common among the pages of early modern books of secrets. In Sforza's case, however, the emphasis assumes additional valence. As a military leader who knew the importance of crafting a public persona, an alchemist who sought not to produce gold but rather to create metals that had the appearance of gold, and a woman who exploited the transformative power of cosmetics on female beauty, Sforza's understanding of the power of simulation was pragmatic and extensive. As Joyce de Vries writes, "Caterina was fully aware that the visual world—encompassing not only art but also spectacle and performance—offered a significant means to exercise power in the princely courts."[33] Describing the careful attention Sforza lavished on her person and on her court, de Vries persuasively argues that Sforza was entirely cognizant of the fact that "… carefully chosen words, deeds, and appearances could nuance or even improve one's position."[34] Certainly, like many figures of her day, Sforza understood that "seeming" was as important as "being."[35] Even in her recipes for producing alchemical gold, Sforza is clear that the most important aspect of the operation is to produce a convincing counterfeit, and specifies that the practitioner should not be deterred by any pangs of conscience at the fraud.[36] Likewise, it is not the actual condition of being a virgin that is important in her *Experimenti*, but rather the practical and convincing imitation of that culturally privileged state. Because virginity itself functions as a commodity that bears value in a circuit of exchange, the manufacture (or counterfeit) of coinage and that of sexual purity are implicitly, and importantly, linked.[37]

Male Performance

Sforza's appreciation of the virtues of simulation are applied not only to recipes for determining or feigning female virginity, but also applied to matters concerning the male body. Although the question of male virginity is virtually nonexistent in Sforza's text (unsurprisingly, given that it did not carry the cultural weight of female virginity), the problem of male potency (or rather, impotency) is very present. Sforza's recipes for reversing impotence propose to combat "that natural defect, whereby a man [or person] is unable to perform with a woman" (*el difecto de natura, in alcuno homo o persona non posente usare cum femina*).[38] To this end, the *Experimenti* offer formulas for simulating or increasing potency, and improving both sexual attractiveness and sexual performance. Various recipes to increase the size of the male member (*ad magnificandum virgam*) assure results that far surpass that organ's natural state in all dimensions (*Modus procedendi ut addatur in longitudine et grossitudine virge ultra misuram naturalem*), or promise a long-lasting effect that guarantees the satisfaction of the female partner. A recipe to make the erection last all night (*a fare stare duro lo membro tutta la notte*) assures its user "[...] you will be able go to bed with a woman and you will see that you will stay erect and be able to do anything you want and enjoy yourself" (*va a letto con la donna vederai che starà duro et potrai fare quanto te piacerà et stare in festa*).[39] Sforza's recipes are based on ingredients considered to have aphrodisiac properties and commonly used for erotic purposes, either when mixed with wine and ingested or made into unguents to be directly applied to the penis. The satyrion root, for example, as Laura Giannetti points out in this volume, was considered a sexual stimulant. It plays a prominent role in Sforza's secrets for improving libido, along with pepper and *stincus marinus*, or skink (a kind of lizard), which in powdered form was especially prized.[40]

It is interesting to note that the explanatory headings attached to many of Sforza's recipes for correcting male impotence are partially encrypted, particularly in the titles that indicate their purpose. Some typical examples read: "A fare *tkrbrf* el menbro," which translates to "A fare *tirare* el menbro" ("To lengthen the member"); or, "A fare *stbrf dxrp lp mfnbrp*," which stands for "A fare *stare duro lo menbro*" ("To make the member erect").[41] Since the code is easily broken—the key is provided in the manuscript—this air of secrecy suggests less a desire to restrict the flow of information than an effort to highlight the unique and precious nature of the remedy.[42] On the other hand, one far more detailed remedy for impotence is offered entirely in Latin—but not encrypted—setting it off from the others. In this case, the use of Latin rather than the *volgare* suggests that the Latin is meant to elevate the recipe, acting as a filter for the reading public while also signaling the particular value of the recipe, which again promises to fully transform the male member in both length and diameter.[43] Significantly, many remedies for impotence work to arouse the female libido as well (*acende la femina a lebidine*): for example, concoctions made from ingredients such as wild boar fat are also said to excite the "desire that women enjoy" (*luxuria delecta a le femine*).[44]

In fact, Sforza places a considerable importance on female sexual pleasure by noting that an equal aim of this recipe for male performance is the satisfaction of the female partner. Sforza's attention to female pleasure seems to exist as an end in itself, beyond the more common Galenic paradigm for generation.[45]

Remedies for male impotence such as those offered by Sforza abounded in medical treatises long before the age of the vernacular *libri di segreti*. Pier Andrea Mattioli's 1544 translation of Discorides, for example, includes numerous aphrodisiacs such as rocket (arugula), which—when eaten raw and in large quantities—is said to "awaken Venus," while its seed was thought to increase the production of sperm as well as stimulate the libido.[46] Ingredients thought to aid not just in awakening desire, but specifically in achieving erection (*drizzar la verga*) include red chickpeas, pine nuts, carrots and pepper: for the most part common and readily available alimentary ingredients, the effects of which were detailed in vernacular reference manuals such as Durante's *Tesoro della sanità*. Often ingredients were chosen according to an external or visual relationship with the problem they were meant to cure: the "law of similars" made ingredients such as ground orchis, for example, called *testiculisvulpis* for its suggestive shape (particularly useful, according to Mattioli, to "prepare for venereal exertions" [*gli fa più pronti ne' gli essercizi venerei*]).[47] The notion of simulation is again central, as the natural ingredient is thought to trigger a physiological reaction that emulates the plant's particular, natural form.

As Emmanuela Renzetti and Rudolfo Taini note, there is a wide range of approaches to the framing of advice about sexual potency among books of secrets.[48] If the very title of Sforza's collection denotes a direct connection to the alchemical tradition of the "experiment" as a process of discovery achieved through observation and experience,[49] other books of secrets vary in the way in which they describe procedures and convey information. Some works simply list ingredients and their preparations—sometimes pages of them—with little or no explication. Bairo's *Secreti medicinali* dedicates an entire section to "Things that cause erection" (*Cose che fanno drizzar la verga*), which includes a cascade of recipes devoid of narrative transitions or flourishes:

> Cut up small pieces of *testiculisvulpis*, smoked and dried, and chew for a while and it will take effect. Another: Take pinenuts, parsley, *testiculis cervis*, spruce turpentine, pepper, mix with honey, and use. Another: Take red chickpeas, pine nuts, arugula seed, white pepper, honey in wine. Smear the member with honey and distilled mustard oil, or linseed with honey and pepper, and … it has miraculous effect.[50]

A book of secrets that was attributed (falsely) to the physician Gabriele Falloppio, by contrast, offers encouragement along with instruction, as well as an admonition:

> Whether you be a little old man or a gallant, enamored youth who finds himself impeded by some unhappy accident—you will truly see a miracle. But fortunate is he who uses it sparingly, for he thus preserves his soul and the health of his person. And so I exhort everyone to seek a remedy for desire, for they will live healthier and happier lives.[51]

The Pseudo-Falloppio addresses his imagined reader(s) directly, paradoxically offering a fail-safe recipe for sexual satisfaction while at the same time exhorting the same reader(s) to moderation, if not to chastity. Like the Pseudo-Falloppio, authors of other books of secrets, including Sforza, provide remedies for curbing desire; but far more attention is paid to ensuring and increasing sexual function, which was, after all, considered to play an important role in overall general health for both men and women.[52] One anonymous 16th-century collection of alchemical recipes compiled in a series of hurried, informal hands and likely passed down among family members, explains both how to facilitate conception and how to avoid it, as well as how to regulate libido. It suggests a concoction of pulverized carnations and cow's milk to make intercourse last longer; while honey and opium thebaicum applied directly to the male member will curb sexual desire.[53] Furthermore, fertility control is also a recognized concern: if a woman drinks the bark of the jabin tree (*sabina corta*)[54] in water for three days she will avoid conceiving; the contraceptive effect is *cosa probatissima*, as the author, points out: a well-proven recipe.

Impotence, Adultery and Abortifacients

While the results of these remedies for impotence and other forms of sexual dysfunction are of primary importance in the *libri di segreti*, the causes of such problems—whether physiological or psychological —go largely unexamined, with a few interesting exceptions. Pietro Bairo's *Secreti medicinali* offers in one instance an explanation for male impotence, along with appropriate remedies. The problem, he explains, may originate with a magic spell. In a section addressed to "Men Who are Victims of Spells and Hexes, and Cannot Lay With Women" (*Di coloro che son legati & maleficiati, sí che non possono usar con donne*), Bairo suggests a variety of treatments:

> The victim should smear his whole body with crow bile and Cleopatra's sesame oil. Eating a woodpecker dissolves spells and generates strength. Inhaling the vapors of a dead man's teeth is an infallible cure for the afflicted. Wearing beryl stones causes love to grow between husband and wife. Put quicksilver in a quill or hollow nut sealed with wax under the bolster of the hexed ones, or at the entrance to the room or the house, and the hex will be undone. Keeping coral in the house undoes every hex. If a man has been magicked or hexed by some woman, in the morning he should put her fresh feces in his shoe or in his right sock, and as soon as he smells the odor, the hex will be undone … .[55]

As Matteo Duni points out, quicksilver, or mercury—the lodestone of alchemical experiment—was symbolically associated with the variability of human sentiment and thus often appears in medical remedies for sexual problems as well as in love magic.[56] Bairo's instructions, in particular, echo a long tradition of similar advice, drawn most notably from Pietro Hispano's 13th-century *Thesaurus Pauperum*, which still circulated in various editions.[57]

Bairo makes no attempt to explain what circumstances might underlay such a hex, instead assuming the reader's acceptance of the possibility that male sexual function might be impaired through magic. Buried within this list of remedies, however, is one possible cause and/or consequence of male impotence: a rift between a wife and her husband. Bairo notes that wearing beryl stones can restore marital intimacy; the subtext here is that sexual dysfunction, left unchecked, can open the door to female sexual dissatisfaction and emotional alienation.

Sforza's text likewise warns of the side effects of impotence. Here, again, the lines between physiological and social function are blurred, with Sforza suggesting—far more explicitly than Bairo—that a further consequence of impotence might be not just a dissatisfied female partner, but even an unfaithful one. Poor sexual performance is seen, quite simply, as leading to cuckoldry. Male anxiety about such a conjugal scenario is implied in recipes meant to ensure "that a woman allows no one to touch her but you" (*A fare che una donna* [the next part is encrypted] *non se lassi toccare ad altri che a te*) or, indeed, that "she will never desire anyone else but you and if you were to ask her for it she would remove her heart from her chest and give it to you" (*a fare che una donna … mai desiderarà altri che te et se tu* [the next part is encrypted] *volessi farla trare te darà el core*).[58]

Sforza's recipes thus promise not just a physiological result, but a lasting emotional one. Here, again, it is significant that the titles of recipes to arouse female desire are partially encrypted, as in certain remedies for male impotence, either to conceal their purpose or (more probably) to highlight their importance.[59] Sforza's remedies again employ a mix of common ingredients thought to have aphrodisiacal qualities, especially spices and oils geared more particularly to the awakening of female desire: for example, the male partner is advised to apply an unguent of musk, civet and ginger to his penis before having relations with his female partner.[60] Such recipes often come with a warning, however, for if the remedy is to work, the man who uses it must apply the unguent without his female partner's knowledge.[61] Similarly, several recipes for impregnating a female partner also specify that they must be employed without the woman's knowledge. Implicit in such instructions is the notion that a reluctant or disinterested female partner may be won over and the heterosexual partnership cemented through sexual intimacy and, ultimately, procreation.[62] As Piero Camporesi notes, these kinds of remedies effect a dual artifice: they are meant to ensure not just the physical union of bodies, but an enduring emotional bond built upon a foundation of sexual satisfaction. Yet, in both cases, the bond is "medically" induced, not spontaneous or genuine.[63]

In terms of the physical and emotional results expected from remedies to impotence, there is an evident anxiety regarding the strength of the heterosexual bond and the fidelity of the female partner. Female sexual desire, while tolerable and even medically desirable in moderation, becomes destabilizing when not regulated or contained. Thus "binding" recipes that act either through a form of love magic or by causing pregnancy require that the female partner be deprived of sexual or reproductive agency in order to work effectively. Such physical and emotional unions are achieved through artificial means—the simulation or repair of sexual function—while the secretive action required by the male partner reposes on the deception that is central to the very notion of simulation.

Over and above a clear interest in protecting and promoting heterosexual, generative unions (thereby diminishing the threat of sexual infidelity), books of secrets also pays a certain amount of attention to non-procreative concerns, such as increasing sexual pleasure for both men and women. In keeping with Galenic thought, sexual pleasure—particularly on the woman's part—was thought to increase the chances of conception, and recipes for achieving this end abound in *libri di segreti*.[64] However, the presence of recipes for contraceptives and abortifacients alongside those meant to facilitate conception complicates a unilateral reading of these works as simply promoting the generation of children. Rather, it supports the supposition that books of secrets sought to offer a guide toward making sexual intercourse into a bodily function as healthy as any other. Sforza's collection abounds with instructions for avoiding pregnancy. Sometimes, the aim of such recipes is implicit, as in instructions for contraception that are couched as a means to determine whether or not a woman is fertile (which can work both to achieve or avoid pregnancy); in other instances, the recipes are transparently described as "impediments to conception" (*Delo impedimentum del concipere e delo impregniare*).[65] Similarly, recipes for abortifacients can be ambiguous, as in those explaining how to bring on menses (*a far venire el mestro*), or explicit, as in one of Sforza's recipes that details how to provoke a miscarriage prior to the third trimester.[66]

Conclusions

Libri di segreti—both those kept for personal use and those that circulated in print—can be said to operate on two levels. On the one hand, they position themselves as collections of useful and pragmatic information, connected by a unifying goal: they aim to teach readers how to care for themselves, whether treating a fever or rectifying a problem with sexual performance or reproductive function. On the other hand, although they are practical handbooks rather than narrative works or prescriptive treatises, these compilations of "secrets" nonetheless reflect the social and sexual concerns of their readership in seeking to promote stable, regulated sexual relationships that would ensure the female partner's fidelity and fertility. Books of secrets thus strive to impart to their readers the idea that they might indeed take control of their own health, sexual relations and emotional bonds. Whether presenting recipes for determining female virginity or formulas for correcting male impotence, these compilations approach matters of sex through the lens of commonplace knowledge, contemporary medical culture and familiar alchemical principles of transformation and simulation in order to enhance healthy physiological function. At the same time they also serve to uphold social and sexual custom by seeking to contain sexual activity—for women at least—within the confines of marriage, thereby protecting men from the prospect of cuckoldry.

Works Cited

Manuscripts and Early Printed Sources (pre-1900)

Bairo, Pietro. *Secreti medicinali*. Venice: Giorgio Valentini, 1629.

Cortese, Isabella. *I secreti della signora Isabella Cortese: ne quali si contengono cose minerali, medicinali, arteficiose, & alchimiche*. Venice: Bariletto, 1574.

Culpepper, Nicholas, *A Directory for Midwives, or a Guide for Women in Their Conception, Bearing, and Suckling Their Children*. London: Printed for George Sawbridge, 1675. [Pseudo-Falloppio]. *Secreti diversi et miracolosi ne' quali si mostra la via facile di risanare le infirmità del corpo humano*. Venice: Appresso Marco di Maria, 1563.

Fioravanti, Leonardo. *De capricci medicinali*. Venice: Lodovico Avanzo, 1573.

Fioravanti, Leonardo. *Del compendio de i secreti rationali*, Venice: Vincenzo Valgrisi, 1564.Fioravanti, Leonardo. *Secreti medicinali*. Venice: Lodovico Avanzo, 1561.

Fondo Magliabecchiano. Biblioteca Comunale Nazionale di Firenze, XV, 38, cc. 45–6.

Gioberti, Lorenzo [Laurent Joubert]. *La prima parte de gli errori popolari, nella quale si contiene l'eccellenza della medicina …* Florence: Giunti, 1592.

Mattioli, Pier Andrea. *I discorsi nei sei libri di Pedacio Discoride Anzarbeo della materia medicinale*. Venice: Vincenzo Valgrisi, 1568.

Rossello, Timoteo. *Della summa de' secreti universali*. Venice: Bariletto, 1565.

[Ruscelli, Girolamo]. *Secreti del reverendo donno Alessio Piemontese*. Pesaro: Appresso gli heredi di Bartolomeo Cesano, 1562.

Ruscelli, Girolamo. *Secreti nuovi*. Venice: Heredi di M. Sessa, 1567.Sforza, Caternina, *Li esperimenti de la exma sra Caterina da Furlj matre de lo inlluxmo sr Giovanni de Medici / copiati dagli autografi di lei dal Conte Lucantonio Cuppano*. University of Delaware Unidel collection, Private archive, Ravenna. MS 095–15; MS 065–16.

Sforza, Caterina. *Li esperimenti de la exma sra Caterina da Furlj matre de lo inlluxmo sr Giovanni de Medici / copiati dagli autografi di lei dal Conte Lucantonio Cuppano*, ed. Pier Desiderio Pasolini. Imola: Tip. D'ignazio Galeati e Figlio, 1894.

Venette, Nicolas. *La génération de l'homme: ou, tableau de l'amour conjugal, considéré dans l'état du mariage*. London, 1751.

Secondary Sources and Modern Editions

Agrimi, Jole and Chiara Crisciani. "Per una ricerca su *experimentum-experimenta:* Riflessione epistemologica e tradizione medica (secoli XIII–XV)." In *Presenza del lessico greco e latino nelle lingue contemporanee*, ed. Pietro Janni and Innocenzo Mazzini. Macerata: Università degli Studi di Macerata, 1990. 9–49.

Arrizabalaga, John, John Henderson and Roger French, eds. *The Great Pox: The French Disease in Renaissance Europe*. New Haven: Yale University Press, 1997.

Bell, Rudolph. *How To Do It: Guides to Good Living for Renaissance Italians*. Chicago: University of Chicago Press, 1999.

Bénézet, Jean-Pierre. *Pharmacie et médicament en Méditerranee occidentale (XIIIe–XIVIe siècles): Sciences, Tecniques et Civilisations du Moyen Âge à l'Aube des Lumières*. Paris: Honoré Champion, 1999.

Berriot-Salvadore, Èvelyne. *Un corps, un destin. La femme dans la médecine de la Renaissance*. Paris: Champion, 1993.

Borris, Kenneth. *Same Sex Desire in the English Renaissance: A Sourcebook of Texts (1470–1650)*. New York/London: Routledge, 2002.

Boylan, Michael. "The Galenic and Hippocratic Challenges to Artistotle's Conception Theory," *Journal of the History of Biology* 17 (Spring 1984): 83–112.

Boylan, Michael."Galen's Conception Theory," *Journal of the History of Biology* 17:1 (Spring, 1986), 47–77.

Breisach, Ernst. *Caterina Sforza: A Renaissance Virago*. Chicago: University of Chicago Press, 1967.

Buttlãn, Ibn and Luisa Cogliati Arano. *Tacuinum Sanitatis: The Medieval Health Handbook*. New York: Braziller, 1976.

Cadden, Joan. *The Meanings of Sex Difference in the Middle Ages: Medicine, Science and Culture*. Cambridge: Cambridge University Press, 1993.

Campbell, Kate Hurd-Mead. "Trotula," *Isis* 14.2 (1930): 340–67.

Camporesi, Piero. *I Balsami di Venere*. Milan: Garzanti, 1989.

Cartwright, Jane. "Virginity and Chastity Tests in Medieval Welsh Prose." In *Medieval Virginities*, Anke Bernau, Ruth Evans and Sarah Salih, eds. Toronto: University of Toronto Press, 2003. 56–79.

Cavaillé, Jean Pierre. *Dis/simulations. Jules-César Vanini, François La Mothe Le Vayer, Gabriel Naudé, Louis Machon et Torquato Accetto. Religion, morale, et politique au XVIe siècle*. Paris: Champion, 2002.

Corsi, Dinora, Lada Hordynsky-Caillat and Redon Odile. "Les secrés des dames, tradition, traductions," *Médiévales* 14 (1988): 47–57.

Crisciani, Chiara. "From the Laboratory to the Library: Alchemy According to Guglielmo Fabri." In *Natural Particulars: Nature and the Disciplines in Renaissance Europe*, ed. Anthony Grafton and Nancy G. Siraisi. Cambridge, MA: MIT Press, 1999. 295–320.

Cross, Tom Peete. "Notes on the Chastity-Testing Horn and Mantle," *Modern Philology* 10.3 (1913): 289–99.

de Vries, Joyce. "Casting Her Widowhood: The Contemporary and Posthumous Portraits of Caterina Sforza." In *Widowhood and Visual Culture in Early Modern Europe*, ed. Allison Levy. Aldershot, UK/Burlington, VT: Ashgate, 2003. 77–92.

de Vries, Joyce. *Caterina Sforza and the Art of Appearances: Gender, Art, and Culture in Early Modern Italy*. Farmham, UK/Burlington, VT: Ashgate, 2010.

Dentzien, Nicole. "Hans Sach's Arthurian Chastity Test," *Arthuriana* 13.1 (2003): 43–65.

Duni, Matteo. *Tra religione e magia, storia del prete modense Guglielmo Campana [1560?–1541]*. Olschki: Firenze, 1999.

Eamon, William. "Arcana Disclosed: The Advent of Printing, the Books of Secrets Tradition, and the Development of Experimental Science in the Sixteenth Century," *History of Science* 22 (1984): 111–50.

Eamon, William. *Science and the Secrets of Nature: Books of Secrets in Medieval and Early Modern Culture*. Princeton, NJ: Princeton University Press, 1994.

Fissell, Mary. "Hairy Women and Naked Truths: Gender and the Politics of Knowledge in *Aristotle's Masterpiece*," *William and Mary Quarterly* 60.1 (2003): 43–74.

Flouret, Jean. *Nicolas Venette: Médecin Rochelais 1633–1698*. La Rochelle: Editions Rupella, 1992.

Galen. *On Semen*, ed. and trans. Phillip de Lacy. Berlin: Akadamie Verlag, 1992.

Gélis, Jacques. *L'Arbre et le Fruit: La naissance dans l'Occident moderne, XVIe–XIXe siècle*. Paris: Fayard, 1984.

Givens, Jean, Karen Reeds and Alain Touwaide, eds. *Visualizing Medieval Medicine and Natural History, 1200–1550*. Aldershot, UK/Burlington, VT: Ashgate, 2006.

Grafton, Anthony and Nancy G. Siraisi. *Natural Particulars and the Disciplines in Early Modern Europe*. Cambridge, MA: MIT Press, 1999.

Green, Monica Helen. "From Diseases of Women to 'Secrets of Women: The Transformation of Gynecological Literature in the Later Middle Ages," *Journal of Medieval and Early Modern Studies* 30 (2000): 5–39.

Green, Monica Helen. *The Trotula: A Medieval Compendium of Women's Medicine*. Philadelphia: University of Pennsylvania Press, 2001.

Gwilliam, Tassie. "Female Fraud: Counterfeit Maidenheads in the Eighteenth Century," *Journal of the History of Sexuality* 6.4 (1996): 518–48.

Hoffman, Kathryn A. "Strange Bodies of Married Women," *Dalhousie French Studies* 56 (2001): 36–45.

Hughes, Jonathan. "Alchemy and the Exploration of Late Medieval Sexuality." In *Medieval Virginities, ed.* Anke Bernau, Ruth Evans, and Sarah Salih. Toronto: University of Toronto Press, 2003, 140–56.

Jacquart, Danielle and Claude Thomasset, eds. *Sexualité et savoir médical au Moyen Age*. Paris: Presses Universitaires, 1985.

Kavey, Allison. *Books of Secrets: Natural Philosophy in England 1550–1600*. Urbana: University of Illinois Press, 2007.

Kelly, Kathleen Coyne. *Performing Virginity and Testing Chastity in the Middle Ages*. London: Routledge, 2000.

Laqueur, Thomas. *The Making of the Modern Body: Sexuality and Society in the Nineteenth Century*. Berkeley: University of California Press, 1987.

Laqueur, Thomas. *Making Sex: Body and Gender From the Greeks to Freud*. Cambridge, MA: Harvard University Press, 1994.

Le May, Helen Rodnite. *Women's Secrets: A Translation of Pseudo-Albertus Magnus'* De Secretis Mulierum *With Commentaries*. Albany: Albany State University, 1992.

Leong, Elaine and Alisha Rankin, eds. *Secrets and Knowledge in Medicine and Science 1500–1800*. Farnham, UK/Burlington, VT: Ashgate, 2011.

Lev, Elizabeth. *The Tigress of Forlì: Renaissance Italy's Most Courageous and Notorious Countess, Caterina Riario Sforza de Medici*. New York: Houghton Mifflin, 2011.

Lochrie, Karma. *Covert Operations: The Medieval Uses of Secrecy*. Philadelphia: University of Pennsylvania Press, 1999.

Lochrie, Karma. *Heterosyncrasies: Female Sexuality When Normal Wasn't*. Minneapolis: University of Minnesota Press, 2005.

Lochrie, Karma, Peggy McCracken and James A. Schultz, eds. *Constructing Medieval Sexuality*. Minneapolis: University of Minnesota Press, 1997.

Maclean, Ian. *The Renaissance Notion of Woman: A Study in the Fortunes of Scholasticism and Medicial Science in European Intellectual Life*. Cambridge: Cambridge University Press, 1983.

McCall, Timothy, Giancarlo Fiorenza and Sean E. Roberts, eds. *Visual Cultures of Secrecy in Early Modern Europe*. Kirksville: Truman State University Press, 2013.

McGough, Laura. *Gender, Sexuality and Syphilis in Early Modern Venice: The Disease That Came To Stay*. New York: Palgrave Macmillan, 2011.

Milanesi, Carlo and Filippo Moise. "Lettere di Giovanni de' Medici, detto delle Bande Nere," *Archivio Storico Italiano*, Nuova Serie, Tomo Nono [IX], Parte 2 [1859]: 127.

Moran, Bruce. *Distilling Knowledge: Alchemy, Chemistry, and the Scientific Revolution*. Cambridge, MA: Harvard University Press, 2005.

Murray, Jaqueline. "On the Origins and Role of 'Wise Women' in Causes for Annulment on the Grounds of Male Impotence," *Journal of Medieval History* 16 (1990): 235–49.

Novielli, Valeria, ed. *Caterina Sforza: Una donna del Cinquecento*. Florence: La Mandragora, 2000.

Nummedal, Tara. *Alchemy and Authority in the Holy Roman Empire*. Chicago: University of Chicago Press, 2007.

Palmero, Giuseppe. "La distillazione: I suoi prodotti ed i suoi usi nell'ambito della 'letteratura dei segreti' tra Quatrrocento e Cinquencento." In *Grappa & Alchimia. Un percorso nella millenaria storia della distillazione* (Atti del convegno "Dall'Alchimia alla grappa: un percorso millenario nella distillazione," Greve in Chianti, 11 settembre 1999), ed. Allen J. Grieco. Rome, 1999. 17–32.

Palmero, Giuseppe. "Ars medica e terapeutica alla fine del Medioevo: Il caso genovese." *Nuova rivista storica* 91:3 (2007): 673–738.

Park, Katharine. "Natural Particulars: Medical Epistemology, Practice, and the Literature of the Healing Springs." In *Natural Particulars and the Disciplines in Early Modern Europe*, ed. Anthony Grafton and Nancy G. Siraisi. Cambridge, MA: MIT Press, 1999. 347–67.

Park, Katherine. *Secrets of Women: Gender, Generation, and the Origins of Human Dissection*. New York: Zone Books, 2006.

Pasolini, Pier Desiderio. *Caterina Sforza*. 3 vols. Rome: Loescher, 1893.

Pomata, Gianna and Nancy G. Siraisi, eds. *Historia: Empiricism and Erudition in Early Modern Europe*. Cambridge, MA: MIT Press, 2005.

Porter, Roy. "Spreading Carnal Knowledge or Selling Dirt Cheap? Nicolas Venette's *Tableau de l'Amour Conjugal* in Eighteenth Century England," *Journal of European Studies* 14 (December 1984): 233–55.

Porter, Roy and Lesley Hall. "Doctors and the Medicalization of Sex in the Enlightenment." In *The Facts of Life: The Creation of Sexual Knowledge in Britain, 1650-1950*, ed. Roy Porter and Lesley Hall. New Haven: Yale University Press, 1995, 65–90.

Preus, Anthony. "Galen's Criticism of Aristotle's Conception Theory," *Journal of the History of Biology* (Spring 1977): 65–85.

Ray, Meredith K. "Experiments with Alchemy: Caterina Sforza in Early Modern Scientific Culture." In *Gender and Scientific Discourse in Early Modern Culture*, ed. Kathleen P. Long. Farnham, UK/Burlington, VT: Ashgate, 2010. 139–64.

Ray, Meredith K. "Prescriptions for Women: Alchemy, Medicine and the Renaissance *Querelle des Femmes*." In *Women Writing Back/Writing Women Back: Transnational Perspectives from the Late Middle Ages to the Dawn of the Modern Era*, ed. Anke Gilleir, Alicia C. Montoya and Suzan van Dijk. Leiden: Brill, 2010. 135–62.

Renzetti, Emmanela and Rodolfo Taini. "Le cure dell'amore: Desiderio e passione in alcuni libri di segreti," *Sanità scienza e storia: rivista del Centro italiano di storia sanitaria e ospitaliera* (1986): 33–86.

Riddle, John M. "Oral contraceptives and Early-Term Abortifacients during Classical Antiquity and the Middle Ages," *Past and Present* 132 (1991): 3–32.

Riddle, John M. *Eve's Herb: A History of Contraception and Abortion in the West*. Cambridge, MA: Harvard University Press, 1997.

Ruggiero, Guido. *Binding Passions; Tales of Magic, Marriage, and Power at the End of the Renaissance*. Oxford: Oxford University Press, 1993.

Sforza, Caterina. *Experimenti de la ex.ma s.ra Caterina da Furlj matre de lo inllux.mo signor Giovanni de Medici*, ed. Paola Gregetti. Ed. fac. Biblioteca Comunale di Imola, 2008.

Simons, Patricia. *The Sex of Men in Premodern Europe: A Cultural History*. Cambridge: Cambridge University Press, 2011.

Siraisi, Nancy G. *Medieval and Early Renaissance Medicine. An Introduction to Knowledge and Practice*. Chicago: University of Chicago Press, 1990.

Synder, Jon R. *Dissimulation and the Culture of Secrecy in Early Modern Europe*. Berkeley: University of California Press, 2009.

Thorndike, Lynn. *A History of Magic and Experimental Science*, 8 vols. New York: Macmillan, 1923–58.

Traub, Valerie. *The Renaissance of Lesbianism*. Cambridge: Cambridge University Press, 2002.

Williams, Steven James. *The Secret of Secrets: The Scholarly Career of a Pseudo-Aristotelian Text in the Latin Middle Ages*. Ann Arbor: University of Michigan Press, 2003.

Witthoft, Brucia. "The *Tacuinum Sanitatis*: A Lombard Panorama," *Gesta* 17.1 (1978): 49–60.

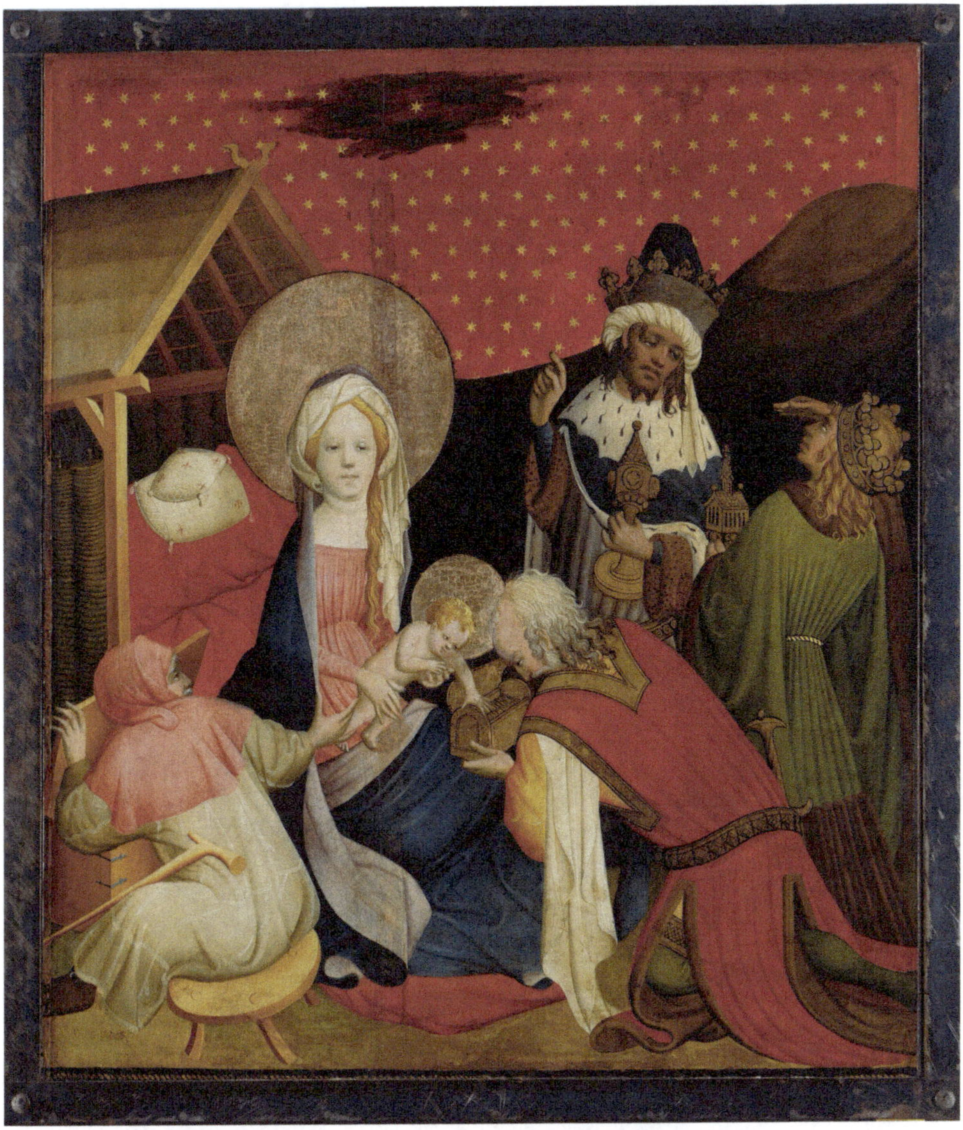

Plate 1 Master Francke, *Adoration of the Magi* fragment of the *Saint Thomas altar*, c. 1424, tempera on oak, 99 × 89.3 cm, Kunsthalle, Hamburg

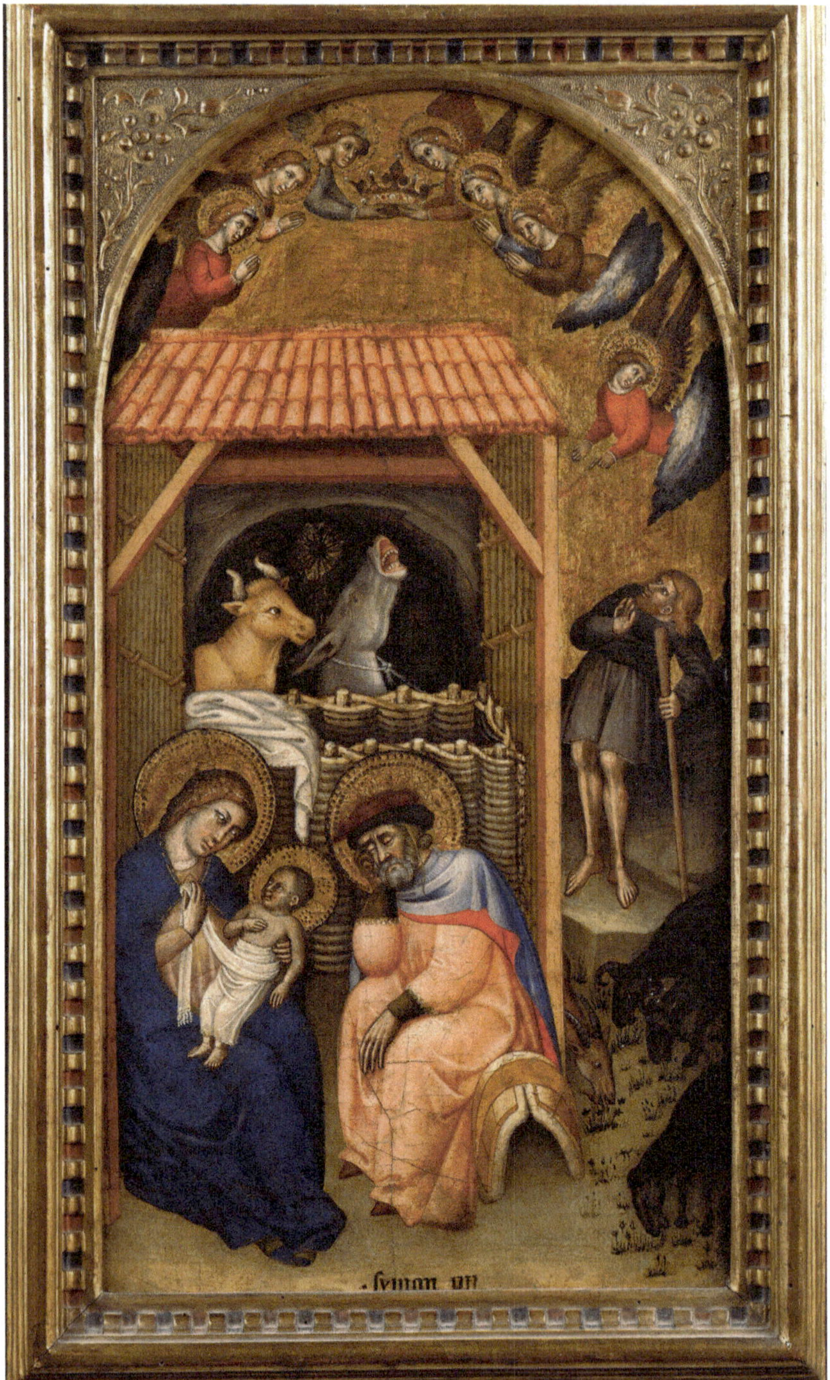

Plate 2 Simone dei Crocifissi, *Nativity of Christ*, c. 1380, tempera on wood, 47 × 25 cm, Uffizi Gallery, Florence

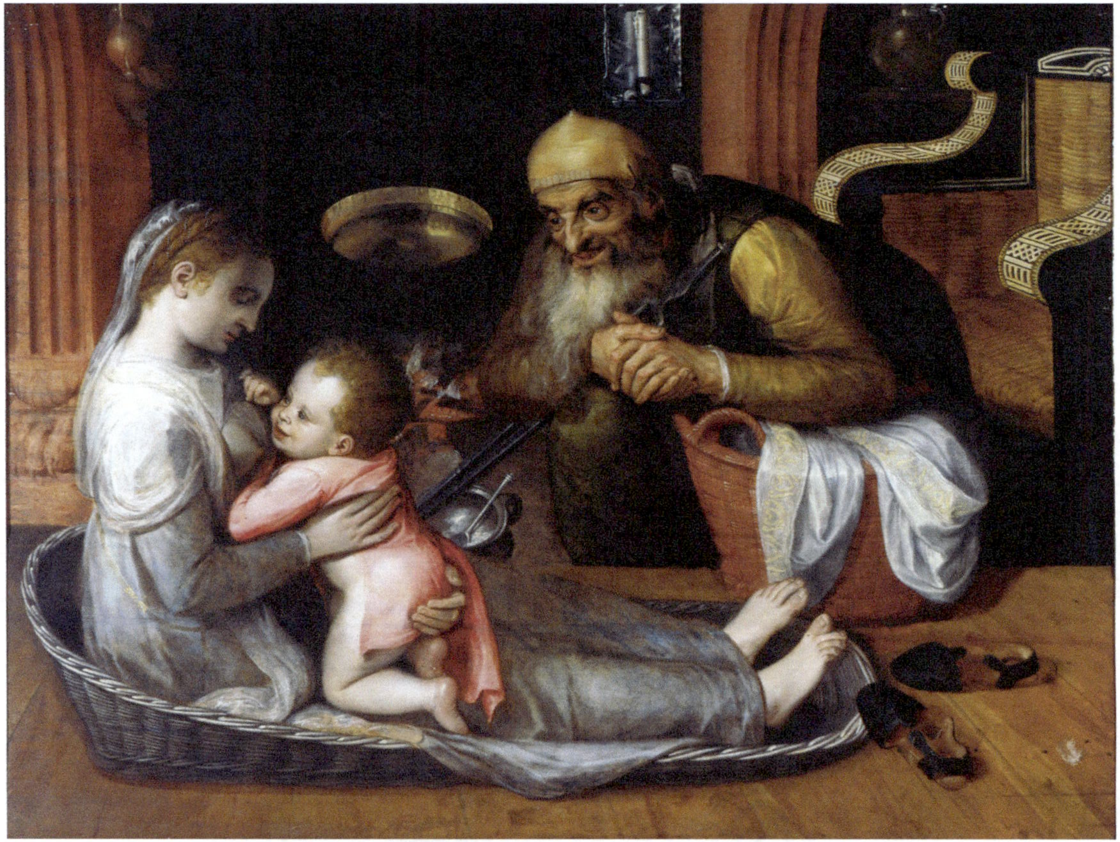

Plate 3 Frans Floris, *The Holy Family*, 16th century, oil on panel, 132 × 166 cm, Musée de la Chartreuse, Douai (inv. 2796) (photo: Hugo Maertens)

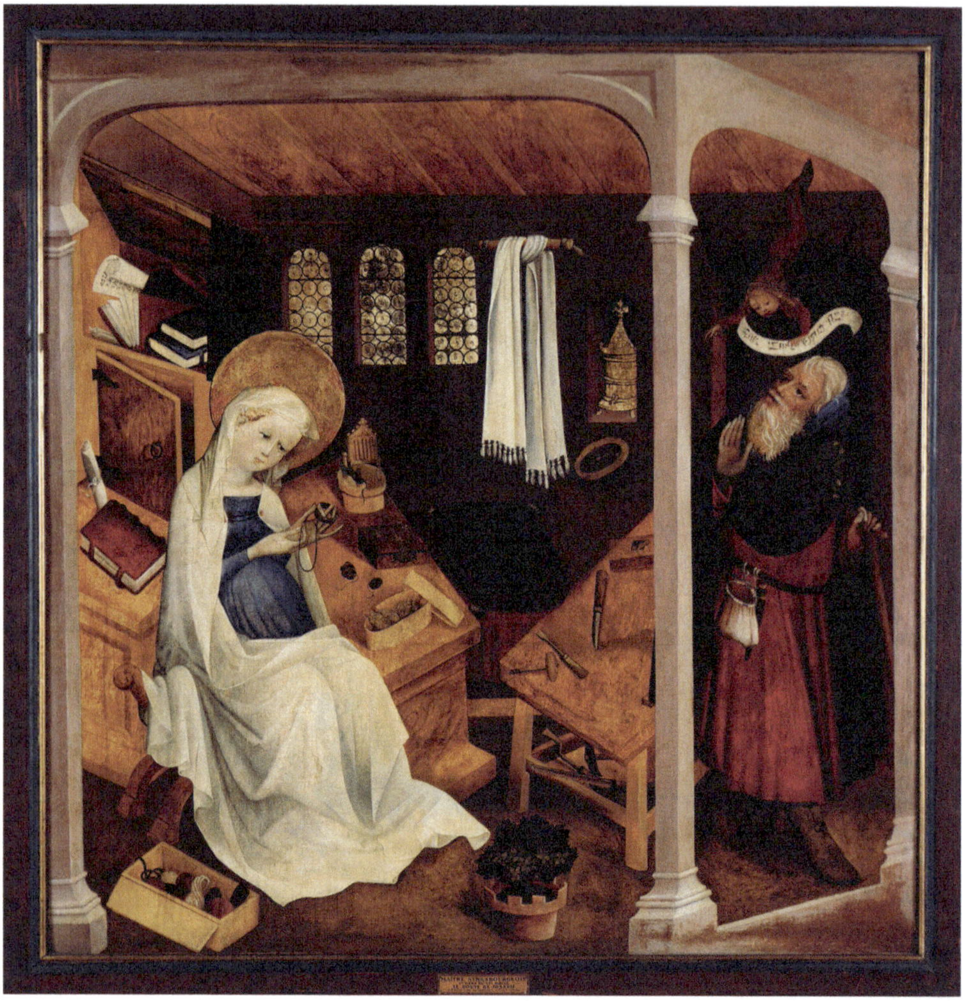

Plate 4 Strasbourg artist, *Joseph's Doubts*, c. 1482, Musée de l'Œuvre Notre-Dame, Strasbourg (© Musée de l'Œuvre Notre Dame de Strasbourg) (photo N. Fussler)

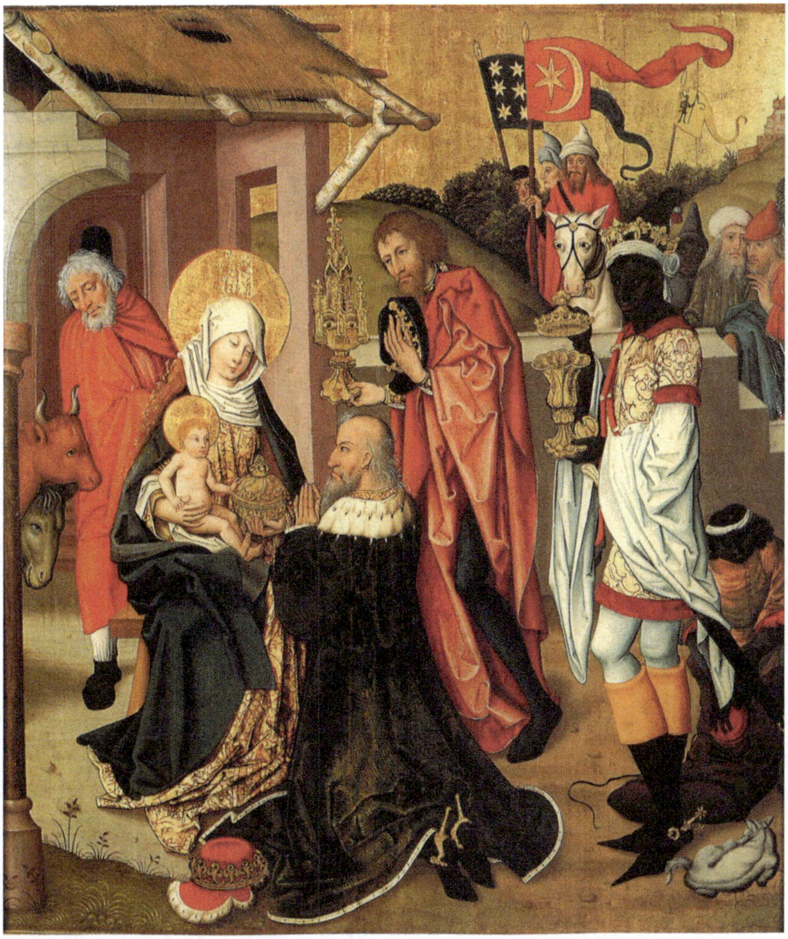

Plate 5 Artist of the School of Schongauer, *Adoration of the Magi*, c. 1475, Musée d'Unterlinden, Colmar (© Musée Unterlinden, Colmar, France)

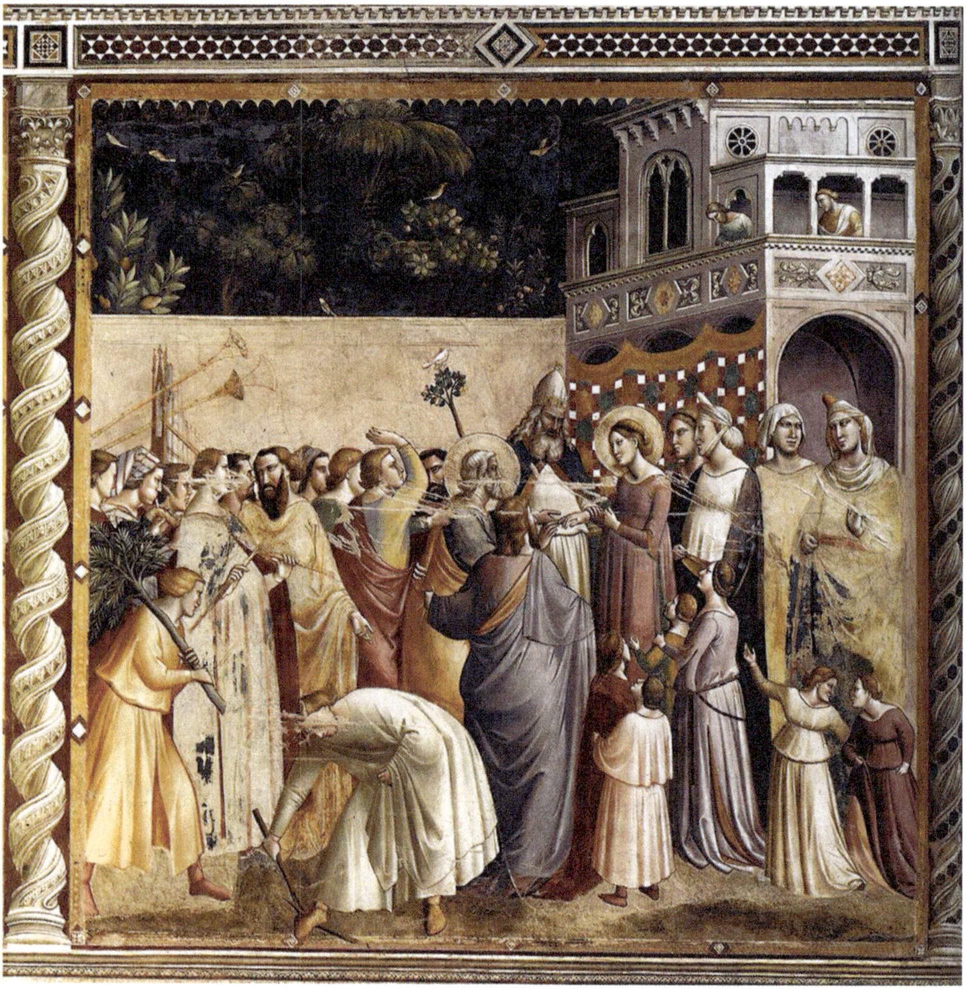

Plate 6 Taddeo Gaddi, *Marriage of the Virgin*, c. 1328–1330, fresco, Florence, Santa Croce, Baroncelli Chapel

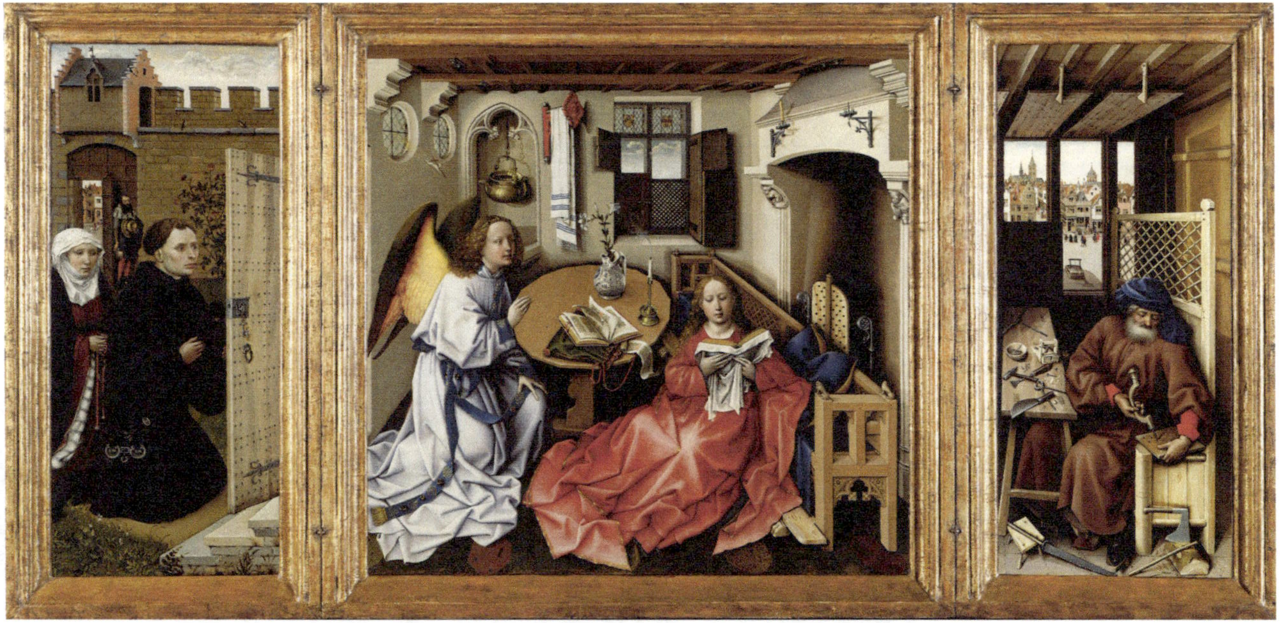

Plate 7 Master of Flémalle (Robert Campin), *The Mérode Altarpiece*, c. 1427, oil on wood, 64.5 × 27 cm; 64 × 63 cm; 64.5 × 28 cm, The Metropolitan Museum of Art, The Cloisters Collection, New York City (1956 [56.70])

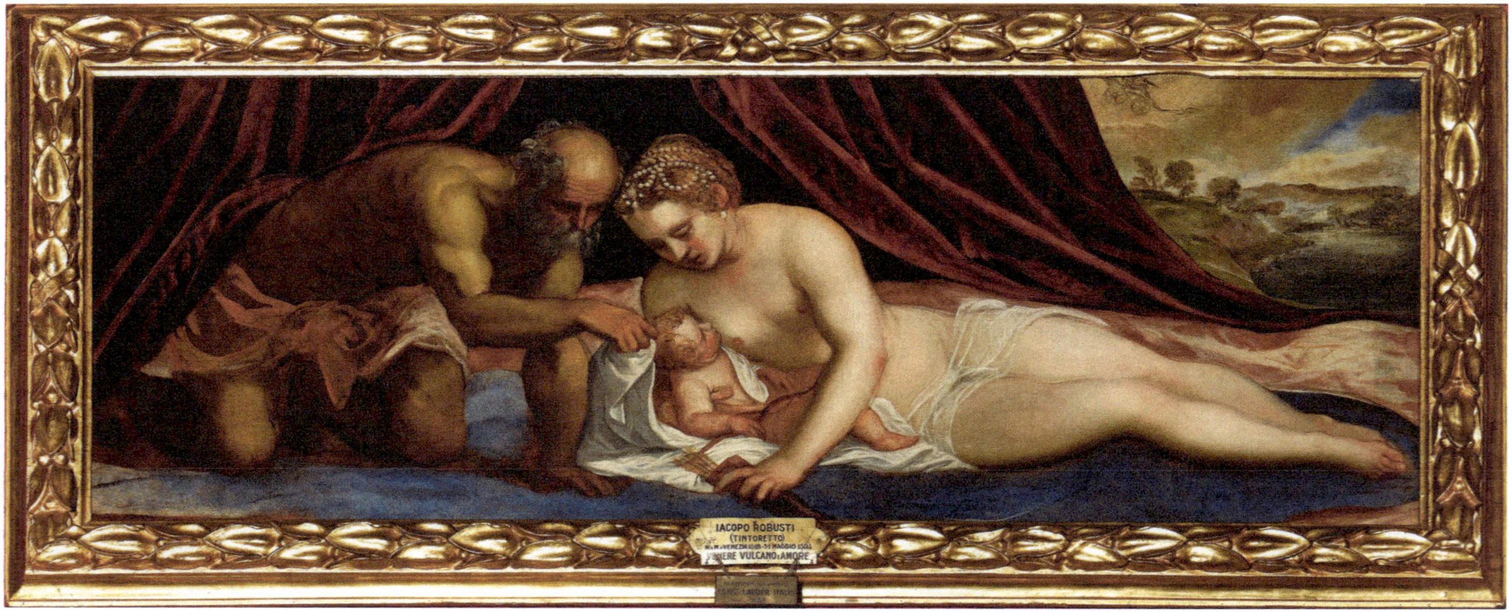

Plate 8 Tintoretto, *Venus, Vulcan and Cupid*, c. 1550–1552, oil on canvas, 85 × 197.4 cm, Galleria Palatina, Palazzo Pitti, Florence (photo: Polo Museale di Firenze)

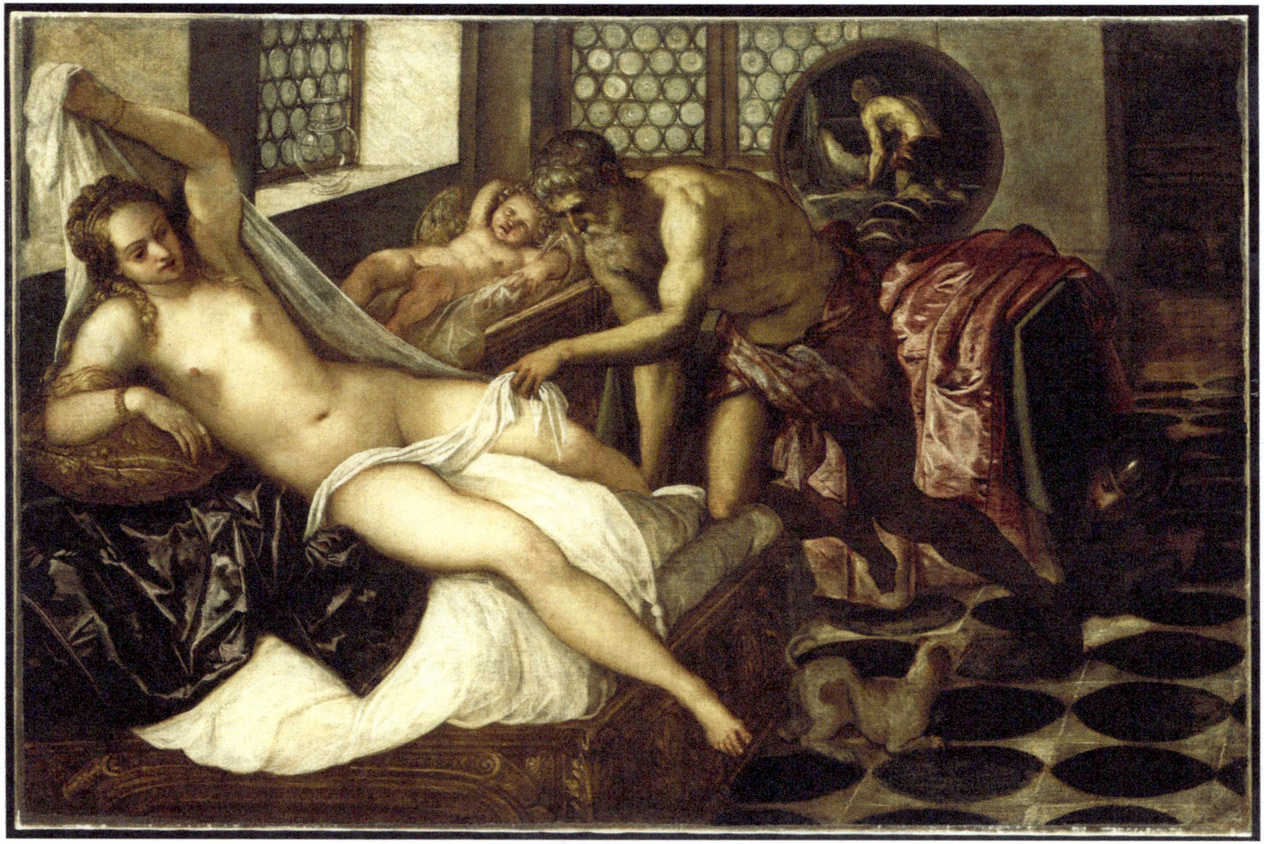

Plate 9 Tintoretto, *Vulcan surprising Venus and Mars*, c. 1548, oil on canvas, 135 × 198 cm, Munich, Alte Pinakothek (inv. 9257) (photo: Bayerische Staatsgemäldesammlungen, Alte Pinakothek München)

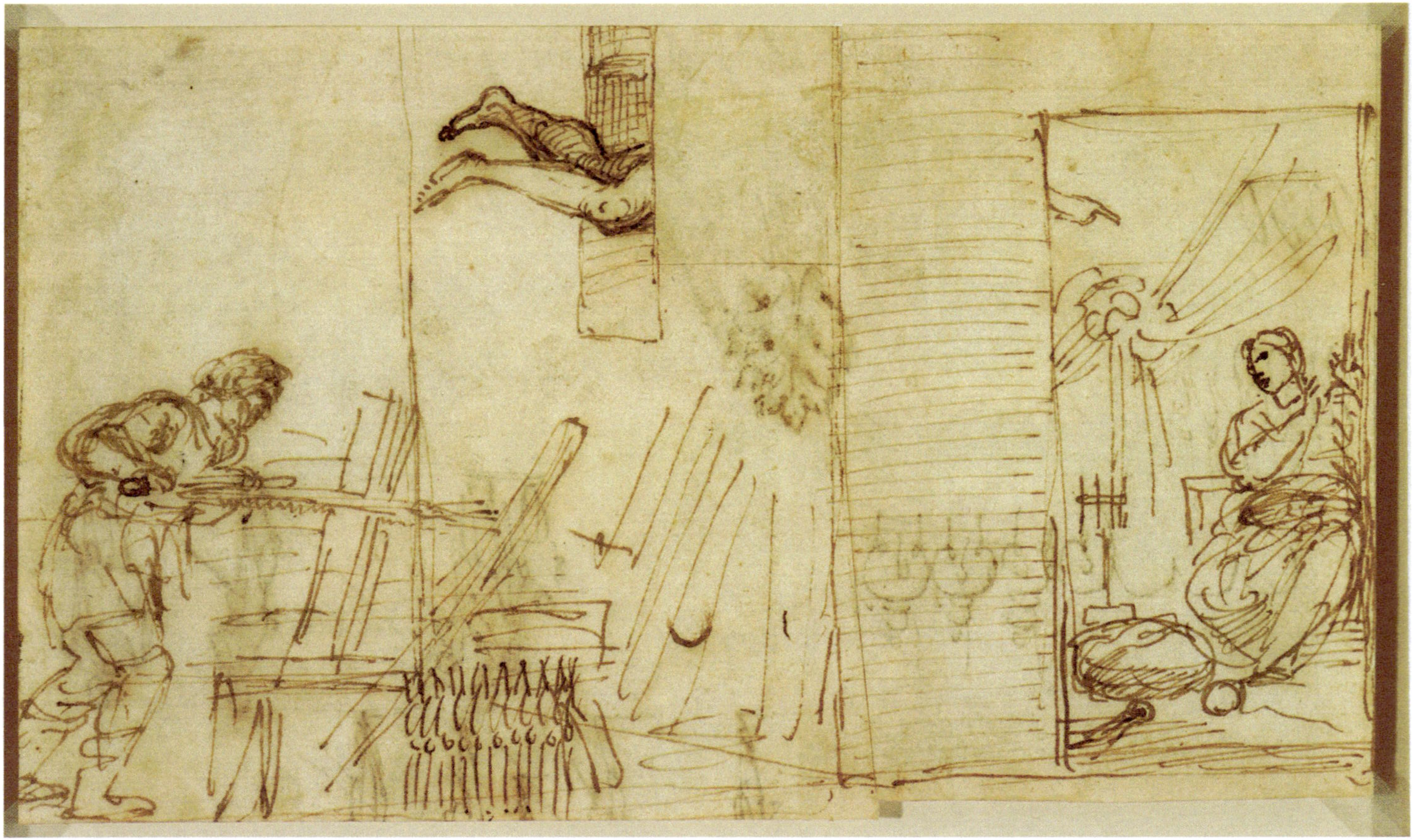

Plate 10 Annibale Carracci, *Parody of Tintoretto's Annunciation in the Scuola di San Rocco*, pen and brown ink, 11.5 × 18.8 cm, Royal Library, Windsor Castle (inv. 1841) (photo: Royal Collection Trust © Her Majesty Queen Elizabeth II 2012)

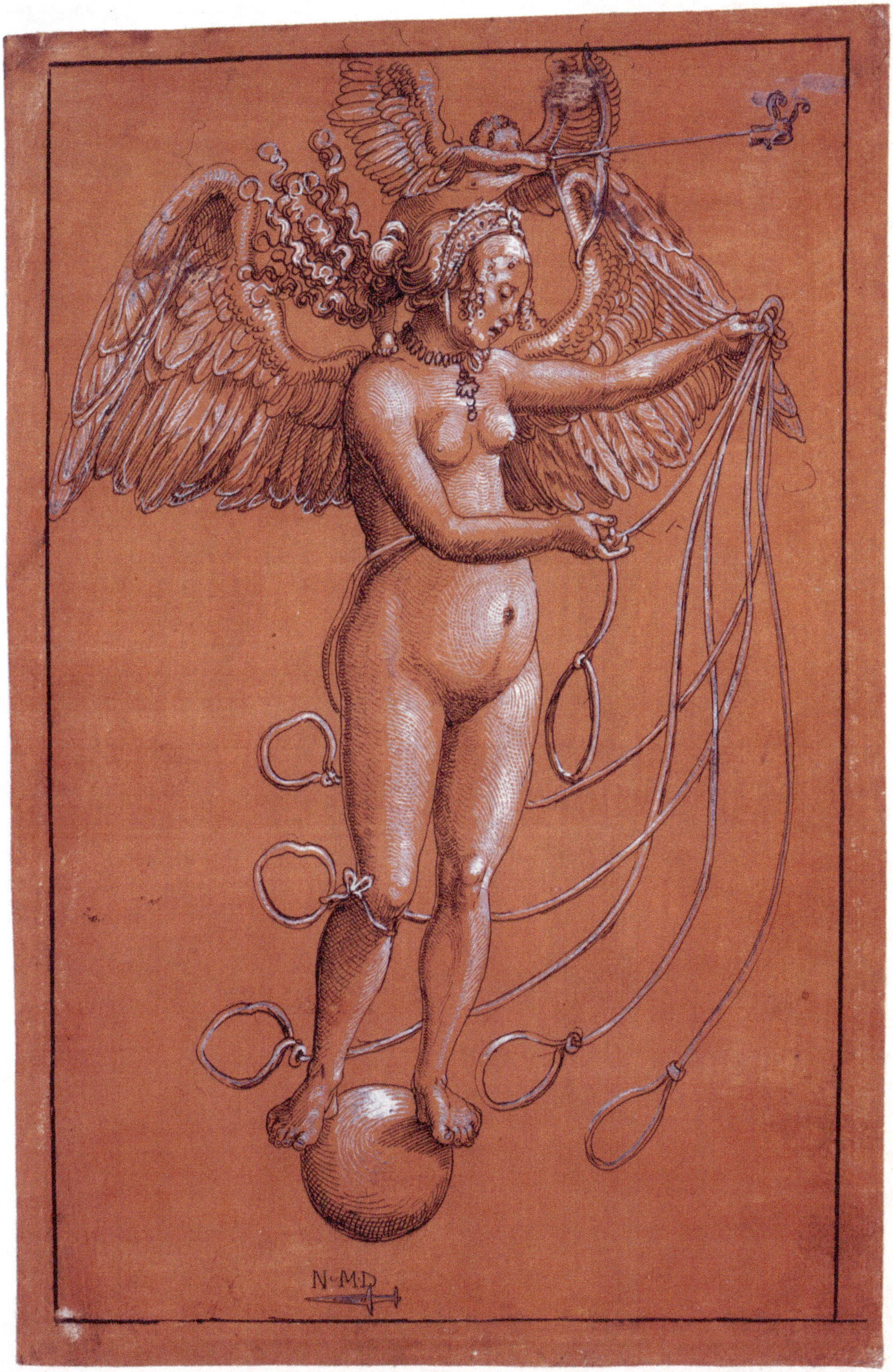

Plate 11 Niklaus Manuel Deutsch, *Venus*, c. 1512, chiaroscuro drawing, 31.4 × 21.7 cm, Kunstmuseum Basel, Kupferstichkabinett (photo: Martin P. Bühler)

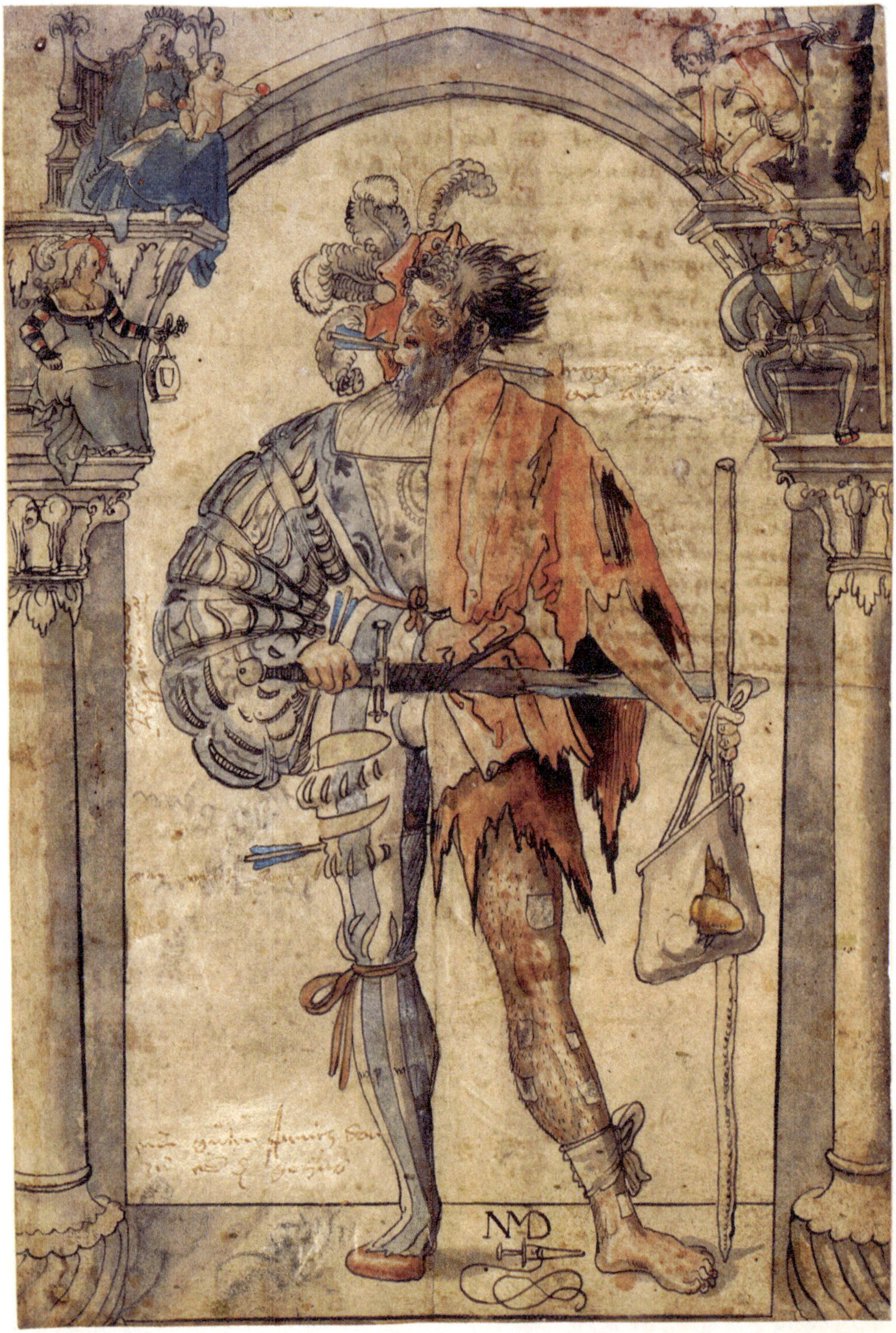

Plate 12 Niklaus Manuel Deutsch, *Allegory on the Transitoriness of Luck in War*, pen in black ink with watercolor on parchment, 31 × 21.3 cm, Kupferstichkabinett, Staatliche Museen zu Berlin (inv. 4287)

Notes

1 On books of secrets and medical culture, see: William Eamon, *Science and the Secrets of Nature: Books of Secrets in Medieval and Early Modern Culture* (Princeton, NJ: Princeton University Press, 1994); Jean-Pierre Bénézet, *Pharmacie et médicament en Méditerranee occidentale (XIII°–XIVI° siècles): Sciences, Tecniques et Civilisations du Moyen Âge à l'Aube des Lumières* (Paris: Honoré Champion, 1999); Giuseppe Palmero, "Ars medica e terapeutica alla fine del Medioevo: Il caso genovese," *Nuova rivista storica* 91.3 (2007): 673–738. See also n. 3 below. On *libri di segreti* and women readers, see: Meredith K. Ray, "Prescriptions for Women: Alchemy, Medicine and the Renaissance *Querelle des Femmes*" in *Women Writing Back/Writing Women Back: Transnational Perspectives from the Late Middle Ages to the Dawn of the Modern Era*, eds. Anke Gilleir, Alicia C. Montoya and Suzan van Dijk (Leiden: Brill, 2010), 135–62. On early modern empirical culture more broadly, see *Historia: Empiricism and Erudition in Early modern Europe*, ed. Gianna Pomata and Nancy G. Siraisi (Cambridge, MA: MIT Press, 2005); *Natural Particulars and the Disciplines in Early Modern Europe*, ed. Anthony Grafton and Nancy G. Siraisi (Cambridge, MA: MIT Press, 1999).

2 As Nancy G. Siraisi points out, recipe collections, among other forms of medical writing, "may be a better guide than more sophisticated medical literature to the kinds of medicines most frequently prescribed" in the early modern period. See *Medieval and Early Renaissance Medicine. An Introduction to Knowledge and Practice* (Chicago: University of Chicago Press, 1990), 148.

3 See Eamon, *Secrets of nature*, and idem, "Arcana Disclosed: The Advent of Printing, the Books of Secrets Tradition, and the Development of Experimental Science in the Sixteenth Century," *History of Science* 22 (1984): 111–50; Allison Kavey, *Books of Secrets: Natural Philosophy in England 1550–1600* (Urbana: University of Illinois Press, 2007); Elaine Leong and Alisha Rankin, eds. *Secrets and Knowledge in Medicine and Science 1500–1800* (Farnham, UK/Burlington, VT: Ashgate, 2011). Piero Camporesi offers a brief overview of the problem in specific regard to the production of aphrodisiacs in *I Balsami di Venere* (Milan: Garzanti, 1989). On the problem of secrecy more generally in medieval and early modern culture, see Karma Lochrie, *Covert Operations: The Medieval Uses of Secrecy* (Philadelphia: University of Pennsylvana Press, 1999) and Timothy McCall, Giancarlo Fiorenza and Sean E. Roberts, eds., *Visual Cultures of Secrecy in Early Modern Europe* (Kirksville: Truman State University Press, 2013).

4 Patricia Simons, *The Sex of Men in Premodern Europe: A Cultural History* (Cambridge: Cambridge University Press, 2011), 126. On early modern understanding of sexual and reproductive function see, among others, Èvelyne Berriot-Salvadore, *Un corps, un destin. La femme dans la médecine de la Renaissance* (Paris: Champion, 1993); Joan Cadden, *The Meanings of Sex Difference in the Middle Ages: Medicine, Science and Culture* (1995); Jacques Gélis, *L'Arbre et le Fruit: La naissance dans l'Occident moderne, XVIe–XIXe siècle* (Paris: Fayard, 1984); Thomas Laqueur, *Making Sex: Body and Gender From the Greeks to Freud* (Cambridge, MA: Harvard University Press, 1994); Ian Maclean, *The Renaissance Notion of Woman: A Study in the Fortunes of Scholasticism and Medicial Science in European Intellectual Life* (Cambridge: Cambridge University Press, 1983); Siraisi, *Medieval and Early Renaissance Medicine, op.cit.*, esp. p. 110 ss; and Danielle Jacquart and Claude Thomasset, eds., *Sexualité et savoir médical au Moyen Age* (Paris: Presses Universitaires, 1985).

5 On the *Tacuinum Sanitatis* see Ibn Buttlān and Luisa Cogliati Arano, *Tacuinum Sanitatis: The Medieval Health Handbook* (New York: Braziller, 1976); Brucia Witthoft, "The *Tacuinum Sanitatis*: A Lombard Panorama," *Gesta* 17.1 (1978): 49–60. On the *De Secretis Mulierum* see Helen Rodnite Le May, *Women's Secrets: A Translation of Pseudo-Albertus Magnus'* De Secretis Mulierum *With Commentaries* (Albany: Albany State University, 1992); Dinora Corsi, Lada Hordynsky-Caillat, Redon Odile, "Les secrés des dames, tradition, traductions," *Médiévales* 14 (1988) 47–57. More generally, see Jean Givens, Karen Reeds and Alain Touwaide, eds., *Visualizing Medieval Medicine and Natural History, 1200–1550* (Farnham, UK/Burlington, VT: Ashgate, 2006).

6 On the *Trotula*, see Monica Helen Green, *The Trotula: A Medieval Compendium of Women's Medicine* (Philadelphia: University of Pennsylvania Press, 2001); see also Kate Campbell Hurd-Mead, "Trotula," *Isis*, 14.2 (1930): 340–67.

7 Nicolas Venette's *La génération de l'homme: ou, tableau de l'amour conjugal, considéré dans l'état du mariage*, first published in 1686, had over 100 editions (see Roy Porter and Lesley Hall, "Doctors and the Medicalization of Sex in the Enlightenment," in *The Facts of Life: The Creation of Sexual Knowledge in Britain, 1650–1950* [eds. Roy Porter and Lesley Hall] (New Haven: Yale University Press, 1995, 65–90, 66); see also Roy Porter, "Spreading Carnal Knowledge or Selling Dirt Cheap? Nicolas Venette's *Tableau de l'Amour Conjugal* in Eighteenth Century England," *Journal of European Studies* 14 (December 1984): 233–55; Jean Flouret, *Nicolas Venette: Médecin Rochelais 1633–1698* (La Rochelle: Editions Rupella, 1992). The pseudo-Aristotelian *Masterpiece* (1684) was pieced together from earlier sources; see Porter and Hall, "Medical Folklore in High and Low Culture: *Aristotle's Masterpiece*" in *The Facts of Life*, 33–64; see also Mary Fissell, "Hairy Women and Naked Truths: Gender and the Politics of Knowledge in *Aristotle's Masterpiece*," *William and Mary Quarterly* 60.1 (2003): 43–74.

8 See Giuseppe Palmero, "La distillazione: I suoi prodotti ed i suoi usi nell'ambito della "letteratura dei segreti" tra Quatrrocento e Cinquencento," in *Grappa & Alchimia. Un percorso nella millenaria storia della distillazione* (Atti del convegno "Dall'Alchimia alla grappa: un percorso millenario nella distillazione," Greve in Chianti, 11 settembre 1999), ed. Allen J. Grieco (Rome, 1999, 17–32).

9 See Palmero, Ibid., 1: "... quelli che noi oggi conosciamo come 'libri di segreti' sono da considerarsi il risultato di alto di quel crogiuolo culturale ... ."

10 Among the earliest examples of books of secrets is the medieval, pseudo-Aristotelian *Secretum Secretorum* (see Steven James Williams, *The Secret of Secrets: The Scholarly Career of a Pseudo-Aristotelian Text in the Latin Middle Ages* [Ann Arbor: University of Michigan Press, 2003]). Pietro Bairo's *Secreti medicinali* was published in Venice in 1561 and had seven editions by 1599; the *Secreti del reverendo donno Alessio Piemontese*, published in Venice in 1555, had 17 editions in the same period (see Eamon, *Science and the Secrets of Nature*, 136). The writer Girolamo Ruscelli was likely behind Piemontese's *Secreti* (ibid., 140). Other books of secrets that circulated in this period include Ruscelli's own *Secreti nuovi* (Venice, 1566); Timoteo Rosello, *Della summa de' secreti universali* (Venice, 1561); Leonardo Fioravanti, *Secreti medicinali* (Venice, 1561), *Capricci medicinali* (Venice, 1561), and idem, *Del compendio de i secreti rationali* (Venice, 1564); and Isabella Cortese, *Secreti* (Venice, 1561), the only printed book of secrets currently attributed to a female author in these years. Caterina Sforza's manuscript collection of *Experimenti* was transcribed by her biographer Pier Desiderio Pasolini in *Caterina Sforza* (Rome: Loescher, 1893, vol. 3) and idem, *Li esperimenti de la exma sra Caterina da Furlj matre de lo inlluxmo sr Giovanni de Medici / copiati dagli autografi di lei dal Conte Lucantonio Cuppano*, ed. Pier Desiderio Pasolini (Imola: Tip. D'ignazio Galeati e Figlio, 1894); a facsimile edition of Pasolini's 1894 transcription was published in 2008 with an introductory essay by Paola Gregetti (*Experimenti de la ex.ma s.ra Caterina da Furlj matre de lo inllux.mo signor Giovanni de Medici*. Ed. fac. Biblioteca Comunale di Imola, 2008). On Sforza and the *Experimenti*, see Meredith K. Ray, "Experiments with Alchemy: Caterina Sforza in Early Modern Scientific Culture," in *Gender and Scientific Discourse in Early Modern Culture*, ed. Kathleen P. Long (Farnham, UK/Burlington, VT: Ashgate, 2010), 139–64. Manuscript collections of "secrets" abound, many of which deal with sexual and reproductive matters: among the numerous compilations housed in Florence's Biblioteca Nazionale, for example, are recipes for regulating menstruation and easing childbirth (BCNF, Fondo Magliabechiano XV, 38, cc. 45–6).

11 Syphilis (often referred to as "mal francese" in books of secrets) was a source of concern for early modern medical writers and recipes aimed at preventing or curing it abound in books of secrets. See John Arrizabalaga, John Henderson and Roger French, eds., *The Great Pox: The French Disease in Renaissance Europe* (New Haven: Yale University Press, 1997); Laura McGough, *Gender, Sexuality and Syphilis in Early Modern Venice: The Disease That Came To Stay* (New York: Palgrave Macmillan, 2011).

12 Jonathan Hughes, "Alchemy and the Exploration of Late Medieval Sexuality," in *Medieval Virginities*, ed. Anke Bernau, Ruth Evans and Sarah Salih (Toronto: University of Toronto Press, 2003), 140. On alchemical and medical culture more generally see Lynn Thorndike's important study, *A History of Magic and Experimental Science* (New York: Macmillan, 1923–58), 8 vols.

13 On alchemical procedures such as these, see Bruce Moran, *Distilling Knowledge: Alchemy, Chemistry, and the Scientific Revolution* (Cambridge, MA: Harvard University Press, 2005); see also Palmero, "La distillazione," *op. cit.*

14 The close connections between alchemical and medical practice in the early modern period have been discussed by many scholars, including Chiara Crisciani, "From the Laboratory to the Library: Alchemy According to Guglielmo Fabri," in *Natural Particulars: Nature and the Disciplines in Renaissance Europe, op. cit.*, 295–320); and Katharine Park, "Natural Particulars: Medical Epistemology, Practice, and the Literature of the Healing Springs," in ibid., 347–67.

15 See Hughes, "Alchemy and the Exploration of Late Medieval Sexuality," 140.

16 Some important medieval and early modern examples include the *Tacuinum Sanitatis* and the Pseudo-Albertus Magnus' *De Secretis Mulierum* (see n. 5 above), sixteenth-century collections such as the Pseudo-Falloppio's *Secreti diversi et miracolosi ne' quali si mostra la via facile di risanare le infirmità del copo humano* (Venice, 1563; see below) and Bairo's *Secreti medicinali*, and later works such as *Aristotle's Masterpiece*, Venette's *Tableau d'amour conjugal*, and Nicholas Culpepper's *Directory for Midwives* (London, 1656) (see nn. 6–7 above). Lorenzo Gioberti's *La prima parte de gli errori popolari, nella quale si contiene l'eccellenza della medicina* ... (Florence, 1592) professed to correct the errors found in many medical advice handbooks. Among many recent contributions to the study of sexuality in the early modern period see Kenneth Borris, *Same Sex Desire in the English Renaissance: A Sourcebook of Texts (1470–1650)* (New York/London: Routledge, 2002); Karma Lochrie, *Heterosyncrasies: Female Sexuality When Normal Wasn't* (Minneapolis: University of Minnesota Press 2005); Karma Lochrie, Peggy McCracken, and James A. Schultz, eds., *Constructing Medieval Sexuality* (Minneapolis: University of Minnesota Press, 1997); Valerie Traub, *The Renaissance of Lesbianism* (Cambridge: Cambridge University Press, 2002).

17 "Il fin di Venere deve essere la procreation dei figliuoli, con la consorte, congiunta per santo matrimonio ..." (Castor Durante, *Tesoro della sanità*, "De Venere" [Venice, Appresso Domenico Farri, 1588], 39).

18 Ibid., 39: "... ma il suo uso deve esser moderato ..." Many authors, including Savonarola and Marinello, echoed the view that sexual intercourse should be practiced in moderation (see Rudolph Bell, *How To Do It: Guides to Good Living for Renaissance Italians* [Chicago: University of Chicago Press, 1999], 26–33; Hughes, "Alchemy and the Exploration of Late Medieval Sexuality," 66).

19 Cf. Katharine Park, *Secrets of Women: Gender, Generation, and the Origins of Human Dissection* (Zone Books, 2006). See also Monica H. Green, "From Diseases of Women to 'Secrets of Women': The Transformation of Gynecological Literature in the Later Middle Ages," in *Journal of Medieval and Early Modern Studies* 30 (2000): 5–39.

20 Park, ibid., 103–4. As Kathryn A. Hoffman points out, attempts by sources dealing with the question of female virginity—such as Jacques Duval's *Traité des hermaphrodites* and Venette's *Tableau de l'amour conjugal*—to "read" the signs of virginity on the female body come to form a "... semiotics of sexual reading where hidden pleasures and guilts traced themselves obsessively on corporeal surfaces" ("Strange Bodies of Married Women," *Dalhousie French Studies* 56 [2001]: 36–45, 37).

21 "Secreto a sapere se la dona pò concipere o non: Prenderai malija (malva) selvatica la farai pissare e sopra della malvia et si in tre giorni non serba pò concipere overo se la serba i tre gorni non pò concipire ..."; the instructions are found in an anonymous manuscript compilation in the University of Delaware Unidel collection (MS 095–15, 33v).

22 Coyne Kelly, *Performing Virginity*, 12. See also Jane Cartwright, "Virginity and Chastity Tests in Medieval Welsh Prose," in *Medieval Virginities, op. cit.*, 56–79.

23 This recipe comes from another anonymous manuscript compilation in the University of Delaware Unidel collection (MS 065–16).

24 See Kathleen Coyne Kelly, *Performing Virginity and Testing Chastity in the Middle Ages* (New York: Routledge, 2000), 12–13.

25 The major biographies of Caterina Sforza remain Pasolini's 1893 *Caterina Sforza* (*op.cit.*) and Ernst Breisach, *Caterina Sforza: A Renaissance Virago* (Chicago: University of Chicago Press, 1967); and now Joyce de Vries's study, *Caterina Sforza and the Art of Appearances: Gender, Art, and Culture in Early Modern Italy* (Farnham, UK/Burlington, VT: Ashgate, 2010); as well as a general biography by Elizabeth Lev, *The Tigress of Forlì: Renaissance Italy's Most Courageous and Notorious Countess, Caterina Riario Sforza de Medici* (New York: Houghton Mifflin, 2011). See also the essays collected in *Caterina Sforza: Una donna del Cinquecento*, ed. Valeria Novielli (Florence: La Mandragora, 2000).

26 Cf. Pasolini, *Caterina Sforza*, 601. While Sforza's original manuscript is lost, scholars agree that the single extant copy, transcribed by Lucantonio Cuppano, in the service of Sforza's son Giovanni de' Medici (known as Giovanni delle Bande Nere), is based on her collection. Giovanni refers to a book left to him by his mother—likely the *Experimenti*—in a letter of 1525 (see Carlo Milanesi and Filippo Moise, "Lettere di Giovanni de' Medici, detto delle Bande Nere" in *Archivio Storico Italiano*, Nuova Serie, Tomo Nono [IX], Parte 2 [1859]: 127); and inventories of Sforza's belongings refer to a book in her hand that is not an account book (DeVries, *Caterina Sforza*, 211 n.118). The Cuppano manuscript now resides in a private collection; I am grateful to the owners (who wish to remain anonymous) for allowing me access to it.

27 "Modo de saper si una dona è vergine o vero Corrupta. Piglia pietra armoniaci et distempera in acqua et dalla a bevere a chi voli se serà vergine non farà nisuna demonstratione, se serà corrutta subito pisciarà ..." (*Experimenti*, 72). I have modernized accents and punctuation for clarity. Page numbers refer to the 2008 facsimile edition of the 1894 Pasolini transcription. All translations are my own.

28 On the motif of the virginity (or chastity) test in Arthurian romance, see Nicole Dentzien, "Hans Sach's Arthurian Chastity Test," *Arthuriana* 13.1 (2003): 43–65 and Tom Peete Cross, "Notes on the Chastity-Testing Horn and Mantle," *Modern Philology* 10.3 (1913): 289–99. The motif appears in medieval and early modern works from Malory's *Morte d'Arthur* to Ariosto's *Orlando furioso*.

29 Ibid., 36. See also Jaqueline Murray, "On the Origins and Role of 'Wise Women' in Causes for Annulment on the Grounds of Male Impotence," *Journal of Medieval History* (1990) v. 16, 239. Park notes that a consequence of the increased encroachment of male medical practitioners into the area of women's medicine after the early 14th century was their growing involvement in consultations on petitions for divorce or inheritance that "hinged on determinations of virginity, pregnancy, and legitimacy," supplementing or replacing formerly all-women juries (*Secrets of Women*, 97).

30 "Piglia della salvia et fanne acqua per lanbicco; poi habbi tre spognette sottili et mettili in ditta acqua. Poi piglia la magior cusí bagnata et mettila in la natura et lassala stare una bona hora; poi piglia la mezzana medemo ... et cusí cavarai questa et metterai la piccola che serà l'ultima in modo

che deventerà strettisima …" ("Take some sage and distill in an alembic; then soak three small sponges in the water. Then take the largest one, soaked in this manner, and place in the vagina and leave it there a good hour; then do the same with the next one … and then remove it and replace it with the smallest one, which will be the last, until [the passage] becomes very narrow …"), *Experimenti*, 71.

31 Cf. *Experimenti*, 71, which calls for ingredients gleaned from various kinds of trees including myrtle, cypress, pine and oak, distilled with alum, water and wine ("Piglia sumachi, grani de mirti … galla de cipresso, galla de guercia perforate an. on. 4 allume de roccho … et fa bollir tutte queste cose in acqua … con la quale doi volte el giorno la natura te lava … fallo per 15 giorni continui che tu vederai quella cosa cusí stretta devenir che tu medesima ne admiraraj" ["Take sumac, myrtle berries … perforated cypress and oak gall, 4 ounces rock alum … boil all these things in water … wash the vagina in the mixture twice daily … do this for 15 days and you will see that it becomes so narrow you yourself will marvel at it"]).

32 Ibid., 71: "Piglia galle on. 3, garofani on. 1, musco on. meza, et fanne sottilmente polvere. Mestica insieme, poi poni in on. una de vino, poi piglia pezza de lino sottile, et molto bene bagiato in ditta copositione pone in la natura quattro volte et poco più se potrai, che demostrarai verissima vergine ("Take 3 ounces gall, 1 once carnation, half an ounce musk, and make a fine powder. Mix together and place in one ounce wine, then take a fine piece of linen and soak it well in this mixture and place in the vagina four times, and a little more if you can, and you will appear to be a true virgin").

33 deVries, *Caterina Sforza and the Art of Appearances*, 1. See also idem, "Casting Her Widowhood: The Contemporary and Posthumous Portraits of Caterina Sforza" in *Widowhood and Visual Culture in Early Modern Europe*, ed. Allison Levy (Farnham, UK/Burlington, VT: Ashgate, 2003), 77–92.

34 Idem., *Caterina Sforza and the Art of Appearances*, 14.

35 See Ibid., 15. Such questions are central to major Renaissance works such as Castiglione's *Libro del cortegiano* (1528) and Machiavelli's *Principe* (1532). On the question of simulation and dissimulation more generally, see for example, Jean Pierre Cavaillé, *Dis/simulations. Jules-César Vanini, François La Mothe Le Vayer, Gabriel Naudé, Louis Machon et Torquato Accetto. Religion, morale, et politique au XVIe siècle* (Paris: Champion, 2002); Jon R. Synder, *Dissimulation and the Culture of Secrecy in Early Modern Europe* (Berkeley: University of California Press, 2009).

36 The recipe bears the heading: "How to lend weight to a scudo or gold ducat without suffering the pangs of conscience" ("A dare gran peso a uno scudo, o ducato de oro senza carigo de coscientia") (Pasolini, *Caterina Sforza*, v. 3, 620). On the issue of alchemical fraud, see Tara Nummedal, *Alchemy and Authority in the Holy Roman Empire* (Chicago: University of Chicago Press, 2007).

37 Tassie Gwilliam draws out the explicit connections between the counterfeit of virginity and that of coinage in the 18th century, when "[t]he implication that counterfeit maidenheads devalue virginity in the same way that fake money devalues coinage—through the debasement created by unauthorized duplication—reflects on the one hand the emotional power of specie in this period and on the other the idea that women's bodies are commodities to be exchanged as well as themselves being tokens of exchange" ("Female Fraud: Counterfeit Maidenheads in the Eighteenth Century," *Journal of the History of Sexuality* 6.4 [1996]: 518–48, 518).

38 *Experimenti*, 146.

39 Ibid., 228, 213.

40 "Ancora dia satirion, dato a bevere molto vale …; la radicata del sati[r]ione bevuta cum vino forte excita …," etc. (ibid., 146). Another "marvelous experiment for indulging in sexual activity as you wish" ("experimento mirabile per [luxuriare] come ti piace") features satyrion, *stincho marino* and saffron and is partially encrypted (ibid., 210). The use of satyrion as an aphrodisiac features not only in medical writing, but in literary works such as Machiavalli's *Clizia* (1525).

41 *Experimenti*, 213. In some cases the instructions for making the remedy are also partially encrypted, for example in the case of another recipe "A fare [stare duro el menbro]," which instructs, "Piglia on. 1 de polvere de stincho marino et bevine … in bon vino mesticato, che sempre *stbrb dxrp* [starà duro] et potrai fare quanto vorrai et la *dpnnb pptrb fbrf fl* [donna potra fare el] fatto suo" ("To [achieve an erection]: Take one ounce powdered *stincus marinus* and drink it … with good wine, and [your erection will be maintained] and you will be able to do as you like, and [likewise your woman])" (ibid.).

42 When applied to the encrypted passages, the key provided on the frontispiece is accurate.

43 "De hijs ingrossant et ellongant virile membrum" (ibid., 228). That the recipe is given entirely in Latin likely also indicates its provenance from another source.

44 Ibid., 146: "Ancora se la verga del homo è unta cum fele de verro et de porco selvaggio excita da fare tosto la luxuria delecta ale femine" ("And if the man's penis is annointed with wild boar's fat [it] quickly leads to that desire women so enjoy").

45 According to Galen's "two-seed" model, female pleasure and orgasm were essential to conception. On the Galenic model see Thomas Laqueur, *The Making of the Modern Body: Sexuality and Society in the Nineteenth Century* (Berkeley: University of California Press, 1987), 5–7; Siraisi, *Medieval and Early Renaissance Medicine, op. cit.*, 110 ss; Simons, *The Sex of Men, op. cit.*, esp. 191–219; Cadden, *Meanings of Sex Difference, op. cit.*, esp. 117–166.

46 Cf. Pier Andrea Mattioli, *I discorsi nei sei libri di Pedacio Discoride Anzarbeo della materia medicinale* (Venice, 1712), 559, 561.

47 Cited in Emmanela Renzetti and Rodolfo Taini, "Le cure dell'amore: Desiderio e passione in alcuni libri di segreti," *Sanità scienza e storia: rivista del Centro italiano di storia sanitaria e ospitaliera* (1986): 33–86, 72.

48 Ibid., 73–4.

49 On the term see Park, *Secrets of Women*, 82, and more extensively, Chiara Crisciani and Jole Agrimi, "Per una ricerca su *experimentum-experimenta:* Riflessione epistemologica e tradizione medica (secoli XIII–XV)" in Pietro Janni and Innocenzo Mazzini, eds. *Presenza del lessico greco e latino nelle lingue contemporanee* (Macerata: Università degli Studi di Macerata, 1990, 9–49); see also Eamon, *Science and the Secrets of Nature*, 53–8.

50 "Taglia in pezzetti verga di lupo, seccata al fumo, et tiene in bocca un pezzetto et farà opera. Un altro. Piglia pignuoli, petroselino, verga di cervo, trementina d'abeto … pepe … ; componi con mele et usa. Un altro. Piglia ceci rossi, pignuoli … seme di rucola, pepe bianco … mele … dà con vino. Unger la verga con mele e con olio di decottion di senapa, o con seme di lino con mele et pepe, … desta mirabilmente …" (Bairo, *Secreti medicinali*, 215–16).

51 "Vederai veramente miracolo tu buon vecchietto, o giovane galante innamorato, et da qualche accidente impedito, ma beato chi poco se ne serve, in salute dell'anima sua e conservation della persona, et sanità. Et cosí esorto ognuno a trovar più tosto rimedio di poter manco lussuriare, che sene viverà pù sano, lieto, e felice" (Pseudo-Falloppio, *Secreti diversi et miracolosi* [Venice, 1563], 116).

52 In addition to being widely considered integral to conception (see n. 45 above), female sexual pleasure was part of a more general picture of health and, especially, an important component of a successful marital partnership, as evidenced by the attention it is given in works such as the *Tacuinum Sanitatis* and in later conjugal "handbooks" such as Venette's *Tableau* or Artistotle's *Masterpiece* (see nns. 5–7 above).

53 "Per augmentare il coito: Rx: garofoli oz. i et meza et cum late bovino dalo a bere … A constrengere la luxuria: Rx: Aqua mela quale sia resulto lo opio tabaico et ungere le membra genitalia …" (University of Delaware Unidel MS 095-15, 43r).

54 The jabin tree (sabina corta) is native to Yucatan; *sabina* may also indicate juniper.

55 "Il legato s'unga tutto il corpo con fiel di corvo, & con olio sesamino di Cleopatra. L'uccello pico mangiato discioglie i legati, & dà fortezza. Suffumigio di dente di huomo morto, discioglie in dubitamente i legati. La pietra berillo portata dà nascare amor tra il marito e la moglie … Metti argento vivo in calamo o in nose straforata stroppanda con cera, & metti sotto il capezzale de maleficiati, overo sotto il sogliaro della porta, per la qual s'entra in camera o incasa, & si disfarà l'incanto. Corallo tenuto in casa, discoglie ogni maleficio … Se qualcuno è legato o maleficiato da qualche femina, metti la mattina del sterco fresco d'essa donna nel suo zoccolo, o calzetta destra del maleficiato, & incontanente ch'egli sentirà il fettore, si disfarà il maleficio …" (Cf. Bairo, *Secreti medicinali*, 271).

56 Duni notes the connections that still existed in the early modern period between some expressions of medicine, astrology, and magic: "… il risultato di una comune visione essenzialmente magica della natura e dei suoi effetti, nella quale l'efficacia terapeutica delle erbe e dei semplici è indiscindibile dagli occulti influssi degli astri sotto il cui segno i farmaci dovevano essere preparati, o dalle formule e preghiere che ne dovevano accompagnare l'uso" (*Tra religione e magia, storia del prete modense Guglielmo Campana [1560?–1541]* [Olschki: Firenze, 1999], 258–9). On love magic and binding spells see also Guido Ruggiero, *Binding Passions; Tales of Magic, Marriage, and Power at the End of the Renaissance* (Oxford: Oxford University Press, 1993).

57 Duni, *Tra religione e magia*, 259. I thank Matteo Duni for directing me to these precedents to Bairo's recipe.

58 *Experimenti*, 215. The bracketed portions are encrypted in the text; see n. 59 below.

59 The example given above, for example—a recipe to ensure that a female partner will desire only her partner and no other man—is partially encrypted; the full heading reads, "Experimenti a fare che una donna non se lassi toccare ad altri che a te ne mai desidererà altri che te et se tu *xplfssk fbrlb trbrf tf dbrb fl cprf* [*volessi farla trare te darà el core*]" ("Experiments to ensure a women does not allow herself to be touched by anyone but you and will never desire anyone but you, and if you were to ask her [*she would cut out her heart and give it to you*]," *Experimenti*, 215). A more general recipe for improving libido, male or female, bears the heading: "A fare *lxxxrkbrf* [*lussuriare*] inestimabile" ("To [*increase libido*] beyond measure," ibid.).

60 Ibid., 215: "Piglia zibetto, uno caratto, muschio uno caratto et fallo impalpabile et impasta omne cosa inseme con siroppo zenzaro verde, poi ugni la testa del membro et usa con donna."

61 "... con questo unguento oneti il [menbro che la donna non lo sappia et usa con essa]" (ibid., 215). This key part of the recipe (in brackets) is again encrypted.

62 See for example recipes to "cause a woman to become pregnant" ("*A far che una se ingravidj*"), which specify placing substances under the woman's pillow or giving them to her to drink, both without her knowledge ("che lei non lo sappia") (ibid., 214–15).

63 "Artificiosi interventi a due livelli: il primo, di pura fruizione carnale ... il secondo, presupponente invece la donazione, oltre che del corpo, anche del cuore" (Camporesi, *I balsami di Venere*, 53).

64 Galen's influential treatise *De Semine* was concerned with the function of male and female "seed" in the processes of conception and reproduction (*On Semen*, ed. and trans. Phillip de Lacy [Berlin: Akadamie Verlag, 1992]). See Laqueur, *Making Sex*, *op. cit.*; Michael Boylan, "The Galenic and Hippocratic Challenges to Artistotle's Conception Theory," *Journal of the History of Biology* 17 (Spring 1984): 83–112 and idem, "Galen's Conception Theory," *Journal of the History of Biology* 19:1 (Spring 1986), 47–77; Anthony Preus, "Galen's Criticism of Aristotle's Conception Theory," *Journal of the History of Biology* (Spring 1977): 65–85.

65 *Experimenti*, 150.

66 "Marvelous experiment to bring on a miscarriage before the fortieth day; must be done in good conscience because after forty days one shouldn't commit such a sin" ("Experimenti mirabile a fare *dfspfrdfrf* [desperdere]: inanti che siano passati li 40 giorni se deve fare respetto la Conscientia che passati non se deve fare per non commettere quell peccato," ibid., 99). The explanatory heading of this recipe is partially encrypted. On abortifacients and contraceptives see John M. Riddle, "Oral contraceptives and Early-Term Abortifacients during Classical Antiquity and the Middle Ages," *Past and Present* 132 (1991): 3–32; idem, *Eve's Herb: A History of Contraception and Abortion in the West* (Cambridge, MA: Harvard University Press, 1999).

PART III
Horns and Visual Innuendo

"Divine cuckolds": Joseph and Vulcan in Renaissance Art and Literature[1]

Francesca Alberti

In Renaissance visual culture, which is heavily indebted to both Christian tradition and classical mythology, two figures incarnate the paradigm of husbands. One is Joseph, who took the young Virgin Mary as his spouse to fulfill God's will.[2] The other is Vulcan, who was given Venus as a wife in recognition of his skill as a blacksmith. While both of these couples are frequently referred to in European art and literature with reference to marriage as a social institution (at least as it was understood in the later Middle Ages and Renaissance), the two figures of husbands have rarely been compared. Yet both these husbands have a lot in common: they were usually represented as unattractive and old while their wives were represented as ideals of female beauty and perfection in both Christian and pagan traditions.[3] Both husbands were thus the less fortunate halves of mismatched couples, according to the logic of contemporary sexual culture, and therefore risked the humiliation of conjugal infidelity on the part of their wives: they risked being cuckolded. This essay examines the two figures separately, starting with Joseph and moving on to Vulcan, in order to demonstrate how both husbands were, in fact, often represented as cuckolds. This comparative analysis will also point out the specific functions and significance of such visual mockery, and will conclude with an examination of Tintoretto's *Vulcan Surprising Venus and Mars* from a new perspective.

Joseph as a Figure of Ridicule

The feast of Saint Joseph first appeared in the Roman breviary in 1480 under Pope Sixtus IV, although it was only officially established by Pope Gregory XV in 1621.[4] Since there is not much information about Joseph in the official Gospels, for a long time artists were free to find inspiration in apocryphal sources and in popular traditions, such as Miracle Plays.[5] Art historians have already noticed how early Renaissance images depict Joseph as an ambiguous and comic character, often ridiculed for his Jewish origins.[6] He could be represented as an ugly old man,[7] or he could be portrayed as being tiny in comparison with his wife. His figure, deprived of a halo, was usually relegated to the background of *Holy Family* pictures and, in images depicting the Nativity or the Adoration of the Magi, he was often represented as being somewhat greedy in that he looks more interested in the kings' rich presents than in the birth of the child (Fig. 7.1 and Plate 1).[8] Joseph was also pictured as someone who was dozing or sleeping so deeply that braying donkeys or nuzzling camels couldn't wake him up: examples are seen in Giotto's fresco in the Arena chapel, and in Simone dei Crocifissi's amusing little panel at the Galleria degli Uffizi (Fig. 7.2 and Plate 2).[9]

During the first decades of 15th century, when the cult of Joseph began to emerge, several Christian authors began to debate how he ought to be represented in pictures. Interestingly enough, the discussion mainly focused on Joseph's advanced age.[10] In a famous sermon preached in Constance in 1416, the theologian Jean Gerson, who was an early advocate of Joseph, openly criticized painters who represented Mary's spouse as being elderly. According to Gerson, if Joseph had been too old he would never have been able to defend the Virgin from the Jews' accusations of adultery and he would simply have been scorned.[11] Although the author concluded his sermon by saying that painters should not be condemned because they share the same freedom as poets,[12] his arguments were relayed by successive defenders of the saint's "youth": first by Isidoro de Isolani, who wrote the *Summa de donis sancti Joseph* (1522), then by Johannes Molanus in his *De Picturis et Imaginibus Sacris* (1570), which appeared in the wake of the Council of Trent. Recalling Gerson, Molanus writes that if Mary had a centenarian husband, her chastity would have been suspect because elderly men were known to be impotent and young women were reputed to be "naturally" lustful. In a chapter dedicated specifically to the representation of Joseph, Molanus also attacks painters for their own lechery, which made them think that only a centenarian husband, a man made impotent by age, would have been able to behave chastely with the Virgin.[13] Moreover, the author writes that painters were guilty for the saint's bad reputation because they represented him as a decrepit figure that was always leaning on his cane or lying on the floor and not paying attention to the baby.

In fact, derogatory or humorous representations of Joseph were common characteristics of his iconography, mainly in the period before Trent. This seems to have been the case with pictures like Hieronymus Bosch's *Adoration of the Magi* (c. 1470–1475) in the Metropolitan Museum of New York.[14] Another example is Frans Floris's *The Holy Family* (c. 1554) in the Musée de la Chartreuse in Douai (Fig. 7.3 and Plate 3).[15] In the Bosch painting, Joseph is depicted as a decrepit, white-haired man supporting himself on a cane. In the Floris picture, Joseph is shown with grotesque features, leering at his young and beautiful wife in an equivocal manner.[16] The real problem related to the

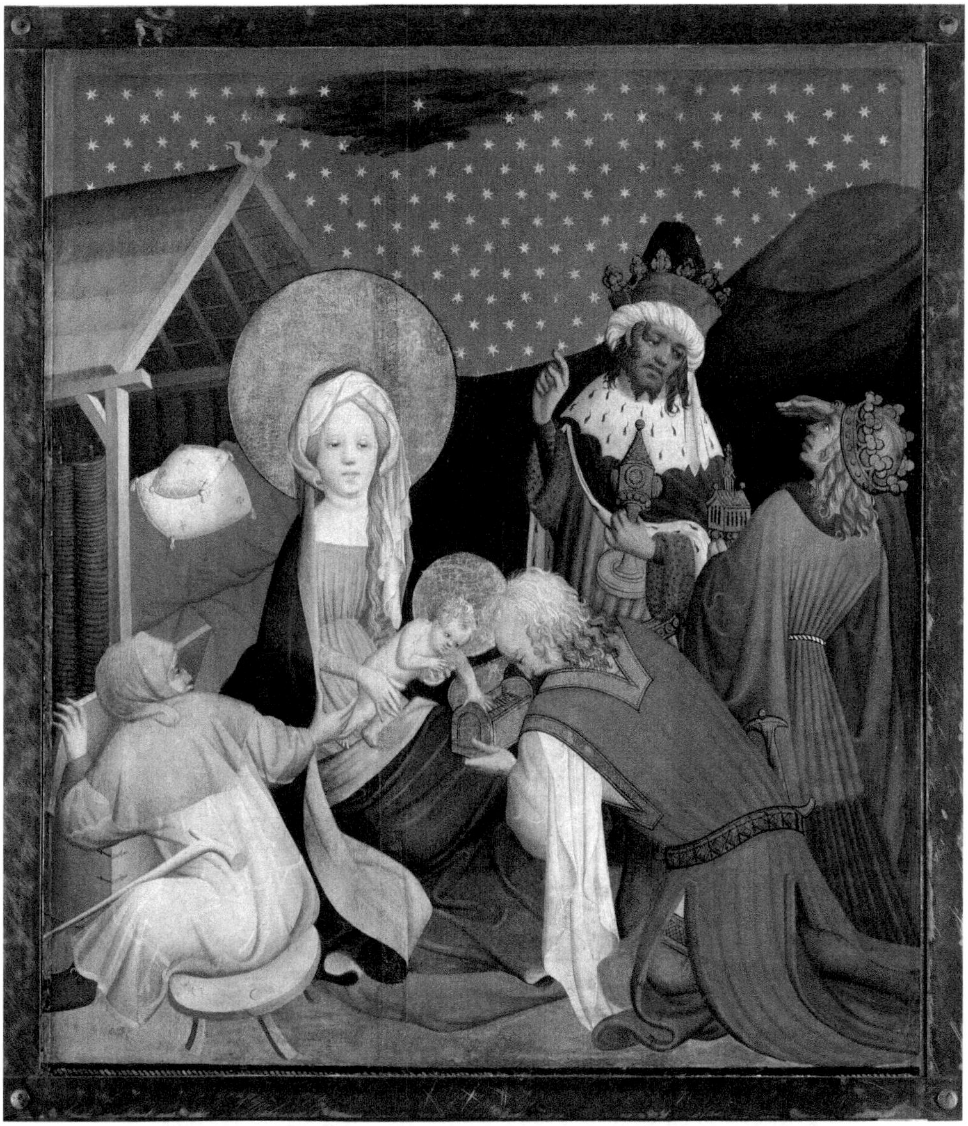

7.1 Master Francke, *Adoration of the Magi* fragment of the *Saint Thomas altar*, c. 1424, tempera on oak, 99 × 89.3 cm, Kunsthalle, Hamburg

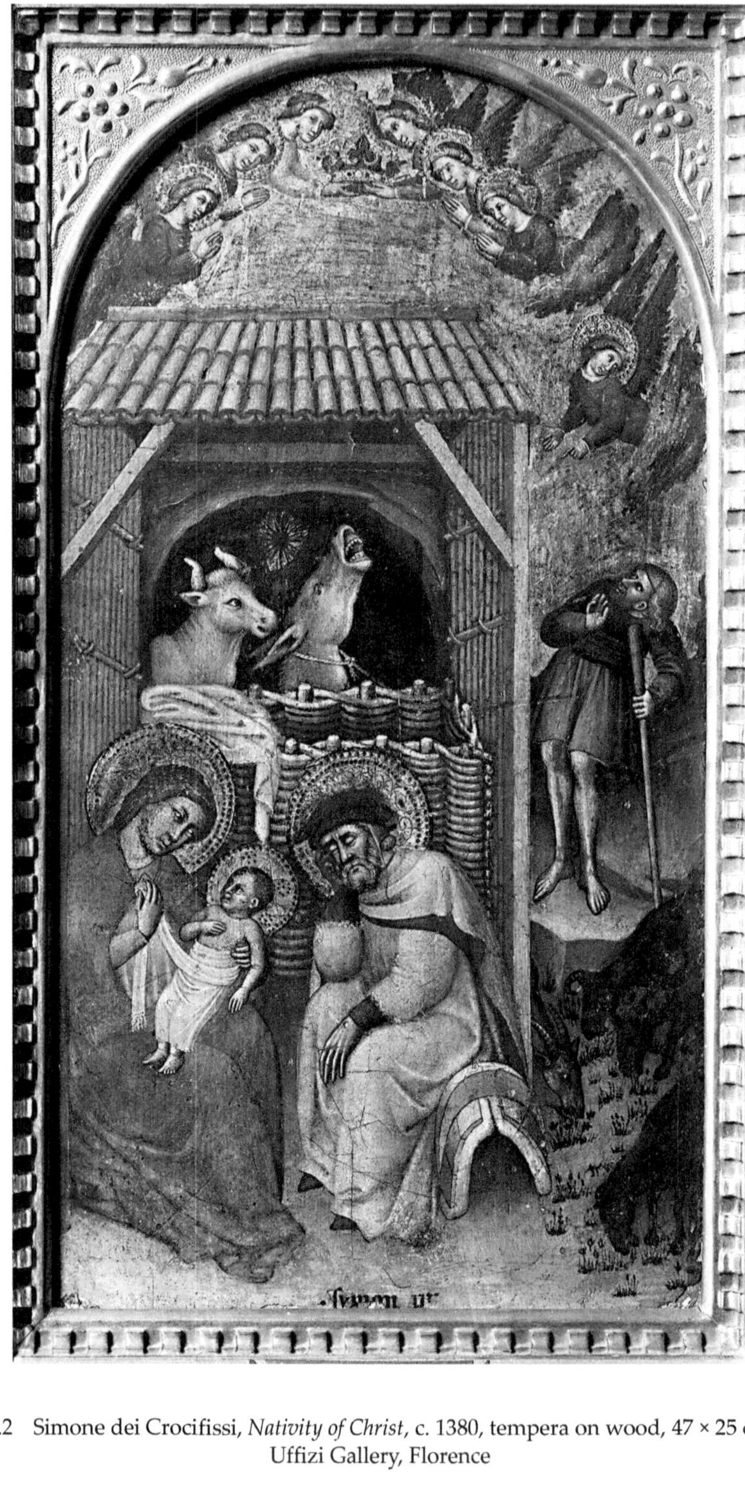

7.2 Simone dei Crocifissi, *Nativity of Christ*, c. 1380, tempera on wood, 47 × 25 cm, Uffizi Gallery, Florence

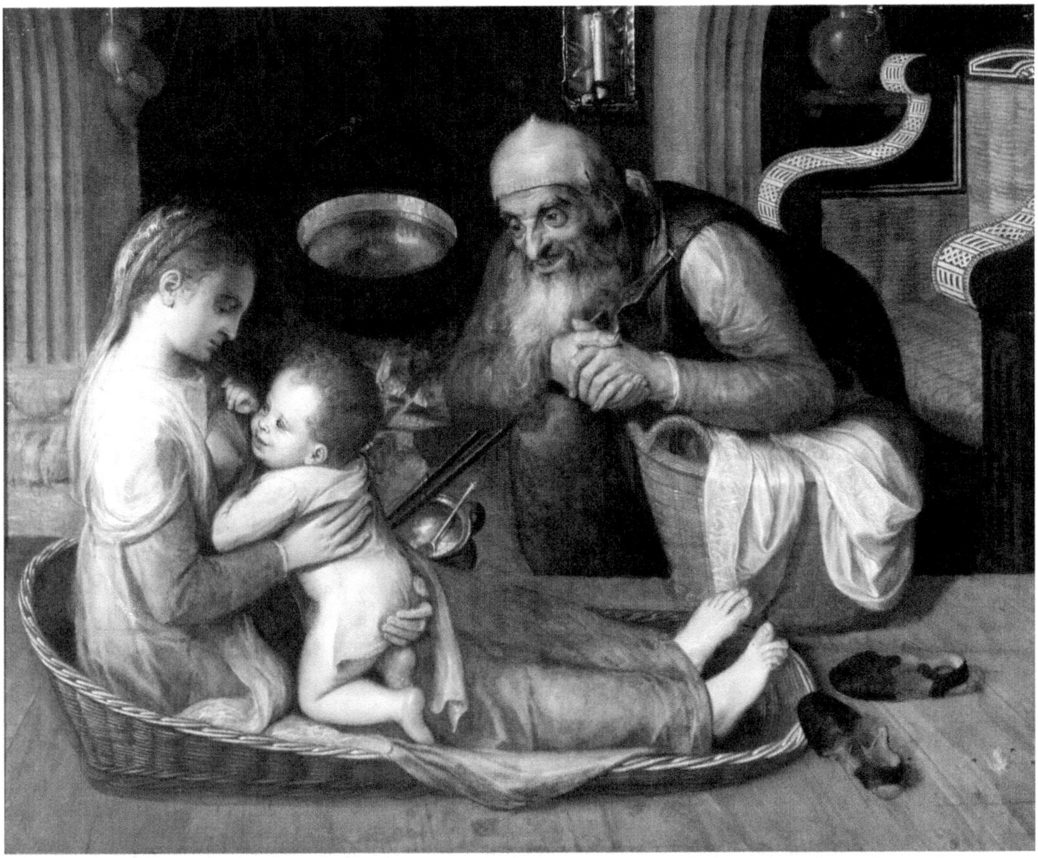

7.3 Frans Floris, *The Holy Family*, 16th century, oil on panel, 132 × 166 cm, Musée de la Chartreuse, Douai (inv. 2796) (photo: Hugo Maertens)

depiction of a geriatric figure was that it evoked the specter of cuckoldry and lechery. Elderly men who married beautiful young girls were major comic characters in Renaissance farces and comedies that embroidered upon the premise that jealous, libidinous and impotent husbands could not satisfy their younger wives, who would therefore easily succumb to younger and more handsome swains.[17]

Did the contemporary commonplaces regarding foolish old age compromise Joseph's reputation? The answer to this question lies in the apocryphal sources that were transposed to both visual culture and Miracle Plays. In these texts, Joseph is portrayed as an old man who is reluctant to marry a young virgin because he is afraid of becoming a laughing stock. In *The Proto-Gospel of James* (IX, 1–2), Joseph protests, saying: "I have sons and am an old man; she is but a child. I do not want to become a laughingstock to the sons of Israel."[18] In the French *Nativité de Notre Jésus Christ*, he appears to be afraid of the traditional *charivari* reserved to re-marrying widowers: "They are going to mock me and call me Sir Riquier [Riquier is a stock name for donkey]; I am ashamed of having come."[19] When Joseph learns about Mary's miraculous pregnancy, his worries inevitably assimilate him with the comic character of the elderly cuckold husband who is betrayed by his wife when he works away from home. In fact, after listening to Mary's account of the Annunciation, Joseph expresses doubts until one of God's messengers, an archangel, appears to reassure him. In *The Gospel of Pseudo-Matthew,* he thinks that archangel Gabriel is a young boy who has tricked his wife.[20] In *The Proto-Gospel of James,* he even wonders if the story of Adam is not repeating itself: "Who has preyed upon me? Who has done this wicked deed in my home and defiled the Virgin? Has not the entire history of Adam been summed up in me? For just as Adam was singing praise to God, when the serpent came and found Eve alone and led here astray, so too has this now happened to me."[21]

In the 15th century, irreverent and humorous representations of Joseph were widespread in liturgical drama—especially in France, Germany and England—and were also common in pictures.[22] The carpenter's working tools can convey allusions to his impotency and, given Mary's miraculous pregnancy, thereby imply his cuckoldry. This occurs, for example, on the right side of a panel painting by the Strasbourg master, dating from around 1482 (Fig. 7.4 and Plate 4). The scene takes place in a room separated into two spaces by a column. A visibly pregnant Mary is engaged in needlework, seated in a chair, while her husband, who seems on the point of leaving the room, is stopped by an angel. The divine messenger points at the Virgin's womb and looks directly at Joseph, reassuring him with the words (indecipherable) that appear on the *banderole.* As if the scene wasn't clear enough, the artist plays on the repetition of a single detail in order to make the subject of Joseph's doubt more evident. While a sheathed knife is hanging from the carpenter's belt, right behind a purse,[23] another knife, in Mary's room, is stuck upright into the wooden table in a rather phallic way. The details of this image symbolically underscore the source of Joseph's anxiety and play on his auxiliary role: aware of his own impotency, he is being informed about who did the job in his place.[24]

Such visual allusions and puns often enhance theological content. In the *Flight from Egypt* of the Master of Frankfurt (1503–1506, Staatsgalerie, Stuttgart), and in a representation of the same subject painted by the Master of 1518 (National Gallery of London), the cradle that Joseph carries on his back (in the first) or the bundles that hang on either side of a stick slung over his shoulder (in the second) could have easily been read in a comic vein.[25] This is certainly the case of the picture representing *Joseph's Repentance of his Doubt* in the Stedelijk Ostmuseum in Hoogstraten,[26] where the giant instruments attached to the carpenter's belt and lying on the floor make fun of his lack of sexual potency. In an *Annunciation* by the Master of the View of Sainte Gudule, today in the Musées Royaux des Beaux-Arts in Brussels (Fig. 7.5), Joseph is shown in the upper background, leaving his home and carrying a huge saw on his back.[27] Here, the sexual belittlement of the saint is not only related to the size of the saw and motion (when used) of such a tool, but is also reinforced by a statue of a horned Moses which decorates the door through which Gabriel enters the Virgin's house. While the statue alludes ostensibly

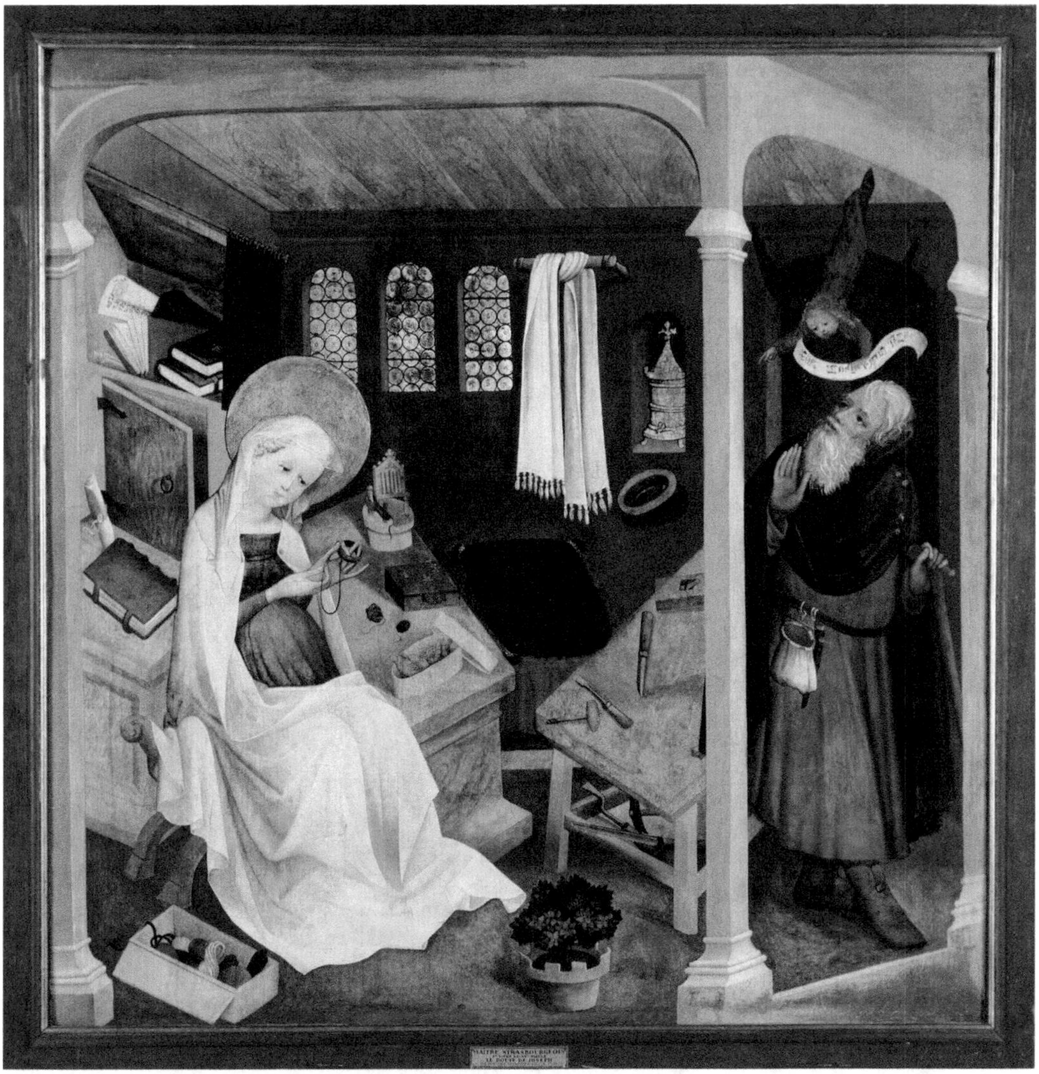

7.4 Strasbourg artist, *Joseph's Doubts*, c. 1482, Musée de l'Œuvre Notre-Dame, Strasbourg (© Musée de l'Œuvre Notre-Dame de Strasbourg) (photo: N. Fussler)

to the passage from the Old Era to the New Era through the Incarnation of Jesus, Moses's horns also underscore the implications of an elderly husband leaving his home and a handsome young angel entering his wife's room.[28] In the background, Joseph is walking next to a small closed garden in which there is a huge fountain with a very allusive shape. This fountain is not just any fountain but recalls the famous *Font dels Pissaïres* in the center of Lacaune in the Pyrenees (completed 1559), which features four small statues of men urinating with disproportionate phalluses. In the painting, the image of this fountain works as a metonym for the Virgin's fertility, but placed right next to the husband it also highlights his impotence (and cuckoldry).[29] In fact, both the phallic fountain and the horned statue function as an ironic—even humorous—commentary on the married couple.

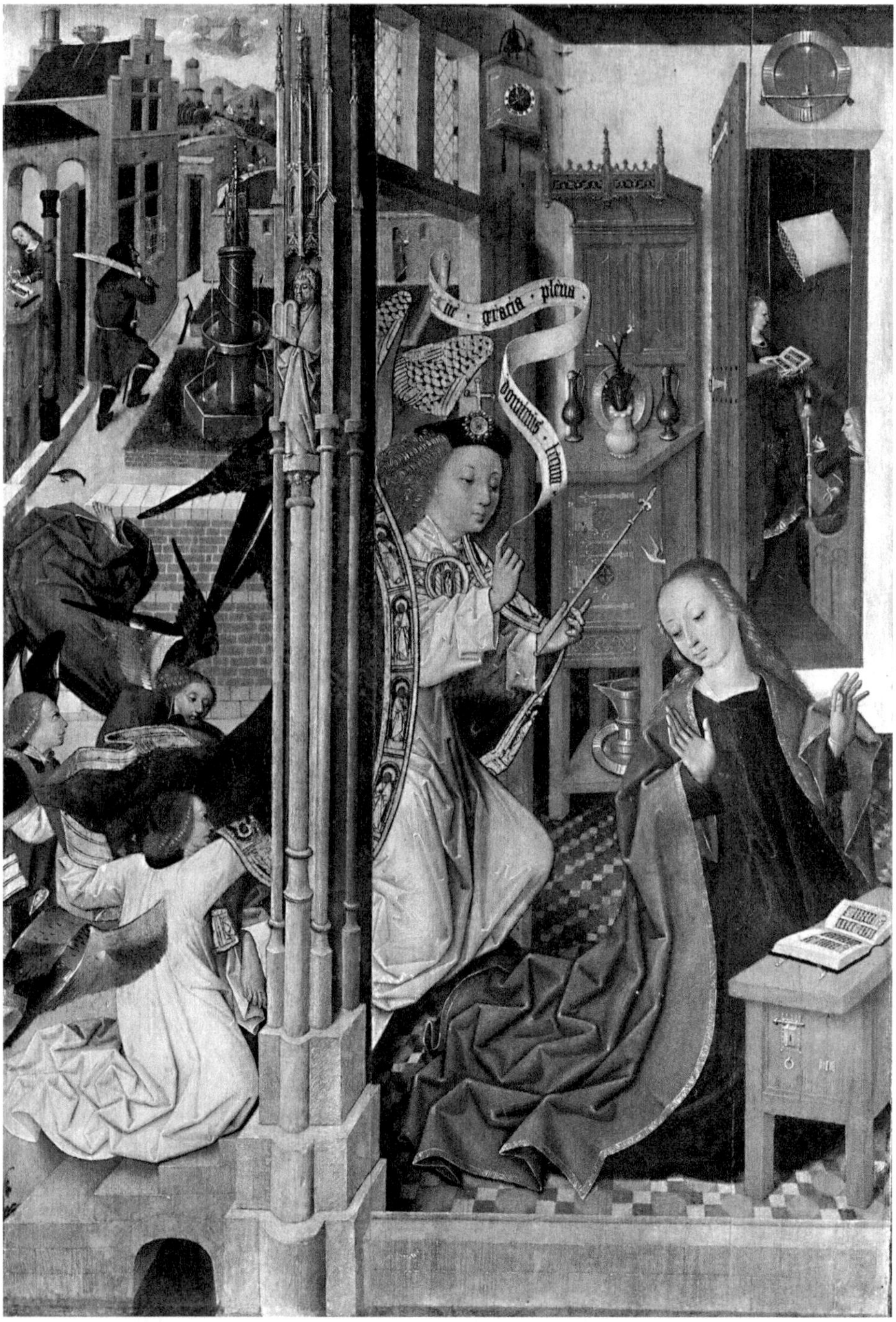

7.5 Master of the View of Sainte-Gudule, *Annunciation*, c. 1480, Musées Royaux des Beaux-Arts, Brussels (© Musée Royaux des Beaux-Arts de Belgique, Bruxelles, photo: Institut royal du Patrimoine artistique)

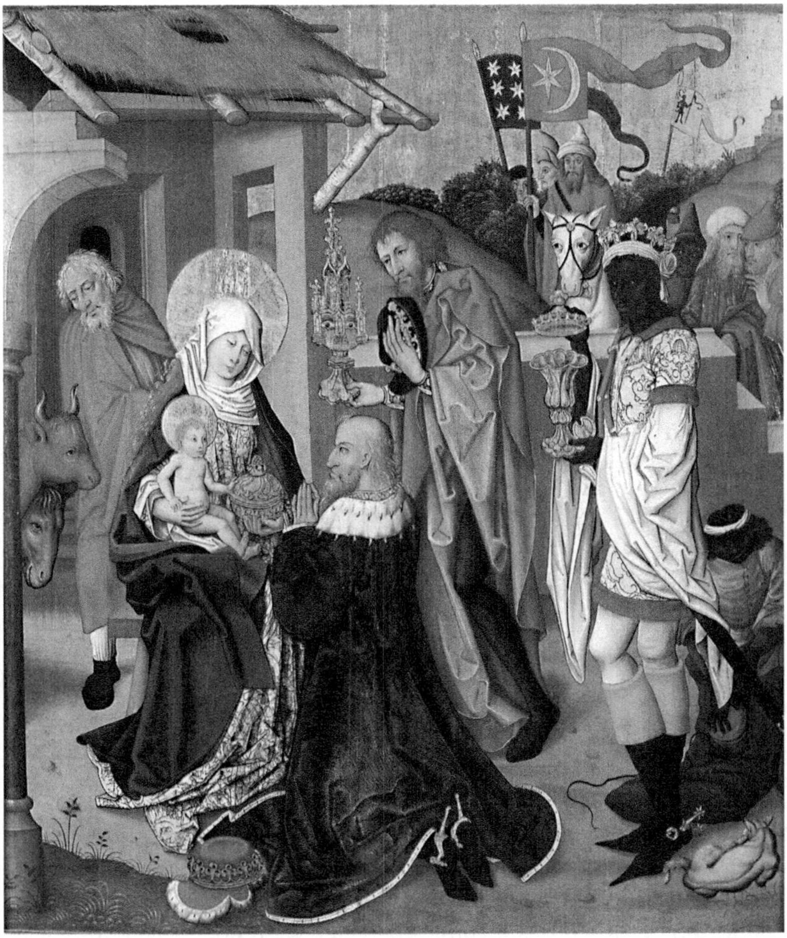

7.6 Artist of the School of Schongauer, *Adoration of the Magi*, c. 1475, Musée d'Unterlinden, Colmar (© Musée Unterlinden, Colmar, France)

Other comic references, such as horned cattle, hens and cocks, were often placed in proximity to Joseph, as can be seen in an *Adoration of the Magi* attributed to an artist of the School of Schongauer, where the carpenter is pictured contemplating the ox's horns while the Magi are paying homage to the Virgin and her son (Fig. 7.6 and Plate 5).[30] It would be rash, however, to interpret these details as a derogatory allusion to the satirical tradition of the willing cuckold, which would certainly not have been appropriate for a saint.[31] On the contrary, by picturing Joseph as God's cuckold, artists underscored the saint's willing acceptance of his role in the history of Salvation. Like Moses, Joseph is *cornutus* because he carries out God's plan. In fact, although Moses's horns made of light had nothing to do with cuckoldry, this did not prevent people from calling him or thinking of him as a *cornutus*. An example of this convention may be found in Gabriel Chappuis Tourangeau's *Monde des cornuz*, written in appendage to the French translation of Anton Francesco Doni's *I Mondi e gli inferni* (1580). In the *Monde des cornuz*, several characters humorously discuss the origins, the types and the effects of horns. Thus, the

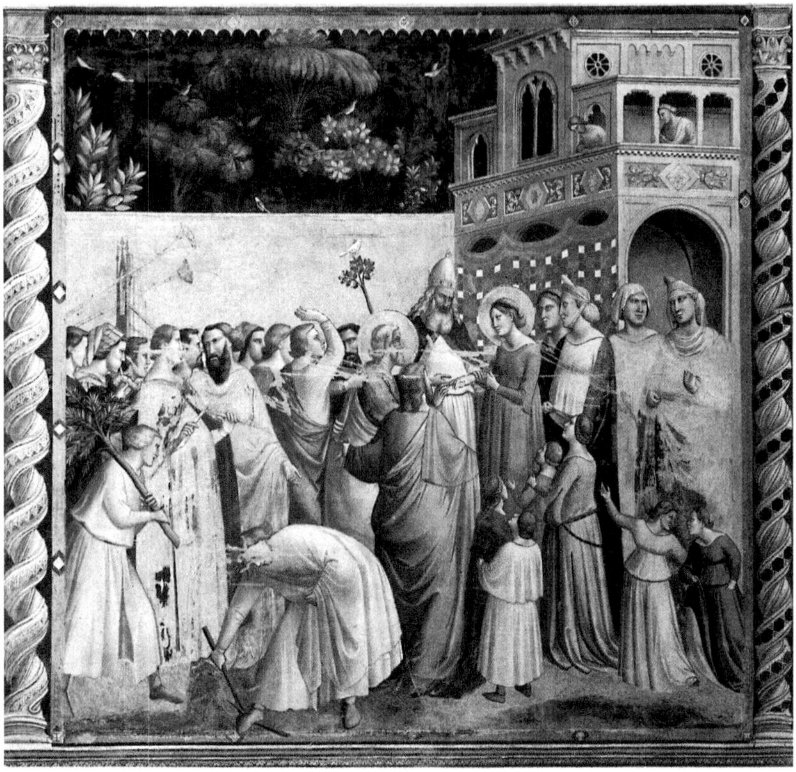

7.7 Taddeo Gaddi, *Marriage of the Virgin*, c. 1328–1330, fresco, Florence, Santa Croce, Baroncelli Chapel

horns of Moses are singled out as an example of dignity and divine favor: "Moses was a good man & lived in the fear of God, his acts were horned in as much as they followed God's will."[32]

Depictions of Joseph as a comic character were not specific to Northern countries. In reference to Giotto's frescos at the Arena Chapel, for example, Andrew Ladis recalls an amusing novella from Franco Sacchetti's *Il Trecentonovelle* which suggests how both the artist and his public may have perceived Mary's husband. In this tale, some of Giotto's friends ask him why this saint is always represented with a melancholic demeanor. Giotto answers: "Why shouldn't he be [melancholy], when he sees his wife is pregnant and he doesn't know by whom?"[33] Ladis connected this kind of humor, which plays on the themes of cuckoldry and impotency, to other, later pictures, such as Taddeo Gaddi's *Marriage of the Virgin* in the Baroncelli chapel at Santa Croce in Florence (Fig. 7.7 and Plate 6).[34] Here, the light-hearted representation of the episode recalls the traditional *mattinata* (charivari or rough music) in which relatives, neighbors and friends celebrated a newlywed couple by making noise, playing loud music and shouting indecencies.[35] Moreover, the artist underscores the saint's age and impotence, not only by contrasting Joseph's elderly physique with that of the young men present, but also by picturing a young man entering the scene with a branch that is much larger than the one held by the holy carpenter. The betrothed does not seem very enthusiastic about his engagement and has to be encouraged by several men who push him and slap his back, engaging in a ritual gesture that has been studied by Christiane Klapisch Zuber.[36] Gaddi here gives an anecdotal character to the earthly marriage ceremony, probably in contrast to the heavenly ceremony between Mary and Christ in the *Coronation of the Virgin* polyptych by Giotto and his assistants, located on the altar of the same chapel.

Joseph as *Pater Familias*

To ignore or underestimate the allusions to Joseph's cuckoldry in the 15th and 16th centuries is to risk neglecting the importance of this figure in pictures representing the mystery of the Incarnation. Joseph's role in the history of Salvation was clear: his marriage to the Virgin was to protect her from scandal and accusations of adultery resulting from signs of her approaching motherhood.[37] But at the same time, especially in pictures, it was important for Joseph's presence not to sow any doubt concerning the miraculous nature of the conception of Jesus. This double perspective is perfectly embodied by the figure of Joseph in the *Mérode Altarpiece* (1490) by Robert Campin (the Master of Flémalle) at the Cloisters Museum in New York (Fig. 7.8 and Plate 7). It is usually assumed that the mousetrap on the edge of the window, represented in the right wing of the triptych, stands as a metaphor of Christ's Incarnation and Death, which served as a type of bait to vanquish the devil.[38] As Meyer Schapiro first noticed, this use of the metaphor of the mousetrap appears several times in Saint Augustine's sermons on redemption.[39] Without diminishing this interpretation, it is also possible that, in the iconographic economy of the picture, this domestic object and its theological symbolism also refer to Joseph's role in the mystery of Incarnation. Panofsky pointed out

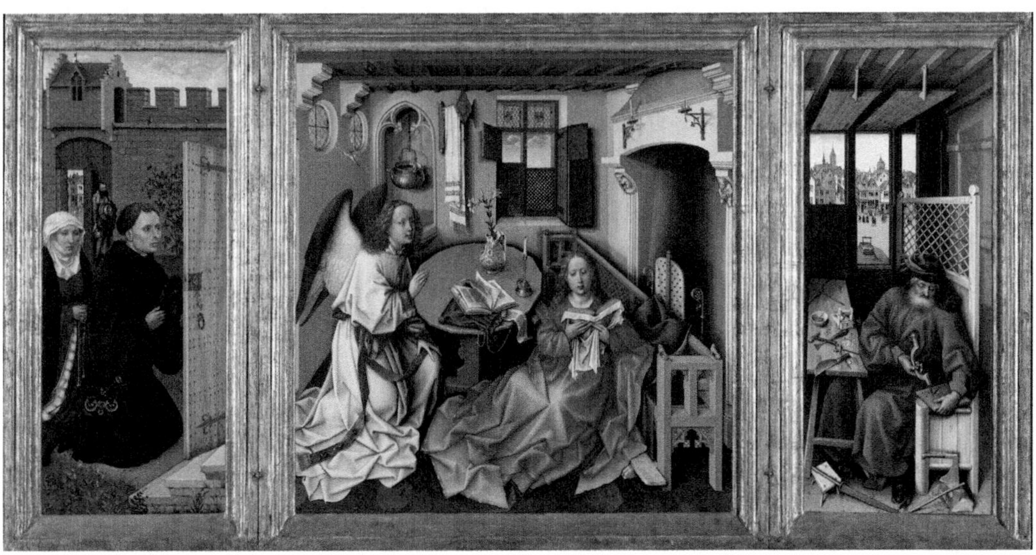

7.8 Master of Flémalle (Robert Campin), *The Mérode Altarpiece*, c. 1427, oil on wood, 64.5 × 27 cm; 64 × 63 cm; 64.5 × 28 cm, The Metropolitan Museum of Art, The Cloisters Collection, New York [1956 (56.70)]

that the object being built by Joseph is probably a *chauferrette*, an instrument used for keeping the feet warm, which underscores Joseph's protective role. Several scholars have noticed that the carpenter's action of piercing holes in a piece of wood was also a well-known erotic metaphor of sexual intercourse, which in this case contrasts amusingly and somewhat wryly with Joseph's impotency and his non-involvement with Mary's pregnancy.[40] Nonetheless, by his presence here, next to the Annunciation,[41] the husband—like a mousetrap—protects the contents of Mary's womb from the devil that might have snatched (like a mouse) the tiny *homunculus* entering the Virgin's room through a closed window. As Shapiro recalls, Joseph's role was also to deceive Satan with respect to the divine plan of redemption.[42] During the Late Middle Ages, Joseph was considered a guardian of the mystery of Incarnation, since thanks to him the devil did not suspect the supernatural origin of Christ.

In Christian literature, Joseph, "the first witness of Incarnation,"[43] was often likened to a shield because he protected the Virgin and her child.[44] While certain authors made fun of his abnegation, evoking the *topos* of the henpecked husband,[45] artists also introduced allusions to the husband's jealousy into their pictures. This would seem to be the case in Giovanni da Asola's *Adoration of the Shepherds* (Fig. 7.9), painted in 1518, and in Titian's *Holy Family with Shepherd* (c. 1510), now at the National Gallery in London: in both cases, Joseph is portrayed giving a warning look to young shepherds, who appear far more interested in admiring the Virgin than in greeting the child.[46] Although this situation may have amused viewers—especially the details such as the forked stick held by Joseph in the painting by Titian, a visual reference to the cuckold's horns—it would certainly not have detracted from the theological message or the devotional function of the painting. Joseph is rightfully protecting his family, and the juxtaposition between the elderly father and the youthful shepherd(s) would surely have attracted the viewer's attention, conveying an admonitory message for all *patres familias*.

In his book *Redeeming Laughter*, Peter L. Berger points out how humor is omnipresent in ordinary people's lives and in everyday experience.[47] By laughing at visual references to Joseph's cuckoldry, spectators might have also recognized the implications of the dogma of Incarnation, which was not always easy to explain pictorially. Humor in this case was not simply a fundamental means to engage the viewer's attention, but also a way to facilitate the interpretation of the scene.[48] In religious images, Joseph represented a link between the sacred world, as represented in the picture space, and the real world, in which the viewers lived. His ridiculed figure thus functioned as a metaphor of man's imperfect and sinful condition before the birth of Jesus, while his acceptance to play a part in the history of Salvation served as a model for worshipers to follow.

Art historians often tend to deny the existence or downplay the importance of ridiculous elements in sacred pictures, as if humor were frivolous and thus reduced the gravity of the painting's theological content. Such an attitude neglects the essential function of comic tropes in visual rhetoric. Christian

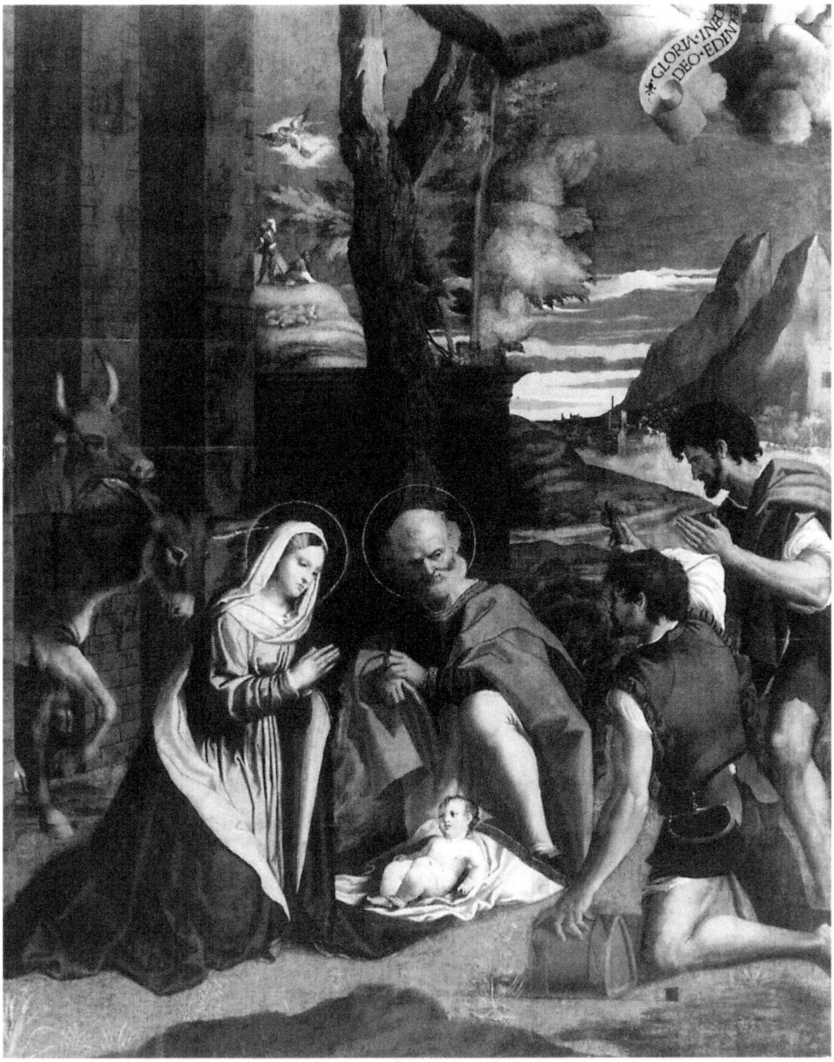

7.9 Giovanni da Asola, *Adoration of the Shepherds*, c. 1516–1520, oil on panel, 280 × 190 cm, Asola, Sant'Andrea Cathedral

believers were repeatedly exposed to humor during homilies, public sermons and sacred representations. Preachers exploited it in their sermons in order to keep the public awake and attentive, or to help their audience better memorize the content of their speeches.[49] Christian authors since Thomas Aquinas celebrated the Aristotelian virtue of *eutrapelia* but condemned the type of raucous laughter (*cum cacchinis*) provoked by mimes and buffoons.[50] Yet, at Eastertime preachers and priests acted as *geloiasés* (buffoons) to make devotees participate, through laughter (*risus paschalis*), in Christ's joyful resurrection,[51] and humorous sexual allusions and metaphors were used to recall the salvific dimension of Incarnation.[52] The comic persona of Joseph played an important role in the theology of Incarnation as it was able to communicate basic doctrine to a large public that was not particularly acquainted with religious matters.

In his *Discorso sopra le immagini sacre e profane*, published in 1582, Gabriele Paleotti invites artists to paint pictures that can satisfy *idioti* (illiterates), who are "the majority of the population, for whose service sacred paintings were principally introduced."[53] He urges painters to use their inventiveness in order to attract the attention of this kind of public, but also to be careful not to represent obscenities or sinful behavior in their pictures.[54] The cardinal's concern is typical of the Counter Reformation attitude towards images, which inevitably influenced the depiction of Joseph and brought about his "rejuvenation," thus rehabilitating the apocryphal version of his biblical figure and admitting him to the pantheon of saints.[55]

Vulcan: a Classical Parallel with the Christian Joseph

The counterpart of Joseph in classical mythology is the god Vulcan, whose far more explicit jealousy and cuckoldry were renowned even in Antiquity.[56] During the Renaissance, these two traditions of celebrated cuckolds reinforced each other. Vasvari is the only author, to my knowledge, who has pointed out a similarity between Joseph and Vulcan: she compared the carpenter's suggestive drilling in the *Mérode Triptych* (c. 1427) to the blacksmith banging on his anvil next to Venus and Mars in a print engraved in 1543 by Enea Vico (Fig. 7.10).[57]

In Vico's engraving, the image of the blacksmith preparing links for a net to catch the adulterous lovers was particularly allusive as it had two sexual connotations: the rhythmic hammering of the anvil and the reference to the well-known use of "nets" used to entrap lovers in late medieval and Renaissance iconography.[58] The display of Vulcan's physical prowess in the

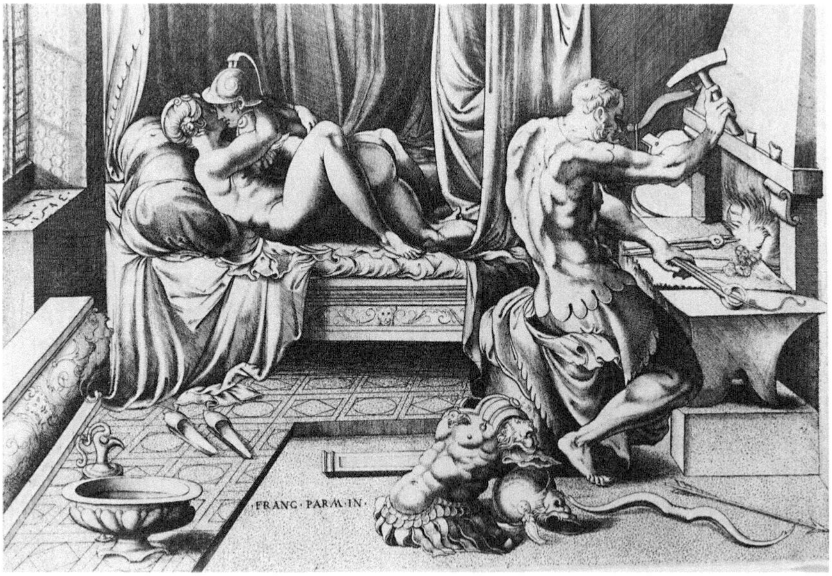

7.10 Enea Vico (after Parmigianino), *Venus and Mars with Vulcan*, 1543, engraving, 20.6 × 37.6 cm, The British Museum, London (© The Trustees of the British Museum)

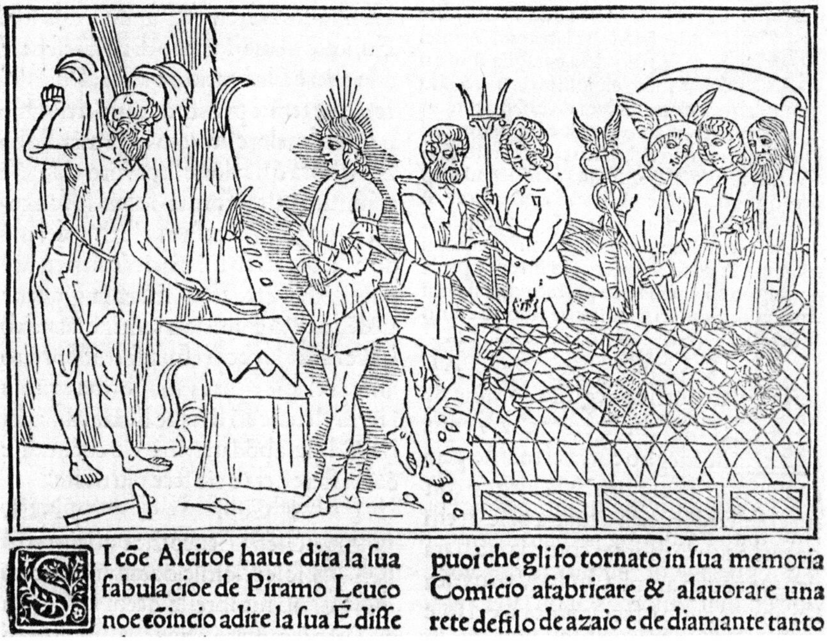
S
I cōe Alcitoe haue dita la ſua
fabula cioe de Piramo Leuco
noe cōincio adire la ſua E diſſe
puoi che gli fo tornato in ſua memoria
Comício afabricare & alauorare una
rete defilo de azaio e de diamante tanto

7.11 Attributed to Jacob of Strasbourg, "Revelation of Venus's adultery by Apollo and Vulcan's subsequent capture of the couple," Giovanni Bonsignori, *Ovidio metamorphoseos vulgare* (Lucantonio Giunta, Venezia, 1497 [second edition 1501, IIII–XXVIII]), woodcut, 29.7 × 20.3 cm, The Metropolitan Museum of Art, New York, Rogers Fund, 1922 (22.16) (© The Metropolitan Museum of Art)

forge metaphorically echoes the scene of amorous concourse being carried out behind him, and thus, once again, serves as a reminder of the cuckolded husband's impotence in the sexual arena. As the Venetian satirical poet Andrea Calmo wrote in a letter: "Mars at the sound of Vulcan's hammering was piercing the pearls of his wife Venus."[59]

With regard to Vulcan's cuckoldry, various iconographic conventions are to be found in Renaissance art. One of these is the type of composition popularized by a woodcut in Giovanni Bonsignori's *Ovidio metamorphoseos vulgare* (1497), which shows both the revelation of the adultery by Apollo and Vulcan's subsequent capture of the couple, shown here (Fig. 7.11).[60] Another convention featured the blacksmith working next to Venus and her son with tools (hammer, anvil, tongs) similar to those of the Holy carpenter working next to the Virgin and Child (hammer, worktable, tongs). In such scenes, artists often introduced allusions to cuckoldry. Palma Giovane's painting at the Staatliche Museen in Kassel, for example, shows Venus suggestively embracing Cupid while Vulcan works in his forge. Similarly, in a drawing by Agostino Carracci (in her Majesty's collection in London), Venus seductively gazes towards the viewer while her husband is hammering the anvil and her son looks bored.[61] As in representations of the Holy family, some painters also arranged the mythological trio into the image of a nuclear family. This is the case of a drawing after Parmigianino[62] and of an intimate family scene by Tintoretto at Palazzo Pitti in Florence (Fig. 7.12 and Plate 8). In such compositions, Venus, Vulcan and Cupid are shown lying outdoors in a tranquil landscape in attitudes similar to those of Joseph, Mary and

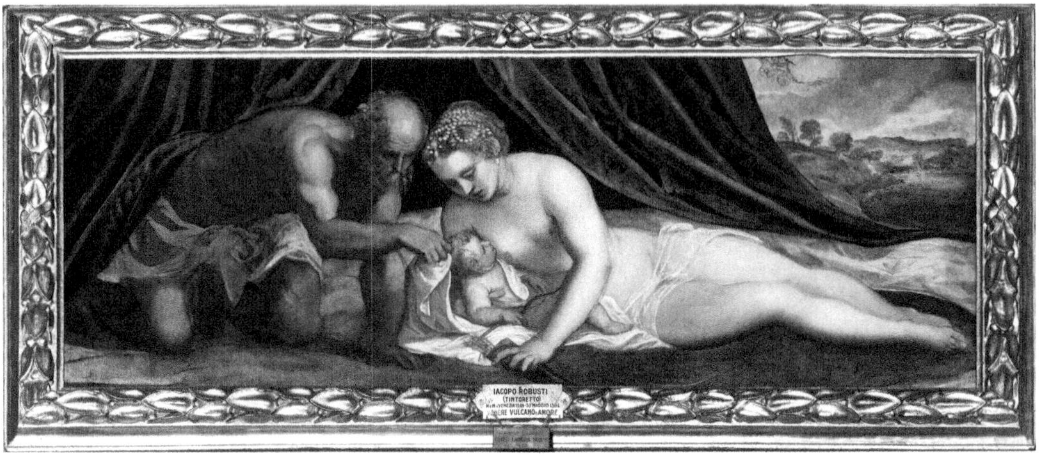

7.12 Tintoretto, *Venus, Vulcan and Cupid*, c. 1550–1552, oil on canvas, 85 × 197.4 cm, Galleria Palatina, Palazzo Pitti, Florence (photo: Polo Museale di Firenze)

Jesus resting on the flight into Egypt.[63] Nevertheless, the idyllic grouping in Tintoretto's painting is disturbed by the appearance of Apollo's chariot in the sky, a presage of the future development of the story and a reminder, to the viewer, that Vulcan is about to have an unpleasant surprise.[64]

Influences between the two traditions worked both ways. It is very likely that some of the images picturing the blacksmith while he is preparing Cupid's or Aeneas's weapons[65] inspired depictions of Joseph shown working with wood next to Jesus and Mary.[66] The two husbands were, in fact, counterparts: not only did they share similar narrative roles, but in many paintings their images were used as doubles of the artist at work.[67]

Vulcan's Doubts: Tintoretto and the Venetian Artistic Context

Tintoretto's *Vulcan surprising Venus and Mars* (c. 1545–1551)[68] at the Alte Pinakothek in Munich (Fig. 7.13 and Plate 9) represents another iconographic equation between Joseph and Vulcan.[69] Tintoretto probably painted this picture after having visited Mantua, where he saw Giulio Romano's fresco, *Jupiter and Olympia* (which inspired his depiction of Venus),[70] and Michelangelo's statue, *Sleeping Cupid* (echoed by the reclining Cupid).[71] The painting clearly does not represent either Vulcan's discovery or his capture of the adulterous couple,[72] but rather a scene located in a contemporary room, a bedroom or more likely a Venetian *anticamera* with an improvised square bed, probably a *lettuccio*. The crippled husband places a knee on his wife's bed and from this awkward position inspects her genitals, attentively lifting the cloth that is covering them. Venus allows her husband to proceed, pulling a light and transparent sheet over her head. Tintoretto makes fun of the husband's curiosity by portraying him in the same position of a satyr discovering a sleeping nymph.[73] Like these half-human, half-animal figures,[74] Vulcan is *cornuto* (horned) but also *beffato* (mocked) because the view of his wife's *pudenda* arouses his desire and distracts him from his jealous search.[75] His blinding passion is also underscored by

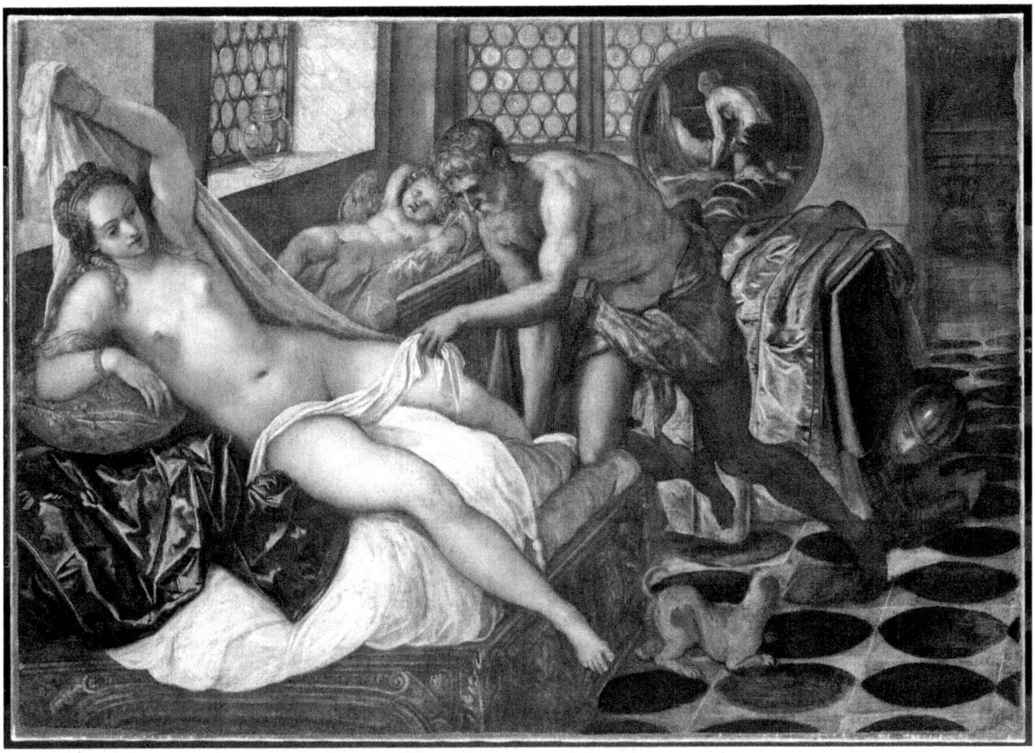

7.13 Tintoretto, *Vulcan surprising Venus and Mars*, c. 1548, oil on canvas, 135 × 198 cm, Munich, Alte Pinakothek (inv. 9257) (photo: Bayerische Staatsgemäldesammlungen, Alte Pinakothek München)

the presence of Cupid, legendary master of deception.[76] Lying with his eyes closed and in a position that recalls that of his mother, Cupid holds an arrow entangled in a veil. The arrow points to the area of his mother's anatomy that is also the object of the blacksmith's gaze.[77] In the meantime, right next to the couple and hidden under the table with only his head sticking out, Mars is waiting for the right moment to escape, pointing at the door from which the jealous husband has just entered.

Tintoretto's contemporaries might easily have associated the proof of adultery sought by Vulcan with a literal *macchio all'honestà* (stain on [her] honor). Adultery was commonly designated as a *macchia* (stain) in trials and archive documentation, and some years after the painting's execution a Venetian law stated that only women who lived *modestamente e senza macchio all'honestà* could marry noble members of the city.[78] Purity and the importance of any stain are social conventions clearly evoked by Vulcan's explicit search. In such an erotic painting, the *macchia* would have surely been perceived also as a more explicit kind of stain, such as the one left by the *coitus* of a young man on Praxiteles's *Aphrodite of Cnidus*.[79] The importance of the *macchia* sought by the husband in this picture should not be underestimated as Tintoretto has also included a transparent glass vase placed on the window ledge above Cupid, on which a spot of light is reflected. This object, which has been interpreted as a parody of a Marian metaphor,[80] needs to be examined more carefully since it provides a key to the picture as a whole. In sacred pictures, glass windows and vases penetrated by rays of light were often used as visual references to Mary's virginity and the mystery by which she remained immaculate although impregnated. Derived from Saint Bernard,[81] this metaphor was also popular among Venetian artists and poets. Titian used it in his *Annunciation* in the church of San Salvatore in Venice, and Pietro Aretino referred to it in a poem dedicated to the King of France, François I: "Oh Virgin after the sweet birth and always / Like solid glass through which the sun enters and exits/ and which remains whole inside and out, / I will praise you with simple words."[82]

Looking carefully at Tintoretto's painting, the white spot of light on the glass vase shares a close resemblance to a white reflection on Mars's helmet.[83] The two reflections are painted in the same way, they are situated on the same plane, behind the suspicious husband, and they are both pointed out by two secondary figures: Cupid and the barking dog.[84] With simple details such as white *macchie*, Tintoretto amusingly associates the *signum* of God's passage through Mary's womb to the presence of Mars in Venus's room and in her body. In both cases, the women are left without a stain: *sine macula*. Mary, of course, remained a virgin, while in the case of Venus, Vulcan's sudden arrival prevented the lovers from full consummation.

The parody of the light-through-glass metaphor of the Incarnation here has another meaning: the light that reveals the invisible presence of the incarnated Word in many Annunciation paintings penetrates into the lover's room to expose an adulterous deity. The invisible presence of God, indicated by a ray of sun, becomes the equivalent of the adulterous lover hidden under the table. Only a small dog, emblem of marital fidelity, can perceive what is going on. The animal barks at the god of war, now prone on the floor, his helmet picked out by a telltale beam of light that creates a small reflection, a *macchia di luce* (spot of light). Described by Stacius as "shining as if it were burning like fiery lightning,"[85] Mars's helmet here becomes a burlesque attribute.

The irreverent reference to Mary's immaculate virginity could have hardily passed unnoticed to an attentive viewer acquainted with sermons and religious imagery, while the reclining position of Cupid, sleeping under the vase, recalls conventional images of the infant Jesus.[86] Parodies of the mystery of the Incarnation and farces that satirized the story of the Annunciation were not rare in this period.[87] Moreover, it is difficult to believe that in a city like Venice, consecrated to the Virgin and often associated with Venus, such parodies would have gone unnoticed.

In a recent article, Zorach formulated the hypothesis that this triangular love story refers directly to the Venetian artistic world and to the competition between Titian and Tintoretto: "Mars represents Tintoretto, the young and fierce artist, while Vulcan stands for his older rival. The bearded god looks very much like some of the self-portraits of the artist. Therefore, the scene could be interpreted as the dramatic competition for the possession of beauty, with Titian in the part of Vulcan, Tintoretto in that of Mars and the *Venus of Urbino* in that of Venus."[88] This hypothesis calls for further exploration.

When Tintoretto made his appearance on the artistic scene, the two main criticisms against him dealt with his *prestezza* (the speed of his artistic production),[89] and with the way he left visible brushstrokes on the canvas—*pennellate galiarde, colpi e macchie* (vigorous brushstrokes, strokes and stains).[90] In a letter written by Aretino in April, 1548, the poet, who had previously congratulated the artist for his wonderful work, warns him not to paint too rapidly.[91] Some years later Ludovico Dolce, another close friend of Titian, writes in his *Dialogo della pittura intitolato l'Aretino* (1557) that certain artists (implying Tintoretto), who have the habit of *macchiare sgarbatamente una tela, o un legno d'un ritratto,* want to be regarded as great masters and think they can surpass Raphael, Michelangelo and Titian.[92]

It is not surprising that Tintoretto answered these malicious attacks with a comic painting challenging the most famous painter of Venus in Venice. The stains (*macchie*) he painted on his canvas, invisible to the elderly Vulcan, implicitly associate him with the rascally young warrior, whose promptness allowed him to escape from the husband's fury. Quite a few Renaissance *novelle,* in fact, describe wives who cheat on their husbands with the "brush" (penis) of young painters.[93] Furthermore, making fun of Vulcan's reaction to his wife's *dolce prospettiva,* Tintoretto explicitly scorned artists who, like Titian,[94] painted pictures to arouse the sexual desire of their patrons.[95]

In her study of the replicas of Titian's erotic paintings, Maria Loh has shown how such paintings where part of a game of one-upmanship, in which the winner was the owner of the most sensuous image.[96] The comic misogyny of Tintoretto's painting ridicules this practice. A couple of documents confirm the competitive context in which this picture was painted. The first is a letter written by Aretino to his friend Jacopo Sansovino in April, 1548, right after he had composed a critical commentary on Tintoretto's *Miracle of the Slave* (Venice: Gallerie dell'Accademia).[97] In this letter, the poet explicitly evokes the painterly competition in which Tintoretto is engaged and says that the young artist, thanks to his *inuentione* (inventiveness), is "close to the prize [*palio*]."[98] The second document is a letter written by the same author to Giovanni Boccamanza, the secretary of the count Bevilacqua, in January 1549, Aretino complains about Titian's overreaction in a dispute with Tintoretto and argues that Titian's behavior is not suitable for a man of his age.[99] The letter does not give any clue about what provoked the elderly painter's anger, nevertheless, the derogatory nickname that Aretino uses for Tintoretto—"Tintorello"—conveys the attitude of disdain that Titian's circle had adopted against the young painter. Might Tintoretto's painting have something to do with this professional rivalry?

In 1548, the Venetian poet Andrea Calmo wrote a facetious *encomium* whose purpose was to defend Tintoretto's *far presto* (speed) against malign and envious critics.[100] Calmo published this piece in a collection of letters entitled *il Rimanente de le pacevole et ingegnose littere,* which also contains a narrative on the *Venus, Vulcan and Mars* story that is close to the scene depicted by Tintoretto. In Calmo's version of the mythological tale, Mars escapes because

Venus protects him. The crippled husband is unable to catch the lovers, for he is too slow, and throws his hammer in their direction. Instead of hitting Mars, however, the weapon strikes Venus, and breaks into two pieces. The fable becomes an etiological explanation for the word *martello,* an expression used by Venetians to refer to passionate love, *"che dà martello al cuore"* (that hammers the heart). In this mythological episode, the hammer refers both to Mars (his name in Italian is *Marte*) and to Vulcan (because the hammer is his tool). The object also has a sexual meaning, which plays on the symbolism of the head of the hammer, called *occhio del martèlo* (the eye of the hammer), the suggestive form of its grip, and the repetitious motion it requires in use.[101] This publication might simply be coincidental or it might help to date Tintoretto's painting of *Venus, Vulcan and Mars* closer to 1548: Tintoretto may have found inspiration in Calmo's text, or the other way around. At any rate, in the vibrant literary and artistic context of 16th-century Venice, the *beffa* (joke) orchestrated against Vulcan on canvas would have easily been recognized as an amusing answer of the young painter to criticisms and unflattering comparisons with Titian.[102] By associating Vulcan with Titian, Tintoretto cleverly compares the "blinding" passion that tricks the husband with the (impotent) envy of the elder artist.

With his figurative *beffa,* Tintoretto not only challenged his major rival in Venice, but through the quotation of the *Sleeping Cupid* he also referred to Michelangelo. The large, round mirror or shield in the background — an emblem of the deceptive power of art to imitate nature — suggests yet another reading of the picture in terms of the current *paragone* debate opposing the art of painting to the art of sculpture. Whereas the picture enables the viewer to observe the situation from different points of view, Vulcan (who also incarnated the archetype of the sculptor) is deceived because he focuses his attention on a desirable object and ignores the rest of the scene. From a single perspective, appearances are deceptive, in life as in art. Thus, rather than answering the *paragone* debate by trying to seduce the viewer, Tintoretto paints a *comedia picta* that makes us aware of the dangers of vision: art is an illusion—an *inganno* (deception)[103]—but if the viewer is not fooled by its seductive power, art can still represent and teach the truth.[104]

Renaissance artists seem to have found in cuckoldry a major artistic topic. Just as Tintoretto made fun of his illustrious predecessors and contemporaries, his own paintings eventually became the objects of parody. His famous *Annunciation* in the Scuola di San Rocco, was clearly mocked by the young Annibale Carracci in a drawing (c. 1597) in the Royal Collection of Windsor Castle (Fig. 7.14 and Plate 10).[105] In it, the graceful figure of the archangel is divided into two parts by the wall of the Virgin's *domuncula,* similar to the two halves of the plank of wood sawn by the carpenter outside the house. It would be difficult not to see in the two pieces of wood placed in a prominent V position anything other than a deliberate reference to horns. Is this a projection of the carpenter's jealous mind? By transforming Tintoretto's humble carpenter into a divine cuckold, Carracci has not only imitated, but also made fun of the Venetian painter—perhaps because, as Leonardo unequivocally stated, "Sad is the disciple who does not surpass his master."[106]

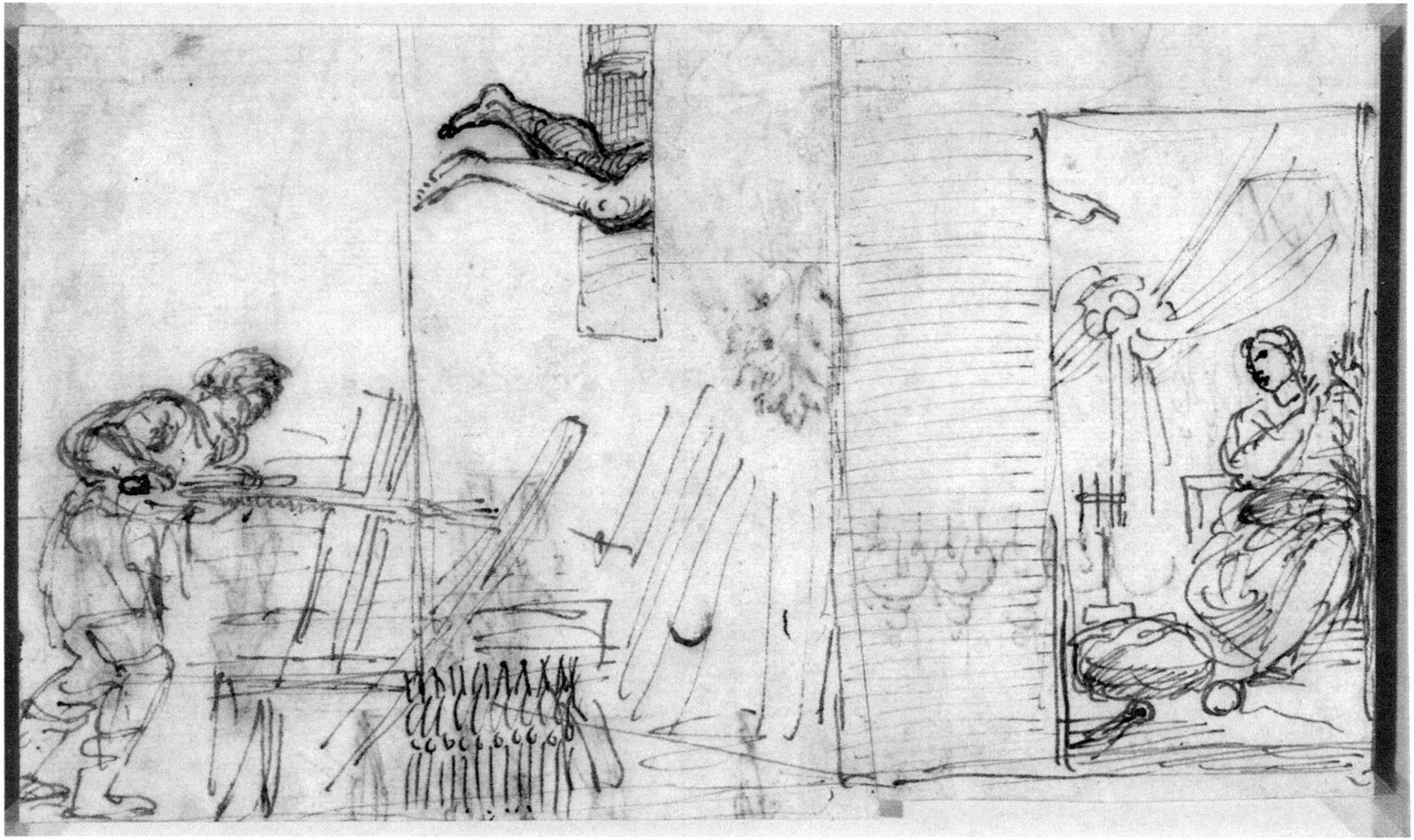

7.14 Annibale Carracci, *Parody of Tintoretto's Annunciation in the Scuola di San Rocco*, pen and brown ink, 11.5 × 18.8 cm, Royal Library, Windsor Castle (inv. 1841) (Royal Collection Trust, © Her Majesty Queen Elizabeth II 2012)

Works Cited

Early Printed Sources (pre-1900)

Boerio Giuseppe, *Dizionario del dialetto veneziano.* Venezia: Reale tipografia di Giovanni Cecchini, 1867.

Calmo, Andrea, *I piacevoli et ingeniosi discorsi in piv lettere compresi, è ne la lingua antica uolgari dechiariti. Ne i qvali se contengono uarij cherebizzi, e fantastiche fantasie philosophiche in uarie materie, pur sempre à le uertu accostate.* Venezia: Comin de Trino di Monferrato, 1547.

Calmo, Andrea, *il Rimanente de le pacevole, et ingegnose lettere indirizzate a diversi, con bellissime argutie. Sotto vaii, et sottilissimi discorsi, dichiarati.* Venezia: Comin da Trino di Monferrato, 1548.

Chappuis Tourangeau, Gabriel, *Les Mondes célestes, terrestres et infernaux ... tirez des œuvres de Doni, ... par Gabriel Chappuis, ... depuis reveuz, corrigez et augmentez du Monde des cornuz, par F. C. T.* [F. Chapuis, Tourangeau.] 1580. Lyon: E. Michel, 1583.

Dolce, Ludovico, *Il marito. Comedia di m. Lodovico Dolce.* Venezia: Gabriele Giolito De Ferrari, 1545.

Gerson, Jean, *Opera omnia, novo ordine digesta, & in V tomos distributa ... quibus accessere Henrici de Hassia, Patri de Alliaco, Joannis Brevicoxa, Joannis de Varenis, scriptorum coaetaneorum, ac insuper Jacobi Almaïni & Joannis Majoris tractatus ... necnon monumenta omnia ad causam Joannis Parvi pertinentia; opera & studio M. Lud. Ellies du Pin ... qui huic novae editioni praefixit Gersoniana, in quibus historia ecclesiastica ... .* Antwerp: sumptibus Societatis, 1706.

Secondary Sources and Modern Editions

Alberti, Francesca, "*Bizzarri componimenti e straordinarie invenzioni.* La *Danaé* de Tintoret, une peinture comique," *Studiolo* 7 (2009): 11–39.

Alberti, Francesca, *Le rire, le ridicule et le comique dans la peinture italienne de la Renaissance. Des facéties de Corrège aux fables burlesques de Tintoret*, Ph.D. Université Paris 1 Panthéon-Sorbonne, 2013.

Anthologie Grecque. Anthologie Palatine, ed. and trans. P. Walt and J. Guillon. Paris: Les Belles Lettres, 1990. 16 vols.

Arasse, Daniel, "À propos de l'article de Meyer Schapiro, *Muscipola diaboli*: le 'réseau figurative' du rétable de Mérode," in *Symboles de la Renaissance.* Paris: Presses de l'Ecole Normale Supérieure, 1976. 47–56.

Arasse, Daniel, *On n'y voit rien, descriptions*, 2000. Paris, Denoël, 2005.

Arasse, Daniel, "Le corps fictif de Sebastien et le coup d'oeil d'Antonello," *Etudes de lettres* 2 (1983): 54–72.

Aretino, Pietro, *La Passione di Gesù* in *Un pronostico satirico di Pietro Aretino (MDXXXIIII)*, 1534, ed. A. Luzio. Bergamo: Instituto italiano d'arti grafiche, 1900.

Aretino, Pietro, *Lettere*, ed. P. Procaccioli, 6 vols. Roma and Salerno: Edizione Nazionale dell'opere di Pietro Aretino, 1999–2002.

Baird, Lorrayne Y., "Fabliau Form and the Hegge 'Joseph's Return,'" *The Chaucer Review* 8 (1973): 159–69.

Bakhtine, Mikhaïl, *L'œuvre de François Rabelais et la culture populaire au Moyen Âge et sous la Renaissance*, trans. A. Robel. Paris: Gallimard, 2012.

Bandello, Matteo, *La terza parte de le Novelle*, 1554. Alessandria: Ed. Dell'Orso, 1995.

Barsella, Susanna, "Il riso dei padri: Il caso di madonna Filippa (Dec., VI 7)," *Humanistica* 4 (2009): 13–22.

Berger, Peter L., *Redeeming laughter: the comic dimension of the human experience*. Berlin/ New York: de Gruyter, 1997.

Boccaccio, Giovanni, *Decamerone*. Novara: Instituto Geografico de Agostini, 1966.

Bodart, Diane H., "Le reflets et l'éclat. Jeux de l'envers dans la peinture vénitienne du XVIe siècle," *Titien, Tintoret, Véronèse: rivalités à Venise*, exhib. cat. Paris: Hazan, 2009. 216–59.

Boggione, Valter and Casalegno Giovanni, *Dizionario storico del lessico erotico italiano: metafore, eufemismi, oscenità, doppi sensi, parole dotte e parole basse in otto secoli di letteratura italiana*. Milano: TEA, 1999.

Bolger Foster Marjory, *The Iconography of Saint Joseph in Netherlandish Art 1400–1550*, Ph.D. University of Kansas, 1978.

Bowen, Barbara C., "Roman Jokes and the Renaissance Prince 1455–1528," *Illinois Classical Studies* 9 (1984): 137–48.

Burke, Peter, "Frontiers of the Comic in Early Modern Italy, c. 1350–1750," in *A Cultural History of Humour*, ed. J. Bremmer and H. Roodenburg, 1997. Cambridge: Polity Press, 2005. 61–75.

Burroughs, Bryson, "A picture by Hieronymus Bosch," *The Metropolitan Museum of Art Bulletin* 8 (1913): 130–33.

Burucùa, José Emilio, *Corderos y Elefantes – La Sacralidad y La Risa En La Modernidad Clasica Siglos XV a XVII*. Buenos Aires, Mino y Davila, 2001.

Carr, Dawson W., *Andrea Mantegna: the Adoration of the Magi*. Los Angeles: J. Paul Getty Museum, 1998.

Casagrande, Carla, "Il peccato di far ridere: derisione, turpiloquio, stultiloquio e scurrilità nei testi teologici e pastorali del secolo XIII," in *Il sorriso dello spirito : riso e comicità nella cultura religiosa dell'Occidente*, ed. R. Alessandrini and M. Borsari. Modena: Fondazione San Carlo & Banca Popolare dell'Emilia Romagna, 2000. 77–105.

Casagrande, Carla, "Ridere in Paradiso. Gaudio, giubilio e riso tra angeli e beati," in *Il Riso. 'Homo risibilis.' Capacità di ridere e pratica del riso nelle città medievali*, ed. F. Mosetti Casaretto. Alessandria: Edizioni dell'Orso, 2005. 177–93.

Cassegrain, Guillaume, *Tintoret*. Paris: Hazan, 2011.

Castelvetro, Ludovico, *Poetica d'Aristotele: volgarizzata e sposta*, 1570. Roma: Laterza, 1978.

Chorpenning, Joseph F., "The Enigma of St Joseph in Poussin's Holy Family on the Steps," *Journal of the Warburg and Courtauld Institutes* 60 (1997): 276–81.

Cieri Via, Claudia, "Venere, Vulcano e Marte: un'allegoria mitologica nella cultura veneta del Cinquecento," in *Die Allegorese des antiken mythos*, ed. H.-J. Horn and H. Walter. Wiesbaden: Harrassowitz Verlag, 1997. 351–94.

Colallucci, Francesco, "*Muscipula diaboli?* Una pseudo-trappola per topi nell'*Adorazione* di Lorenzo Lotto a Washington," *Artibus et Historiae* 21 (1990): 71–88.

Cowan, Alexander F., *Marriage, manners and mobility in early modern Venice*. Farnham, UK/Burlington, VT: Ashgate, 2007.

Cropper, Elizabeth, "The Place of Beauty in the High Renaissance and Its Displacement in the History of Art," in *Place and Displacement in the Renaissance*. Binghamton, NY: Center for Medieval and Renaissance Studies, 1995. 159–205.

Dautreme, Baptiste, "Image du père éternel et image du père terrestre: l'iconographie de saint Joseph entre le Quattrocento et le Cinquecento," *Vivens Homo* 17 (2006), XVII: 147-78.

De Lorris Guillaume and De Meung Jean, *The Romance of the Rose*, trans. C. Dahlberg. Princeton, NJ: Princeton University Press, 1971.

Dufeil, Michel-Marie, "Risus in theologia sancti Thome," in *Le rire au Moyen Âge dans la littérature et dans les arts*. Bordeaux: Presses universitaires de Bordeaux, 1990. 147–63.

Ekserdjian, David, *Parmigianino*. New Haven: Yale University Press, 2006.

'El più soave et dolce et dilectevole et gratioso bochone'. Amore e sesso al tempo dei Gonzaga, ed. C. Cipolla and G. Malacarne. Milano: Franco Angeli, 2006.

Fumagalli, Elena and Rossi, Massimiliano, *Florence au Grand siècle entre peinture et littérature*, exhib. cat. Milano: Silvana Editoriale, 2011.

Ginzburg, Carlo, "Titian, Ovid and the sixteenth century codes for erotic illustration," in *Titian's Venus of Urbino*, ed. R. Goffen. Cambridge, Cambridge University Press, 1997. 23–36.

Grimkowski, Rüdiger, "Testis et custos virginitatis – Zur Josephsikonographie bis um 1400," *Das Munster* 55:3 (2002): 194–9.

Grimkowski, Rüdiger, "Nutritor Domini – Fidelis servus et prudens Aspekte spätmittelalterlicher Josephsikonographie," *Das Munster* 55/4 (2002): 292–302.

Hahn, Cynthia, "Joseph as Ambrose's 'Artisan of Soul' in the *Holy Family in Egypt* by Albrecht Durer," *Zeitschrift für Kunstgeschichte* 47/4 (1984): 515–22.

Hahn, Cynthia, '"Joseph will perfect, Mary enlighten and Jesus save Thee': The Holy family as marriage model in the Mérode Triptych," *The Art Bulletin* 68 (1986): 54–66.

Herrick, Marvin T., *Comic theory in Sixteenth Century*. Urbana, University of Illinois Press, 1964.

Hills, Paul, "Ray, line, vision and traces in Renaissance art," *Word & Image* 6/3 (1990): 217–25.

Jacobelli, Maria Caterina, *Il* Risus Paschalis, *e il fondamento teologico del piacere sessuale*, 1990. Verona: Querinina, 2004.

Jacobs, Fredrika H., "Aretino and Michelangelo, Dolce and Titian: Femmina, Masculo, Grazia," *Art Bulletin* 82/1 (2000): 51–67.

Jacobsen, Michael A., "Vulcan forging Cupid's wing," *The Art Bulletin* 54/4 (1972): 418–29.

Jacopo Titoretto nel quarto centenario della morte, eds. P. Rossi and P. Lionello. Padova: il Poligrafo, 1996.

Klapisch Zuber, Christiane, "Zacharias or the ousted father: Nuptial rites in Tuscany between Giotto and the Council of Trent," in *Woman, family and ritual in Renaissance Italy*. Chicago, London: The University of Chicago Press, 1985. 178–212.

Krischel, Roland, "*L'armamento di Amore*: un'opera giovanile di Jacopo Tintoretto," *Venezia Cinquecento* 3/5 (1993): 79–96.

Krischel, Roland, "Jacopo Tintoretto and Giulio Romano," in *Jacopo Tintoretto*, M. Falomir, B. Aikema, eds. Madrid: M. Falomir, 2009. 58–65.

Krohm, Hartmut, "Alter Daedalus- Zum Begriff künstlerischer Tätigkeit in Dürers "Marienleben," in *Aus Albrecht Dürers Welt*. Turnhout: Brepols, 2001. 77–90.

Kubovy, Michael, *The Psychology of Perspective and Renaissance Art*. Cambridge/New York: Cambridge University Press, 1986.

Ladis, Andrew, "The legend of Giotto's wit and the Arena Chapel," *The Art Bulletin* 68/4 (1986): 581–96.

Le Goff, Jacques, *Un autre Moyen Âge*. Paris: Gallimard, 1999.

Lemée François, *Traité des statües*, eds. D. H. Bodart and H. Ziegler. Weimar: VDG, 2010.

Loh, Maria H., *Titian remade: repetition and the transformation of Early Modern Italian Art*. Los Angeles: Getty Research Institute, 2007.

Margolin, Jean Claude, "Charivari et mariage ridicule," in *Les fêtes de la Renaissance*, ed. J. Jacquot. Paris: C.N.R.S., 1960, III: 580–601.

Matthews-Grieco, Sara, "Satyrs and sausages: erotic strategies and the print market in Cinquecento Italy", in *Erotic cultures of Renaissance Italy*, ed. S. Matthews-Grieco. Farnham, UK/Burlington, VT: Ashgate, 2010). 19–60.

Mauriello, Adriana, "Artisti e beffe in alcune novelle del'500 (Lasca, Doni, Fortini)," *Letteratura & arte* 3, 2005 (2006): 81–91.

Meiss, Millard, "Light as Form and Symbol in Some Fifteenth-Century Paintings," *The Art Bulletin* 27/3 (1945): 175–81.

Mellinkoff, Ruth, *The Horned Moses in Medieval Art and Thought*. Berkeley/Los Angeles/ London: University of California Press, 1970.

Mellinkoff Ruth, *Outcasts: Signs of Otherness in Northern European Art of the Late Middle Ages*, 2 vols. Berkeley: University of California Press, 1993.

Minois, Georges, *Histoire du rire et de la dérision*. Paris: Fayard, 2000.

Molanus, Jean, *Traité des saintes images*. Paris: les Éd. du Cerf, 1996.

Moretti, Felice, "Sorridere sul pulpito, ridere in piazza: gli *exempla* nella predicazione del XIII secolo," *Studi francescani* XCVIII (2001): 131–78.

Nichols, Tom, "Price, *Prestezza* and Production in Jacopo Tintoretto's Business Strategy," *Venezia Cinquecento* 4:12 (1996): 207–33.

Nichols, Tom, *Understanding Tintoretto's "prestezza": literary and other approaches to the contested artistic culture of mid-Cinquecento Venice, Officine del nuovo*, ed. H. Hendrix and P. Procaccioli. Manziana: Vecchiarelli, 2008. 51–64.

Norton, Paul F., "The lost sleeping Cupid of Michelangelo," *The Art Bulletin* 39 (1957): 251–7.

O'Connell, Michael, "Mockery, Farce, and *Risus Paschalis* in the York *Christ before Herod*," in *Ludus. Medieval and Early Renaissance Theatre and Drama, Farce and Farcical Elements*, ed. W. Hüsken, K. Schoell, L. Søndergaard. Amsterdam: Rodopi, 2002. 45–58.

Paleotti, Gabriele, *Discourse on sacred and profane images*, trans. W. McCuaig. Los Angeles: The Getty Research Institute, 2012.

Panofsky, Erwin, *Early Netherlandish Painting, its origin and Character*. Cambridge, MA: Harvard University Press, 1953.

Pardo, Mary, "Artifice as seduction in Titian," in *Sexuality and Gender in Early Modern Europe: Institutions, Texts, Images*, ed. J. Grantham Turner. Cambridge: Cambridge University Press, 1993. 55–89.

Parker, Deborah, "Towards a Reading of Bronzino's Burlesque Poetry," *Renaissance Quarterly* 50:4 (1997): 1011–44.

Payan, Paul, "Ridicule? L'image ambiguë de saint Joseph à la fin du Moyen Âge," *Médiévales* 39 (2000): 96–111.

Peacock, Martha, "*Hoorndragers* and *Hennetasters*: the old impotent cuckold as "Other" in Sixteenth- and Seventeenth-century Netherlandish Art," in *Old Age in the Middle Ages and the Renaissance. Interdisciplinary approaches to a Neglected topic*, ed. A. Classen. Berlin: de Gruyter, 2007. 485–516.

Petrucci, Armando et al., *Scrittura e popolo nella Roma Barocca: 1585–1721*. Roma: Quasar, 1982.

Popham, Arthur E., *Catalogue of the drawings of Parmigianino*. New Haven: Yale University Press, 1971.

Réau, Louis, *Iconographie de l'art Chrétien*, 3 vols. Paris: Presses Universitaires de France, 1955–1958.

Riso e comicità nel cristianesimo antico, ed. C. Mazzucco. Torino: dell'Orso, 2007.

Robertson, Clare, "Annibale Carracci and *Invenzione*: Medium and function in the Early Drawings," *Master Drawings* 35:1 (1997): 3–42.

Romani, Vittoria, *Daniele da Volterra amico di Michelangelo*, exhib. cat. Firenze: Mandragora, 2003.

Roskill, Mark W., *Dolce's Aretino and Venetian art theory of the Cinquecento*. Toronto: University of Toronto, 2000.

Ruiz, Juan, *Libro de buen amor*, c. 1322. Madrid: Espasa-Calpe, 1997.

Sacchetti, Franco, *Il Trecentonovelle*. Torino: UTET, 2004.

Schapiro, Meyer, '"Muscipula diaboli,' the Symbolism of the Mérode Altarpiece," *The Art Bulletin* 27:3 (1945): 182–7.

Schapiro, Meyer, *Style, artiste et société*. Paris: Gallimard, 1982.

Schwarzenberg, Erkinger, "La gelosia di Vulcano alle corti di Mantova e di Ferrara," *Mitteilungen des Kunsthistorischen Institutes in Florenz* 49:3 (2005): 289–322.

Sframeli, Maria, *The Myth of Venus*, exhib. cat. Milano/Cinisello Balsamo: Silvana, Arthemisia, 2003.

Simons, Patricia, *The Sex of Men in Premodern Europe: A Cultural History*. Cambridge: Cambridge University Press, 2011.

Singleton, Charles S., *Canti Carnascialeschi del Rinascimento*. Bari: Laterza, 1932.

Sohm, Philippe L., *Pittoresco: Marco Boschini, his critics, and their critiques of painterly brushwork in seventeenth and eighteenth century Italy*. Cambridge: Cambridge Studies in the History of Art, 1991.

Taddeo Gaddi: critical reappraisal and catalogue raisonné, exhib. cat. London: University of Missouri Press, 1982.

The Apocryphal Gospels: texts and translations, trans. and ed. Bart D. Ehrman and Zlatko Plese. Oxford: Oxford University Press, 2011.

Thürlemann Félix, "Das Lukas-Triptychon in Stolzenhain, Ein verlorenes Hauptewerk von Robert Campin in einer Kopie aus des Werkstatt Derick Baegerts," *Zeitschrift für Kunstgeschichte* 61 (1992): 524–64.

Tintoretto, exhib. cat. Madrid: Museo nacional del Prado, 2007.

Titian's Venus of Urbino, ed. R. Goffen. Cambridge: Cambridge University Press, 1997.

Vasari, Giorgio, *Les vite de' più eccellenti pittori, scultori e architettori nelle redazioni del 1550 e del 1568*, ed. R. Bettarini, P. Barocchi. Firenze: Sansoni, 1966–1987.

Vasvari, Louise O., "Joseph on the Margin: the Mérode Tryptic and Medieval Spectacle," *Mediaevalia, a Journal of Medieval Studies* 18 (1995): 163–89.

Venere e amore: Michelangelo e la nuova bellezza ideale, exhib. cat. Firenze: Giunti, 2002.

Viscardi, Giuseppe Maria, *Tra Europa e "Indie di quaggiù." Chiesa, religiosità e cultura popolare nel Mezzogiorno (secoli XV–XIX)*. Roma: Edizioni di Storia e Letteratura, 2005.

Walsh, Martin W., "Divine Cuckold/Holy Fool: The Comic Imagery of Joseph in the English 'Troubles' Play," in *England in the Fourteenth Century*, ed. W. M. Ormond. Woodbridge: Boydell Press, 1986. 278–97.

Wilson, Carolyn C., *Saint Joseph in Italian Renaissance Society and Art: New Directions and Interpretations*. Philadelphia: St. Joseph's University Press, 2001.

Woolf, Rosemary, *The English Mystery Play*. London: Swindell, 1972.

Yates, Francis, *L'Art de la Mémoire*, trans. D. Arasse. Paris: Gallimard, 1975.

Zorach, Rebecca, "Passioni triangolari," in *Sesso nel Rinascimento. Pratica, perversione e punizione nell'Italia Rinascimentale*, ed. Allison Levy. Firenze: Le lettere, 2009. 159–70.

Zuccaro, Federico, *Il Lamento della pittura su l'onde venete*, 1605, *Scritti d'arte di Federico Zuccari*. Firenze: L. S. Olschki, 1961.

Notes

1 The phrase "Divine cuckolds" is taken from Martin W. Walsh, "Divine Cuckold/Holy Fool: The Comic Imagery of Joseph in the English "Troubles' Play," in *England in the Fourteenth Century*, ed. W. M. Ormond (Woodbridge: Boydell Press, 1986), 278–97. I wish to express my gratitude to Eglé de Richemont and Sara F. Matthews-Grieco for their precious help and stimulating comments.

2 Homer, *Odyssey*, VIII, vv. 306–21.

3 Mary and Venus share many attributes and their representations influenced each other. Bronzino's painting of *Time revealing Deception* at the National Gallery in London is one of the most notorious examples of how a sacred composition (Michelangelo's *Tondo Doni*) could be transformed into an erotic mythological allegory.

4 On the iconography of Joseph see Louis Réau, *Iconographie de l'art Chrétien*, 3 vols. (Paris: Presses Universitaires de France, 1955–1958), II, 753–60; Marjory Bolger Foster, *The Iconography of Saint Joseph in Netherlandish Art 1400–1550*, PhD University of Kansas, 1978; Carolyn C. Wilson, *Saint Joseph in Italian Renaissance Society and Art: New Directions and Interpretations* (Philadelphia: St. Joseph's University Press, 2001). For studies that focused on the theme of Joseph as cuckold see Walsh, 1986; Ruth Mellinkoff, *Outcasts: Signs of Otherness in Northern European Art of the Late Middle Ages*, 2 vols. (Berkeley: University of California Press, 1993), I, 79–82, 142–4, 222–6; Louise O. Vasvari, "Joseph on the Margin: the Mérode Tryptic and Medieval Spectacle," *Mediaevalia, a Journal of Medieval Studies* 18 (1995): 163–89; Paul Payan, "Ridicule? L'image ambiguë de saint Joseph à la fin du Moyen Âge," *Médiévales* 39 (2000): 96–111.

5 Rosemary Woolf, *The English Mystery Play* (London: Swindell, 1972), 170–77; Lorrayne Y. Baird, "Fabliau Form and the Hegge "Joseph's Return," *The Chaucer Review* 8 (1973): 159–69; Rüdiger Grimkowski, "Testis et custos virginitatis—Zur Josephsikonographie bis um 1400," *Das Munster* 55/3 (2002): 194–9; *Idem*, "Nutritor Domini—Fidelis servus et prudens Aspekte spätmittelalterlicher Josephsikonographie," *Das Munster* 55/4 (2002): 292–302.

6 For the examples that follow see Mellinkoff's controversial (but still useful) study: 1993, I, 222–4, II, iii.89–101, vi.71–7, xi.15–41.

7 See also Joseph's stereotyped features painted by Michelangelo in the Sistine Chapel.

8 See also what Vasari writes about Joseph in Spinello Aretino's *Adoration of the Magi*: "allegro fuori di modo per la venuta di que're, da lui considerati con maniera bellissima mentre aprivano i vasi del loro tesoro e gl'offerivano," Giorgio Vasari, *Les vite de' più eccellenti pittori, scultori e architettori nelle redazioni del 1550 e del 1568*, ed. R. Bettarini and P. Barocchi (Firenze: Sansoni, 1966–1987), II, 282.

9 Wilson associates Joseph's sleep to the rest of the philosopher and of the righteous (see Wilson, 2001, 35–9), but when a loud sound reverberates close to him, it becomes an amusing feature. A braying donkey appears next to the saint in a preparatory sketch for the *Adoration of the shepherds* of Pellegrino Tibaldi, see *Daniele da Volterra amico di Michelangelo*, exhib. cat. (Firenze: Mandragora, 2003), 64–5.

10 Joseph is described simply as being *vecchio* in many documents. As Ladis pointed out, Joseph became a-popular *exemplum* of old age very early in Italian medieval drama. In one play, a wife says to her husband "Non vedi tu che pari un Giuseppo / Con questa barba già canuta e bianca?" See Andrew Ladis, "The legend of Giotto's wit and the Arena Chapel," *The Art Bulletin* 68/4 (1986), 598.

11 Jean Gerson had already insisted on this argument in a sermon of 1413 entitled *Considérations sur saint Joseph*. "Si convenoit pour les dits offices deubment faire que saint Joseph ne fust point viel, lait, deffectueux et febble et comme impotent au labeur et qui eust eu gregner besoing d'estre servi que de servir," see by Payan, 2000, 106, note 43.

12 "Pictoribus atque poetis / Quidlibet audendi semper fuit aequa potestas," ibid., 106–7.

13 Molanus dedicates two chapters to the representation of Joseph in pictures, Jean Molanus, *Traité des saintes images* (Paris: les Éd. du Cerf, 1996), II, 29, 109–111, III, 12, 368–71. It is important to notice how in his arguments against Joseph's representation as an old man, the author introduces a possible overlap of the artist in general with the saint's figure.

14 Bryson Burroughs, "A picture by Hieronymus Bosch," *The Metropolitan Museum of Art Bulletin* 8 (1913), 132.

15 Mellinkoff, 1993, I, 143, II, vi.74.

16 Frans Floris plays with the comic motif of the unmatched couple. The food that Joseph is preparing refers to his role as Christ's *nutritor*, but the expression on his face underlines his lecherous desire.

17 See for example the essay by Laura Gianetti "The Satyr in the Kitchen Pantry" in this volume.

18 *The Apocryphal Gospels: texts and translations*, trans. and ed. Bart D. Ehrman and Zlatko Plese (Oxford University Press, 2011), 51.

19 "De moy se devroient bien moquer/ Et loy appeler dam Riquier / Honteux suy d'y estre venu," quoted by Vasvari, 1995, 170–71. The author also quotes the wit in the N-Town *Marriage of Mary and Joseph*.

20 *The Gospel of Pseudo-Matthew* might have inspired Giovanni Boccaccio's amusing parody of the Annunciation. In one of the *Decameron* novels a Franciscan friar, Frate Alberto da Imola, takes advantage of rich venetian lady, Lisetta da ca'Quirino, by making her think he is the archangel Gabriel, who comes to visit her every night because he has fallen in love with her beauty, see Giovanni Boccaccio, *Decamerone* (Novara: Instituto Geografico de Agostini, 1966), I, IV/2, 406–18. I thank Paul Barolsky for this reference.

21 *The Gospel of Pseudo-Matthew* 13 (1), in *The Apocryphal Gospels*, 2000, 55. Payan notes that Joseph also complains of being a new Adam in the *Ludus Coventriae* and in the Towneley cycle, see Payan, 2000, 105, note 39.

22 *Cfr. supra*, note 4–5, also Ladis, 1986, 581–96. The best synthesis on the topic is in Payan's article.

23 On the purse and the moneybag as metaphors of the testicles see Vasvari, 1995, 177; Francesca Alberti, "*Bizzarri componimenti e straordinarie invenzioni*. La *Danaé* de Tintoret, une peinture comique," *Studiolo* 7 (2009): 22–39; Patricia Simons, *The Sex of Men in Premodern Europe: A Cultural History* (Cambridge: Cambridge University Press, 2011), 169–86.

24 For this interpretation see Vasvari, 1995, 176–8. In the apocryphal sources Joseph's impotency is implicitly due to his age, see *The Gospel of Pseudo-Matthew*.

25 In these paintings, the shape of the bundle carried by Joseph explicitly recalls men's testicles (both pictures are reproduced in Mellinkoff, 1993, II, vi.73). The bundle also resembles the main attribute of the *Ture Läng* colossal statue, two balls hanging from a chain, carried on a staff over the figure's shoulder. This statue was erected in Sweden in "honor" of cuckold husbands, see Olaus Magnus, *Historia de Gentium Septentrionalibus*, 1555 quoted in François Lemée, *Traité des statües*, ed. D.H. Bodart and H. Ziegler (Weimar, 2010), 315–17.

26 This painting is reproduced and discussed by Vasvari, 1995, 179.

27 The satirical character of Joseph's enormous saw has been noticed by Vasvari, 1995, 178–80. For tools and weapons as metaphors of sexual attributes see Valter Boggione and Giovanni Casalegno, *Dizionario storico del lessico erotico italiano: metafore, eufemismi, oscenità, doppi sensi, parole dotte e parole basse in otto secoli di letteratura italiana* (Milano: TEA, 1999), 240.

28 Thürlemann has identified the fountain pictured next to Joseph with the *Font dels Pissaïres* in the centre of Lacaune, see Félix Thürlemann, "Das Lukas-Triptychon in Stolzenhain, Ein verlorenes Hauptewerk von Robert Campin in einer Kopie aus des Werkstatt Derick Baegerts," 55 (1992), 544–6.

29 The garden and the fountain metaphors are studied by Simons, 2011, 238, see also the following pages.

30 Another important examples of horns related to Joseph's cuckoldry might be found in Correggio's *Adoration of the shepherds*, also called "the Night," at the Gemäldegalerie in Dresden. In the painting, the younger shepherd looks at his older companion while making the sign of the horns with his hand. Consequently the older peasant looks in direction of Joseph (God's cuckold) depicted in the background of the picture. Through the shepherds' attitude, Correggio might have wanted to make evident how the simple men were incapable of understanding the mystery of Incarnation.

31 For a specific study on these motifs and their relation to cuckoldry, see Martha Peacock, "*Hoorndragers* and *Hennetasters*: the old impotent cuckold as 'Other' in Sixteenth- and Seventeenth-century Netherlandish Art," in *Old Age in the Middle Ages and the Renaissance. Interdisciplinary approaches to a Neglected topic*, ed. A. Classen (Berlin: de Gruyter, 2007), 485–516. One of the most widespread defamatory epithets during the 16th century is *cornuto*, see Armando Petrucci et al., *Scrittura e popolo nella Roma Barocca: 1585–1721* (Roma: Quasar, 1982), cat. 73–6. For other examples of horned cuckolds see also Baccio del Bianco's drawings in *Florence au Grand siècle entre peinture et littérature*, exhib. cat. (Milano: Silvana Editoriale, 2011), 252–7. See also the essay in this volume by Louise Rice, chapter 9.

32 Gabriel Chappuis Tourangeau, *Le monde des cornuz …*, 1580 (Lyon: E. Michel, 1583), 687. See also Ruth Mellinkoff, *The Horned Moses in Medieval Art and Thought*, (Berkeley/Los Angeles/London: University of California Press, 1970), ch. X, "Ambiguity of the Meaning of Horns: Horns of Dishonour as well as Horns of Honour," 121–37.

33 "Deh dimmi, Giotto, perché é dipinto Iosepf cosi sempre maliconoso?" E Giotto rispose: "Non ha egli ragione, che vede pregna la moglie, e non sa di cui?" Franco Sacchetti, *Il Trecentonovelle* (Torino: UTET, 2004), LXXV, 225.

34 Ladis described Taddeo Gaddi's picture as one the most "light-hearted, humour-filled paintings of the Trecento," *Taddeo Gaddi: critical reappraisal and catalogue raisonné*, exhib. cat. (London: University of Missouri Press, 1982), 27–8. He also states that "Joseph fulfills an important narrative and theological role by acting as a foil for the supernatural."

35 Jean Claude Margolin, "Charivari et mariage ridicule," in *Les fêtes de la Renaissance*, ed. J. Jacquot (Paris: C.N.R.S., 1960), III, 580–601; see also all the carnavalesque songs on old cuckold husbands in Charles S. Singleton, *Canti Carnascialeschi del Rinascimento* (Bari: Laterza, 1932), 74, 112–15, 243. On the *charivari* and noisy confusion in public space related to sexual *mores*, see also the essay in this volume by M. A. Katritzky, "Historical and Literary Contexts for the Skimmington: Impotence and Samuel Butler's *Hudibras*."

36 Christiane Klapisch Zuber, "Zacharias or the ousted father: Nuptial rites in Tuscany between Giotto and the Council of Trent," in *Woman, family and ritual in Renaissance Italy* (Chicago/London: The University of Chicago Press, 1985), 178–212.

37 Gerson speaks of this problem in his sermon of 1416, *cfr. supra* note 11.

38 Meyer Schapiro, "'Muscipula diabolic,' the Symbolism of the Mérode Altarpiece," *The Art Bulletin*, 27/3 (1945), 182–7; Erwin Panofsky, *Early Netherlandish Painting, its origin and Character* (Cambridge, MA: Harvard University Press, 1953), 164; Daniel Arasse, "À propos de l'article de Meyer Schapiro, *Muscipola Diaboli*: le 'réseau figurative' du rétable de Mérode," in *Symboles de la Renaissance* (Paris: Presses de l'Ecole Normale Supérieure, 1976), 47–63; Meyer Schapiro, *Style, artiste et société* (Paris: Gallimard, 1982), 147–70; Cynthia Hahn, "'Joseph will perfect, Mary enlighten and Jesus save Thee': The Holy family as marriage model in the Mérode Triptych," *The Art Bulletin* 68 (1986): 54–66.

39 Schapiro, 1945, 182, notes 4 and 6.

40 Ibid., 186; Vasvari, 1995, 167–9.

41 Joseph is here painted as a model for the husband, pictured on the triptych's left wing, see ibid., 184–6; Hahn, 1986.

42 The *homunculus* and the mousetrap are both placed next to a window. Gerson thought that Joseph was deeply involved in the divine plan of redemption. Ignetius also writes that the Virgin was married to Joseph in order to conceal the birth of Christ from the devil, who thought that the child was begotten by Joseph, see Gerson, *Opera Omnia*, the sermons dates of 1417 (Antwerp: 1706), 3, col. 1352.

43 Bernard of Clairvaux describes Joseph as, "carefully watching … during the whole time she was in his custody, Joseph became the most faithful witness of her purity," Hahn, 1986, 62, note 59.

44 Joseph F. Chorpenning, "The Enigma of St Joseph in Poussin's Holy Family on the Steps," *Journal of the Warburg and Courtauld Institutes* 60 (1997): 278–9.

45 In the *Louanges de saint Joseph*, Eustache Deschamps compares old men that are victims of their young and beautiful wives to Joseph: "Vous qui servez à femme et a enfant/ aiez Joseph toudis en remembrance; / Femmes servit toujours tristes, dolans, / Et Jhesu Crist garda en son enfance; / A pié trotoit, son fardel sur sa lance; / En plusieurs lieux est figuré ainsi, / Lez un mulet, pour leur faire plaisance, / Et si n'ot oncques feste en ce monde ci,'" quoted by Payan, 2000, 107–8. See also Tristan de Lescagne and Molanus, who criticize painters for picturing Joseph as a *veillard chenu* or as a *vieillard débile*, in *Traité des saintes images*, 1570 (Paris: les Éd. du Cerf, 1996), I, 366.

46 In the painting of Giovanni da Asola Joseph looks at the shepherds while pointing at baby Jesus with his index finger, while in Titian's painting Joseph protects his family by placing his cane in front of the young shepherd. I disagree with Wilson who thinks that during the Renaissance Joseph's figure was never considered to be amusing, see Wilson, 2001, 10, 182. The source for Joseph's warning gaze might be Andrea Mantegna's *Adoration of the Magi* at the Getty Museum in Los Angeles (c. 1500), about which Dawson M. Carr writes: "Indeed, here he scrutinizes the exotic strangers with a mixture of curiosity and suspicion. In contrast to the Virgin's contemplative humility, Joseph is the image of the active, probing side of human experience," *Andrea Mantegna: the Adoration of the Magi* (Los Angeles: J. Paul Getty Museum, 1998), 76–7.

47 Peter L. Berger, *Redeeming laughter: the comic dimension of the human experience* (Berlin/New York: de Gruyter, 1997).

48 On the admonitory function of humor and its relation to the art of memory see Francis Yates, *L'Art de la Mémoire*, 1966, trans. D. Arasse (Paris: Gallimard, 1975), 22–5.

49 See Georges Minois, *Histoire du rire et de la dérision* (Paris: Fayard, 2000), 189–98; Carla Casagrande, "Il peccato di far ridere: derisione, turpiloquio, stultiloquio e scurrilità nei testi teologici e pastorali del secolo XIII," in *Il sorriso dello spirito: riso e comicità nella cultura religiosa dell'Occidente*, eds. R. Alessandrini and M. Borsari (Modena: Fondazione San Carlo & Banca Popolare dell'Emilia Romagna, 2000), 77–105; Felice Moretti, "Sorridere sul pulpito, ridere in piazza: gli *exempla* nella predicazione del XIII secolo," *Studi francescani*, XCVIII (2001): 131–78; José Emilio Burucùa, *Corderos y Elefantes–La Sacralidad y La Risa En La Modernidad Clasica Siglos XV a XVII* (Buenos Aires: Mino y Davila, 2001); *Il Riso. "Homo risibilis." Capacità di ridere e pratica del riso nelle città medievali*, ed. F. Mosetti Casaretto (Alessandria: Edizioni dell'Orso, 2002); *Riso e comicità nel cristianesimo antico*, ed. C. Mazzucco (Torino: dell'Orso, 2007); Susanna Barsella, "Il riso dei padri: Il caso di madonna Filippa (Dec., VI 7)," *Humanistica* 4 (2009): 13–18. For more bibliography on this subject, see Alberti Francesca, *Le rire, le ridicule et le comique dans la peinture italienne de la Renaissance. Des facéties de Corrège aux fables burlesques de Tintoret*, PhD Université Paris 1 Panthéon-Sorbonne, 2013.

50 On *eutrapelia*, see Aristotle, *Ethics* (IV, 6). Thomas Aquinas translated this book into Latin; on his own thoughts about laughter and religion see Jacques Le Goff, *Un autre Moyen Âge* (Paris:

Gallimard, 1999), 1343–68, particularly 1360, n. 6; Minois, 2000, 923; Carla Casagrande, "Ridere in Paradiso. Gaudio, giubilio e riso tra angeli e beati," in *Il riso. "Homo risibilis,"* 2005, 187–9; Michel-Marie Dufeil, "Risus in theologia sancti Thome," in *Le rire au Moyen Âge dans la littérature et dans les arts* (Bordeaux: Presses universitaires de Bordeaux, 1990), 147–63.

51 Mikhaïl Bakhtine, *L'œuvre de François Rabelais et la culture populaire au Moyen Âge et sous la Renaissance*, trans. A. Robel (Paris: Gallimard, 2012), 86; Maria Caterina Jacobelli, *Il Risus Paschalis, e il fondamento teologico del piacere sessuale*, 1990 (Verona: Querinina, 2004), 16–27; Micheal O'Connell, "Mockery, Farce, and *Risus Paschalis* in the York *Christ before Herod*," in *Ludus. Medieval and Early Renaissance Theatre and Drama*, ed. W. Hüsken, K. Schoell and L. Søndergaard (Amsterdam: Rodopi, 2002), 45–58; Giuseppe Maria Viscardi, *Tra Europa e "Indie di quaggiù." Chiesa, religiosità e cultura popolare nel Mezzogiorno (secoli XV–XIX)* (Roma: Edizioni di Storia e Letteratura, 2005), 295–304.

52 Jacobelli, 2004, 16–27; Barsella, 2009, 15–16.

53 Gabriele Paleotti, *Discourse on sacred and profane images* (Los Angeles: trans. W. McCuaig, The Getty Research Institute, 2012), 312.

54 Ibid., 313.

55 Derogatory images of Joseph are rare during the XVIIth century, yet his figure can sometimes appear ambiguous as in Orazio Gentileschi's *Rest from the Flight into Egypt*, 1628, Paris, Musée du Louvre. Burke recalls the opinion of several leading figure of the Counter-Reformation, such as Carlo Borromeo or Robert Bellarmine, who were against revealing details about the lives of saints that might encourage laughter rather than edification (*quae risum potis quam aedificationem pariant*). Peter Burke, "Frontiers of the Comic in Early Modern Italy, c. 1350–1750," in *A Cultural History of Humour*, ed. J. Bremmer and H. Roodenburg, 1997 (Cambridge: Polity Press, 2005), 69.

56 Erkinger Schwarzenberg, "La gelosia di Vulcano alle corti di Mantova e di Ferrara," *Mitteilungen des Kunsthistorischen Institutes in Florenz* 49:3 (2005), 290–318.

57 Vasvari, 1995, 168.

58 Matthews-Grieco, Sara, "*Satyrs and sausages: erotic strategies and the print market in Cinquecento Italy*," in *Erotic cultures of Renaissance Italy*, ed. S. Matthews-Grieco (Farnham, UK/Burlington, VT: Ashgate, 2010), 19–60; Rebecca Zorach, "Passioni triangolari," in *Sesso nel Rinascimento. Pratica, perversione e punizione nell'Italia Rinascimentale*, ed. A. Levy (Firenze: Le lettere, 2009), 166–7.

59 "Marte al son de l'ancuzene de Vulcan sbusava le perle de so muier Venere," in *Le Lettere di Messer Andrea Calmo*, ed. Andrea Calmo, 4 vols. (1547), I, 45.

60 The *Allegory of September* in Schifanoia's Sala dei Mesi in Ferrara is one of the rare antecedents to this two-part composition.

61 In Palma Giovane's painting, the kiss of Venus and Cupid anticipates the goddess' amorous exchanges with Mars, painted in another picture at the National Gallery in London. In Agostino Carracci's drawing (Royal Library Windsor Castle), the bored attitude of Cupid parodies the efforts of the blacksmith who, although he is working hardily, does not manage to capture his wife's attention.

62 In a private collection: see Arthur E. Popham, *Catalogue of the drawings of Parmigianino* (New Haven: Yale University Press, 1971), III, plate 365; David Ekserdjian, *Parmigianino* (New Haven: Yale University Press, 2006), 114.

63 Tintoretto's picture at Palazzo Pitti in Florence has already been associated with the iconography of the *Rest from the flight into Egypt* in *The Myth of Venus*, exhib. cat. (Cinisello Balsamo: Silvana, Arthemisia 2003), 92–3.

64 Picture at the Alte Pinakothek in Munich. Although the paintings have never been interpreted as *pendants*, it should be noticed that Vulcan's position, his gesture and the cloth he is wearing around his hips are exactly the same in both pictures.

65 See examples in Michael A. Jacobsen, "Vulcan forging Cupid's wing," *The Art Bulletin* 54:4 (1972): 418–29; Roland Krischel, "*L'armamento di Amore*: un'opera giovanile di Jacopo Tintoretto," *Venezia Cinquecento* 3:5 (1993): 79–96.

66 For example see Bernhard Strigel, *Holy Family* (c. 1505) at the Germanisches Nationalmuseum in Nuremberg, or Johann Sadelern, *Holy Family before St. Michael's Church*, engraved as a frontispiece for *Trophea Bavarica Sancto Micheali Archangelo* (Munich: 1597). During the XVIIth century, the two iconographies might easily have been confused. One might compare, for example, Bartolomeo Esteban Murillo, *Holy Family with Saint John the Baptist* (1655–1660) with David Teniers (the elder), *Venus visiting Vulcan's forge* (1638).

67 See Cynthia Hahn, "Joseph as Ambrose's 'Artisan of Soul' in the *Holy Family in Egypt* by Albrecht Durer," *Zeitschrift für Kunstgeschichte* 47:4 (1984): 515–22; Francesco Colallucci, "*Muscipula diaboli?* Una pseudo-trappola per topi nell'*Adorazione* di Lorenzo Lotto a Washington," *Artibus et Historiae*, 21 (1990): 71–88; Hartmut Krohm, "Alter Daedalus- Zum Begriff künstlerischer Tätigkeit in Dürers 'Marienleben,' in *Aus Albrecht Dürers Welt* (Turnhout: Brepols, 2001), 77–90; Baptiste Dautreme "Image du père éternel et image du père terrestre: l'iconographie de saint Joseph entre le Quattrocento et le Cinquecento," *Vivens Homo* 17 (2006), XVII: 147–78.

68 There is a controversy on the dating of the painting, see *Tintoretto*, exhib. cat. (Madrid: Museo nacional del Prado, 2007), cat. 5, 200.

69 For an extensive bibliography on this painting see ibid., 200; also see Louise Beverly Brown and Erasmus Weddigen articles in *Jacopo Tintoretto nel quarto centenario della morte*, eds. P. Rossi and L. Puppi (Padova: il Poligrafo, 1996); Claudia Cieri Via, "Venere, Vulcano e Marte: un'allegoria mitologica nella cultura veneta del Cinquecento," in *Die Allegorese des antiken mythos*, ed. H.-J. Horn and H. Walter (Wiesbaden: Harrassowitz Verlag, 1997), 351–94; Daniel Arasse, *On n'y voit rien, descriptions*, 2000 (Paris: Denoël, 2005), 11–23; Zorach, 2009.

70 Roland Krischel, "Jacopo Tintoretto and Giulio Romano" in *Jacopo Tintoretto*, ed. M. Falomir and B. Aikema (Madrid: M. Falomir, 2009), 58–65.

71 Paul F. Norton, "The lost sleeping Cupid of Michelangelo," *The Art Bulletin* 39 (1957): 254–6.

72 Therefore, I think that the title of the painting could be changed to *Vulcan's doubt*.

73 The connection between Tintoretto's painting and the iconography of a satyr discovering a nymph has been noticed first by Claudia Cieri Via, who gives many examples to support her hypothesis, starting with the illustration of Francesco Colonna's *Hypnerothomachia Poliphili* (1499) (Cieri Via, 1997).

74 Vulcan, on the point of capturing the lovers under the net, looks like the satyr in a drawing by Frans Floris dating c. 1550.

75 Venus's shameful gesture of lifting the transparent and flimsy *velamen* may also be interpreted as a way to seduce her husband. The same action is one of Armida's deceptive tricks, which is described by Torquato Tasso in the following way: "Vela il soverchio ardir con la vergogna / E fa' manto del vero a la menzogna', Torquato Tasso," *Gerusalemme liberata*, IV, vv. 199–200.

76 Even though he is sleeping, Cupid exercises his power, see *Anthologie Grecque. Anthologie Palatine*, ed. and trans. P. Walt, J. Guillon (Paris: Les Belles Lettres, 1990), 16 vols., 211–12. On Cupid as an image of deception: *Venere e amore: Michelangelo e la nuova bellezza ideale*, exhib. cat. (Firenze: Giunti, 2002), 90–108.

77 In the *De Pictura*, Alberti compares the act of painting to archery. The same idea appears in Filarete's *Trattato di architettura* (1465). Kubovy and Arasse have shown how artists conceived rays of light as arrows, see Michael Kubovy, *The psychology of perspective and Renaissance art* (Cambridge: Cambridge University Press, 1986), 8–16; Daniel Arasse, "Le corps fictif de Sebastien et le coup d'oeil d'Antonello," *Études de lettres* 2 (1983): 54–72.

78 For mentions of the word *macchia* in adulterous documents and trials see "El più soave et dolce et dilectevole et gratioso bochone." *Amore e sesso al tempo dei Gonzaga*, ed. Costantino Cipolla and Giancarlo Malacarne (Milano: Franco Angeli, 2006), 243. The law was promulgated June 30, 1589, see Alexander F. Cowan, *Marriage, manners and mobility in early modern Venice* (Farnham, UK/Burlington, VT: Ashgate, 2007), 137. When referring to a woman, the phrase "senza macchio all'honestà" meant "without any stain on her honourable reputation."

79 For the story of the Cnidian Venus, see Pliny, *Natural History*, 36.21. Renaissance references to the ancient *macchia* are discussed by Elizabeth Cropper, "The Place of Beauty in the High Renaissance and Its Displacement in the History of Art," in *Place and Displacement in the Renaissance* (Binghamton, New York: Center for Medieval and Renaissance Studies, 1995), 188; Fredrika H. Jacobs, "Aretino and Michelangelo, Dolce and Titian: Femmina, Masculo, Grazia," *Art Bulletin*, 82:1 (2000): 52; Philippe L. Sohm, *Pittoresco: Marco Boschini, his critics, and their critiques of painterly brushwork in seventeenth and eighteenth century Italy* (Cambridge: Cambridge Studies in the History of Art, 1991), 36–42.

80 Daniel Arasse, *On n'y voit rien. Descriptions* (Paris: Gallimard, 2005), 20: "le vase de verre posé sur le rebord de la fenêtre est plus subtil, parce que plus irrévérencieux sans doute: il fait sourire car il évoque irrésistiblement la transparence du vase virginal de Marie 'qui n'a-jamais-connu-d'homme.'"

81 "Just as the brilliance of the sun fills and penetrates a glass window without damaging it, and pierces the solid form with imperceptible subtlety, neither hurting it when entering nor destroying it when emerging: thus the word of God, the splendour of the Father, entered the virgin chamber and then came forth the closed womb," quoted in Millard Meiss, "Light as Form and Symbol in Some Fifteenth-Century Paintings," *The Art Bulletin* 27:3 (1945): 176.

82 "Vergine doppo il gentil parto e sempre / Qual saldo vetro ov'entra e esce il sole / Che intero si riman dentro e di fore, / Ti loderò con semplici parole," Pietro Aretino, *La Passione di Gesù*, quoted in *Un pronostico satirico di Pietro Aretino (MDXXXIIII)*, 1534, ed. A. Luzio (Bergamo: Instituto italiano d'arti grafiche, 1900), 120.

83 On the relation between reflections and armour see Diane H. Bodart, "Le reflets et l'éclat. Jeux de l'envers dans la peinture vénitienne du XVIe siècle," *Titien, Tintoret, Véronèse: rivalités à Venise*, exhib. cat. (Paris: Hazan, 2009), 232, "l'insistance sur le traitement lumineux des armures fait écho au thème du *lustro*, le lustre en tant qu'éclat de la lumière réfléchie comme l'avait définie Leonard en opposition au *lume*, l'illumination diffuse venant de la lumière indirecte." On light reflection in Venetian art see also Paul Hills, "Ray, line, vision and traces in Renaissance art," *Word & Image* 6:3 (1990): 217–25.

84 The barking dog is a *leitmotif* of comic literature quoted by Cicero and Castiglione, see Barbara C. Bowen, "Roman Jokes and the Renaissance Prince 1455–1528," *Illinois Classical Studies* 9 (1984): 137–48.

85 Stacius's description of the armour is quoted by Bodart, 2009, note 20.

86 For example, Raphael's *Madonna of the Blue Diadem*, v. 1510–1512, oil on wood, 68 × 49 cm, Paris, Musée du Louvre.

87 *Cfr. Supra*, note 19.

88 Zorach, 2009, 168.

89 Tom Nichols, "Price, Prestezza and Production in Jacopo Tintoretto's Business Strategy," Venezia Cinquecento 4:12 (1996): 207–33; Idem, Understanding Tintoretto's "prestezza": literary and other approaches to the contested artistic culture of mid-Cinquecento Venice, in Officine del nuovo, eds. H. Hendrix and P. Procaccioli (Manziana: Vecchiarelli, 2008), 51–64.

90 Boschini speaks of "colpi mortali" see Sohm, 1991, 146–52; Guillaume Cassegrain, *Tintoret* (Paris: Hazan, 2011), ch. II.

91 "E beato il nome vostro, se reduceste la prestezza del fatto in la pazienza del fare. Benché a poco a poco a ciò provvederanno gli anni. Conciosia ch'essi, e non altri, sono bastati a raffrenare il corso de la trascuratezza, di che tanto si prevale a gioventù volenterosa e veloce," in Pietro Aretino, *Lettere* ed. P. Procaccioli, (Roma and Salerno: Edizione Nazionale dell'opere di Pietro Aretino, 1999–2002), IV, no. 429, 266.

92 Mark W. Roskill, *Dolce's Aretino and Venetian art theory of the Cinquecento*, (Toronto: University of Toronto, 2000), 210. Also see Federico Zuccaro's *Lamento della pittura*, writes that Tintoretto has stained the robe of Art: "questa veste é macchiata é gran dolore, che il cor m'afligge, e mi tormenta l'alma" and "cadei, misera me, per un tentore, che di far cose grandi mi dié segno, mentre ne gli anni suoi era nel fiore," Federico Zuccaro, *Il Lamento della pittura su l'onde venete*, 1605, *Scritti d'arte di Federico Zuccari* (Firenze: L. S. Olschki, 1961), 126–7.

93 See Juan Ruiz, *Libro de buen amor*, c. 1322 (Madrid: Espasa-Calpe, 1997), vv. 474–84; Matteo Bandello, *La terza parte de le Novelle*, 1554 (Alessandria, ed. Dell'Orso, 1995), 277–82.

94 On Titian see Mary Pardo, "Artifice as seduction in Titian," in *Sexuality and Gender in Early Modern Europe: Institutions, Texts, Images*, ed. J. Grantham Turner (Cambridge: Cambridge University Press, 1993), 55–89; *Titian's* Venus of Urbino, ed. R. Goffen (Cambridge: Cambridge University Press, 1997).

95 During the 16th century, the "sexualization" of perspective in painting was a current phenomenon. Alberti's triangular perspective system was metaphorically associated to women's *pudenda* and the artist's brush became a well know substitute for the phallus. Many examples testify to this tradition, from the famous expression of Paolo Uccello "oh che dolce cosa è questa prospettiva!" to Bronzino's burlesque poems, in which *pennello, prospettiva* and *scorcio* become metaphors of sexual intercourse as in many carnavalesque songs (see Deborah Parker, "Towards a Reading of Bronzino's Burlesque Poetry," *Renaissance Quarterly* 50:4 (1997): 1011–44; Alberti, 2009, 22–3). To illustrate his treatise on perspective, Durer chose the image of an artist tracing the foreshortening of a lascivious naked female model using a *grille* and a long prism with a phallic shape, which gave the act of looking at and creating an erotic connotation (see Zorach, 2009, 163).

96 Maria H. Loh, *Titian remade: repetition and the transformation of Early Modern Italian Art* (Los Angeles: Getty Research Institute, 2007), 23, 33–7, 38–42: "The artistic strategy of serial repetition, therefore, functioned as a sociological strategy for crafting artistic hegemony, ideology, and taste"; also Carlo Ginzburg, "Titian, Ovid and the sixteenth century codes for erotic illustration," in *Titian's* Venus of Urbino, 23–36.

97 Cfr. Supra, 88.

98 "Per non essere la più laudabile pace, che la guerra che in gara della virtù fà l'uomo virtuoso, contra l'altro: quella del Tintoretto, et ciascun pittore, che insieme contendano per la perminenza; puo chiamarsi fraternal amistade infra loro; in tanto attenda quello, et questo studiare il disegno,

et il colorire, se nella inuentine, et nella pratica costui vuole auanzar'colui, et colui, costui; et cosi tutti rimarrano famosi, se bene Iacopo nel corso è si puo dir' presso il palio, ma solo voi siete senza il fastidio della emulazione," Venice, April, 1548, see *Documentation* in *Tintoretto*, 2007, 420.

99 "È atto degno del suo errore il pentirsi che fa Tiziano circa la furia che gli sciolse in mio pregiudizio a punto allora la lingua che doveva essercitarla in ringraziarmi del ciò che sempre feci per grado de la sua fama e del commodo. Io, oltra che ognuno sa il quanto è salito in suso la sua virtù per mio mezo, ne chiamo in testimonio la conscienza di lui solo, e il vero; e, quando pure il Tintorello, per tristizia o pazzia, fusse mancato a la promessa, che colpa ne ho io ? Sì che, se ben merito che mi chiegga perdono, come di voler far dice, non voglio. Imperoché altri non dimanda perdono del fallo a se stesso. Bastami assai che mi abbia per quel fratel ch'io gli sono ; confessando essere uscito dei termini convenienti ad uomo come lui grave di età e di senno. Di genaio, in Vinezia, M.D.XLVIII 1548," Aretino, 2000, V, 132.

100 Andrea Calmo, *il Rimanente de le pacevole, et ingegnose lettere indirizzate a diversi, con bellissime argutie. Sotto vaii, et sottilissimi discorsi, dichiarati* (Venezia: Comin da Trino di Monferrato, 1548), 37.

101 Calmo, 1548, 21; for the eye of the hammer, *occhio del martèlo*, see Giuseppe Boerio, *Dizionario del dialetto veneziano* (Venezia: Reale tipografia di Giovanni Cecchini, 1867). Mars is also able to escape in the *Roman de la Rose*, where, although the husband surprises the lovers, the wife refuses to face up to the facts and by telling a bunch of lies enables her lover to escape, see Guillaume de Lorris and Jean de Meung, *The Romance of the Rose*, trans. C. Dahlberg (Princeton, NJ: Princeton University Press, 1971), vv. 18031–100.

102 For the *beffe* in 16th-century artistic context see Adriana Mauriello, "Artisti e beffe in alcune novelle del'500 (Lasca, Doni, Fortini)," *Letteratura & arte* 3 2005 (2006): 81–91.

103 "Gl'nganni altrui, et ci dilettano e ci costringono per l'allegrezza a ridere, essendo cagione la natura nostra corrotta per lo peccato de' nostri primi parenti." As Ludovico Castelvetro writes in his *Poetic*, deceit (*inganno*) was a well know ingredient for laughter, Ludovico Castelvetro, *Poetica d'Aristotele: volgarizzata e sposta*, 1570 (Roma: Laterza, 1978), 131.

104 The presence of the large mirror relates the satirical content of the picture to comedies published in that period. For 16th-century authors, comedies were conceived as polished mirrors capable of reflecting contemporary society. "Onde la scena si può dire un lucido specchio: nel qual ciscuno puote discernere quello che in questa vita incerta e misera per l'uomo seguir si debba, e quel che fugire," Ludovico Dolce, *Il Marito* (Venezia: G. Giolito de' Ferrari, 1545), v. 17–21. See Marvin T. Herrick, *Comic theory in Sixteenth Century* (Urbana: University of Illinois Press, 1964).

105 Windsor Castle, Royal Library inv. RL 1841. The drawing is briefly discussed by Clare Robertson, "Annibale Carracci and *Invenzione:* Medium and function in the Early Drawings," *Master Drawings* 35:1 (1997): 26–7.

106 "Tristo è quel discepolo che non avanza il suo maestro" (Codice Forster, III, f. 66 v).

Niklaus Manuel and Urs Graf: Cuckolds, Impotence and Sex Workers in Swiss Renaissance Art (c. 1510–1517)[1]

Christiane Andersson

Rapid social change and economic turmoil in the early 16th century produced new and unusual images in the history of northern Swiss art, especially drawings of a sexual nature, amongst which are depictions of cuckolds and references to impotence that had not previously been part of the pictorial tradition in this area. These new images were produced in the urban centers of Bern and Basel during the second decade of the century, during the last few years before another source of great upheaval, the Protestant Reformation, would take hold. Although expressions of discontent with the practices of the Catholic Church were already widespread, the religious struggles that were to dominate the rest of the 16th century had not yet appeared in full force.

In the late 15th and early 16th centuries, the Swiss Confederacy, which by 1513 consisted of 13 cantons, had become a society founded on a culture of mercenary warfare. War determined economic life, politics, religion and even art, and the mercenary lifestyle led to pervasive and rapid social and economic change. The two most important Swiss artists of this period whose work will be studied here, Niklaus Manuel Deutsch of Bern and Urs Graf of Basel, both served as mercenary soldiers numerous times.[2] They experienced firsthand this type of temporary military service that was then considered the most important, and for many the most lucrative—occupation, so it is hardly surprising that the major social and political issues of the time also became prominent themes in their artistic production. In their drawings, these two artists focused particularly on the lives of mercenaries and their women, on the transitoriness of life, love and military success and on the conflicts between the sexes. For the purposes of this volume, I will here concentrate on the drawings representing the fragility of men's honor lost through war, cuckoldry or impotence, and on the vulnerability of men with respect to lustful and domineering women. Conflicts that arose in Switzerland between cantons, between social classes and between the sexes thus constitute the historical context in which these images of cuckolds and impotence should be interpreted and understood.

Niklaus Manuel Deutsch

Niklaus Manuel Deutsch was a painter, draughtsman, designer of woodcuts and stained glass panels, playwright and statesman active in Bern between about 1510 and 1530, the year of his death. He was the most important artist of the early 16th century in Bern, best known for his paintings—altarpieces, portraits, mythological and biblical scenes—and for his fine drawings.[3] He served on the city council and was an active supporter of the Reformation in his native city. His plays all focus on antipapal issues from the point of view of the "common man,"[4] while his artwork encompasses the major religious and secular themes current in his time.

Manuel's drawing of a cuckold (Fig. 8.1) created with black chalk or charcoal on an unusually large sheet of paper (31 × 21 cm) depicts an almost nude man wearing on his head a cock or rooster and a curved ram's horn, attributes that were universally understood in early 16th-century Switzerland (and in most of Europe, as the essays in this volume make abundantly clear) as identifying a cuckold. The facial expression of this no-longer young man suggests displeasure or disappointment. His beard, a traditional sign of manhood, is short and skimpy, not what was expected of a mature adult, while his bare torso and near total nudity give him a certain vulnerability. He wears only a single, very curious garment: frilly pants that both reveal and draw attention to the diminutive size of his genitals, perhaps implying his impotence. In Swiss art of this period, such a frivolous garment is found only in Manuel's work, and as we will see further on, is always used in a sexually suggestive context. Here it is held together at the left side with a ribbon forming a bow. The decorative bow, something usually worn by women in this period,[5] and therefore "unmanly," is repeated at his knees, where two ribbons resemble garters but hold up nothing. The cuckold clutches in his hands a symbolic object to which we will return, a double rope, weighted at one end with two large balls.

The banderole fluttering above his head is a common Renaissance device used to add elucidating inscriptions to images. Here it bears both the artist's signature and an inscription that provides some clues for the interpretation of the work. Four words, slightly trimmed at the middle but quite legible, read: *NIEMMAN.KANSS.(A)LSS.WV̈SSE(N)* or "no one can know it all," meaning that no one can anticipate how things will turn out and implying, in this context, that the man's cuckoldry was certainly an unexpected state of affairs. This phrase was the artist's favorite motto, and should be interpreted as an expression of the uncertainty and turmoil of life and of a certain resignation when confronted with powers beyond his control. Manuel inscribed this saying, especially in its abbreviated form *NKAW*, on a number of his drawings between c. 1510 and 1515, and most often on images illustrating the power of women over men, a fraught topic also implied in this drawing of a cuckold. The pictures that bear this motto[6] thus emphasize the uncertainty and dangers of love.

In two such drawings, created about 1510 and inscribed with the acronym *NKAW*, attractive young women carry hearts impaled on a Swiss sword and on a mercenary's pike, as a kind of trophy.[7] In another, later drawing of about 1517 in Manuel's silverpoint model book, a nude woman holds a heart that she is about to stab with a Swiss dagger.[8] In the 1510 drawing with the heart pierced by a pike, the artist makes it clear that it is to be understood as his own heart.[9] The woman holding the weapon looks down at Niklaus Manuel's monogram and at the dagger, which both identify (as we shall soon see) the artist himself in this sketch. The women in all of these works are clearly in control of (men's) hearts and the men, as the images imply, have fallen prey to female wiles and thereby lost their hearts. And, as the artist's own motto points out, none of them could anticipate the suffering that giving their heart to a woman would cause them—NKAW, "no-one can know it all."

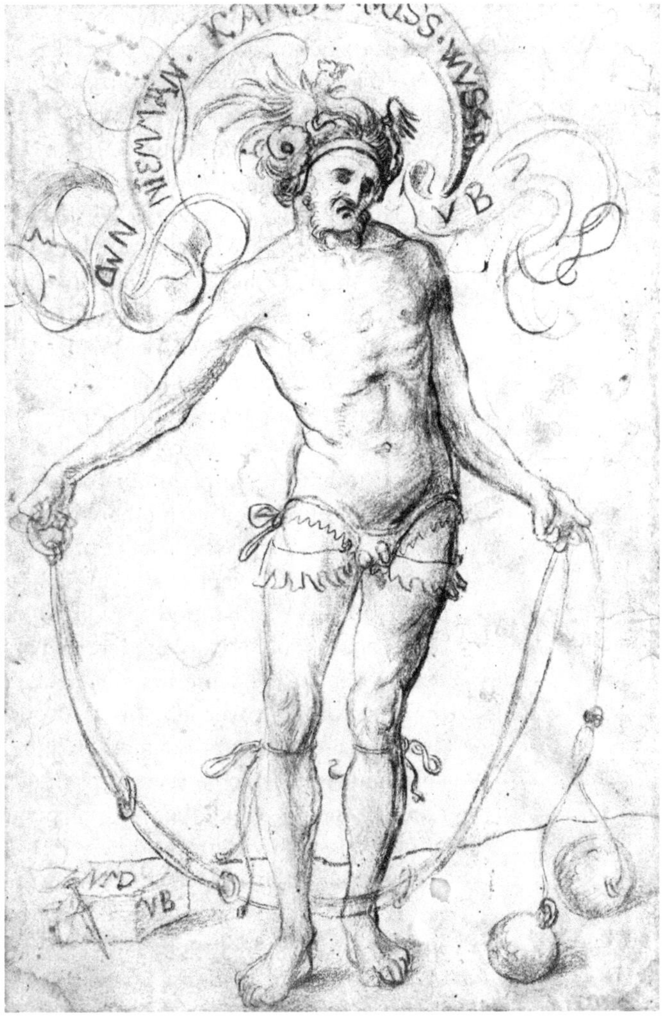

8.1 Niklaus Manuel Deutsch, *Cuckold*, c. 1514, black chalk, 31.2 × 21.1 cm, Kunstmuseum Basel, Kupferstichkabinett (photo: Martin P. Bühler)

Returning to Manuel's drawing of a cuckold (Fig. 8.1), the inscription "*NIEMMAN.KANSS.(A)LSS.WV̈SSE(N)*" refers to the cuckold himself: having given his heart to a woman who has betrayed and cuckolded him, he appears vulnerable, perplexed, helpless and, in the value system of this period, worthy only of scorn and ridicule. The fluttering banderole over the cuckold also bears the artist's signature, inscribed in the form of his initials shown upside down (*NMD* for Niklaus Manuel Deutsch), and it identifies his home town at the right (*VB* meaning "von Bern"). The artist signed his work with the same initials a second time on the stone at the lower left: *NMD* and *VB*. Propped up against the stone is a Swiss dagger, a weapon so ubiquitous among the Swiss that it came to be understood as a national symbol. The artist consistently added it to his monogram as a part of his signature. The shape and length of this typically Swiss weapon changed over the course of the first decades of the 16th century, and its shape evolved correspondingly in the artist's signature as well. This formal evolution helps to date the drawing to about 1514.

The unusually large size of this drawing of a hapless cuckold, the artist's double signature and the work's high degree of finish and artistic refinement suggest that Niklaus Manuel created this drawing as an independent work of art. This purpose distinguishes it clearly from other drawings by this artist, made as preparatory sketches for works of art to be executed in other mediums, such as stained glass.[10] The special status of this drawing as an independent work of art on a par with a small painting gives it greater importance and meaning within the artist's oeuvre. It is a self-conscious, intentional and highly crafted visual statement, albeit one with a very unusual subject. Perhaps it was made for a patron with a sense of humor? Much more likely, however, is that the artist showed it to his friends as an amusement,[11] and it would appear to have remained in his possession: after Manuel's death it seems to have been purchased with other contents of his studio by the Basel collector, Basilius Amerbach, whose large holdings formed the foundation of the Basel Kunstmuseum's exceptionally fine collection of old masters.[12]

The NKAW motto found on Niklaus Manuel's drawing of a cuckold appears on yet another of his drawings created around the same time, c. 1514 (Fig. 8.2). It is signed in the same manner, with his initials and the Swiss dagger on the stone at the lower left. *NIEMAN. KANS. ALS. WV̈SSEN* is inscribed on this sketch of a young woman looking down at an overturned lamp in her left hand from which a few drops of oil trickle down. The overturned lamp identifies her as one of the five foolish virgins from the biblical parable of the wise and foolish virgins (Matthew 25:1–13), an allegorical story about how to enter the kingdom of Heaven. Having foolishly not planned ahead—contrary to the prudent wise virgins—and having no oil to light the way to welcome Christ—their "bridegroom"—the foolish virgins remained excluded from Christ's presence, meaning from Heaven.

In Swiss culture around 1510–1520, the foolish virgins' transgression was considered to have been a sexual one. This explains why, in Niklaus Manuel's drawing, the foolish virgin's skirt is hitched up to show her legs in a way no proper woman would have done in 1514. This detail reveals that the artist intended the drawing to be understood on two levels of meaning: she is not only a biblical, foolish virgin who has lost her oil, but also a sex worker who has lost her virginity.[13] Her appearance is typical of the camp followers and prostitutes who customarily accompanied mercenary campaigns and who appear often in drawings by Niklaus Manuel and Urs Graf. Once a woman had lost her virginity, she was required to wear a matron's bonnet (as shown here), a custom that applied not only to married women but also to sex workers. During this era, the loss of virginity outside of marriage generally meant that a woman had no other choice but to become a prostitute, and many women in the countryside became rape victims of marauding mercenary soldiers. With their farms plundered, the livestock stolen, the fields burned and their virginity lost, women had no other option than to join their abusers and accompany the military campaigns, where they cooked, washed and performed sexual services for the mercenaries.[14]

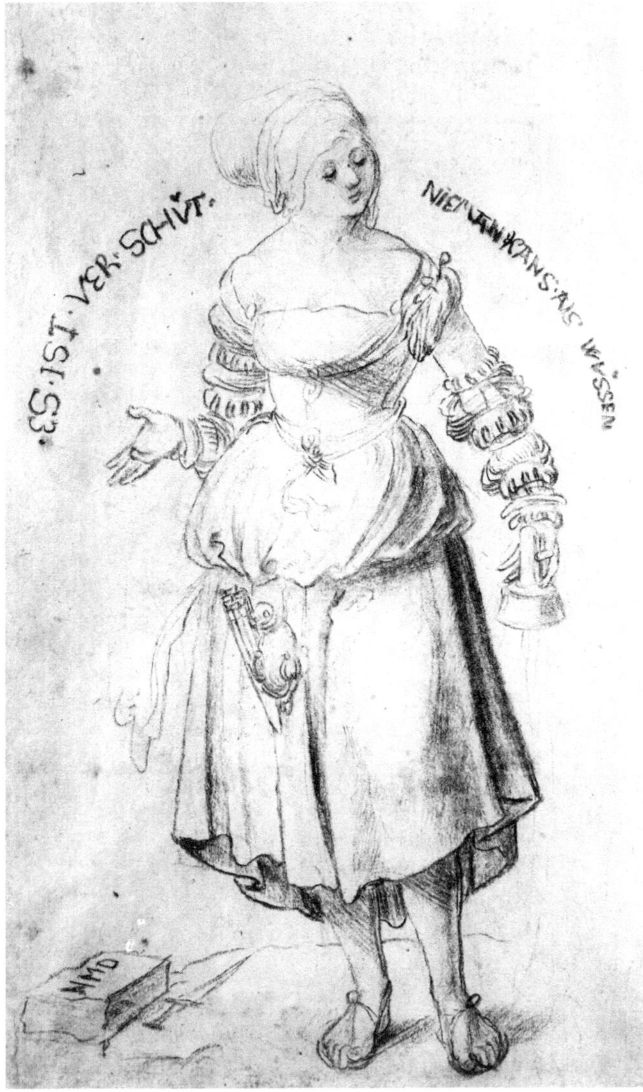

8.2 Niklaus Manuel Deutsch, *Foolish Virgin*, c. 1514, black chalk, 30.9 × 20.2 cm, Kunstmuseum Basel, Kupferstichkabinett (photo: Martin P. Bühler)

Manuel's foolish virgin is dressed in the latest fashion from northern Italy transmitted via the mercenary armies and their camp followers. Contemporary commentators like the Bernese chronicler Valerius Anshelm condemned such new trends in clothing for their expense and vanity. Wearing the new slashed sleeves and fashionable Italian-style sandals,[15] as well as a dagger and money purse dangling from a sash around her hips, Manuel's foolish virgin would appear to be successful in her current line of work. She makes an open gesture with her right hand, while with the left she pours the remaining oil from her lamp, saying, as the inscription states: "It is gone; no one can know everything" (*.ES. IST.VERSCHV̈T. NIEMAN.KANS. ALS.WV̈SSEN*). The term *verschütt* can refer to a loss of any kind, but here the lost oil refers both to the foolish virgin *topos* and to her lost virginity. Niklaus Manuel makes her seem to shrug it off, accepting her situation as inevitable.

Both drawings by Niklaus Manuel with these inscriptions convey a fatalistic sense of loss of control, a real and metaphorical sexual disorder that echoes the general turmoil of the times. Things just seem to go wrong; the cuckold and the sex worker could not have anticipated or prevented what happened to them: events beyond their control have inexorably, cruelly and radically changed their lives. And in both images, their difficulties are primarily erotic ones. The artist makes both figures endure the worst criticism that could be leveled at anyone during this age: the man has been cuckolded and the woman has lost her "honor." Both experience degradation to what this society considered

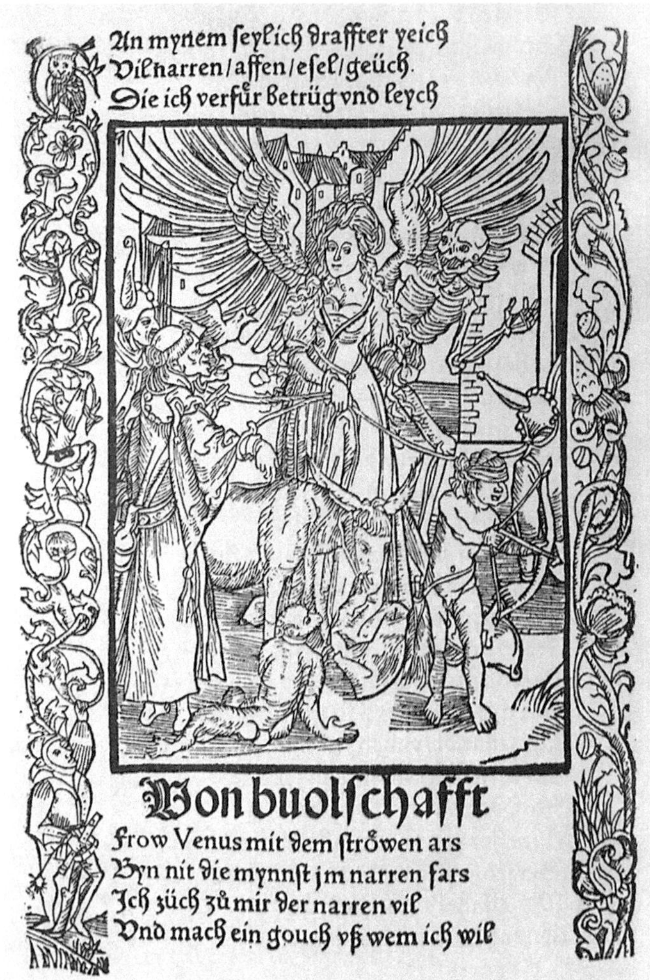
Von buolschafft
Frow Venus mit dem ströwen ars
Byn nit die mynnst jm narren fars
Ich züch zů mir der narren vil
Vnd mach ein gouch vß wem ich wil

8.3 "On Adultery," from Sebastian Brant, *Ship of Fools*, 1494, anonymous woodcut illustration, octavo size (photo: Andersson)

to be the lowest possible status among their sex.

Manuel's drawing of a cuckold (Fig. 8.1) suggests that the man's predicament was caused by falling in love with a woman and losing control. This meaning is specifically conveyed by a heretofore unstudied detail, the double cord that he holds in both hands and that passes between his legs. The two strands of rope are held together by rings and are anchored by two round weights on the ground. The pair of heavy balls, to the modern viewer reminiscent of a ball and chain, might also suggest a reflection with respect to his own, compromised virility—he has (metaphorically) lost his "balls." Furthermore, the cord he holds is a little known but not uncommon symbol in northern Switzerland and Germany during this period, with an extensive visual and literary tradition. It signifies and makes visible the emotional bond of the lovelorn, and often appears in comic or satirical contexts to poke fun at foolishly amorous men who have fallen prey to domineering women. Shown bound by ropes symbolizing both emotional dependence and physical subjugation to their beloved, lovers are frequent objects of ridicule in the satirical fool's literature so popular in northern Switzerland in the late 15th and the beginning of the 16th centuries. The first and best-known work of fool's literature (that spawned countless later imitations) was *The Ship of Fools*, written by Sebastian Brant and published—not by chance—on Carnival Day in 1494 in Basel.[16] Brant devised a litany of cautionary tales about the failings and foibles of his fellow men and women. In each chapter, illustrated by an allegorical woodcut, he discusses and warns against a particular human weakness, each presented by the author as a particular type of fool.

Symbolic ropes appear in the woodcut vignette illustrating Brant's chapter on adultery and illicit courtship entitled *Von buolschafft* (Fig. 8.3). The central figure of Venus is shown restraining various figures by ropes that encircle

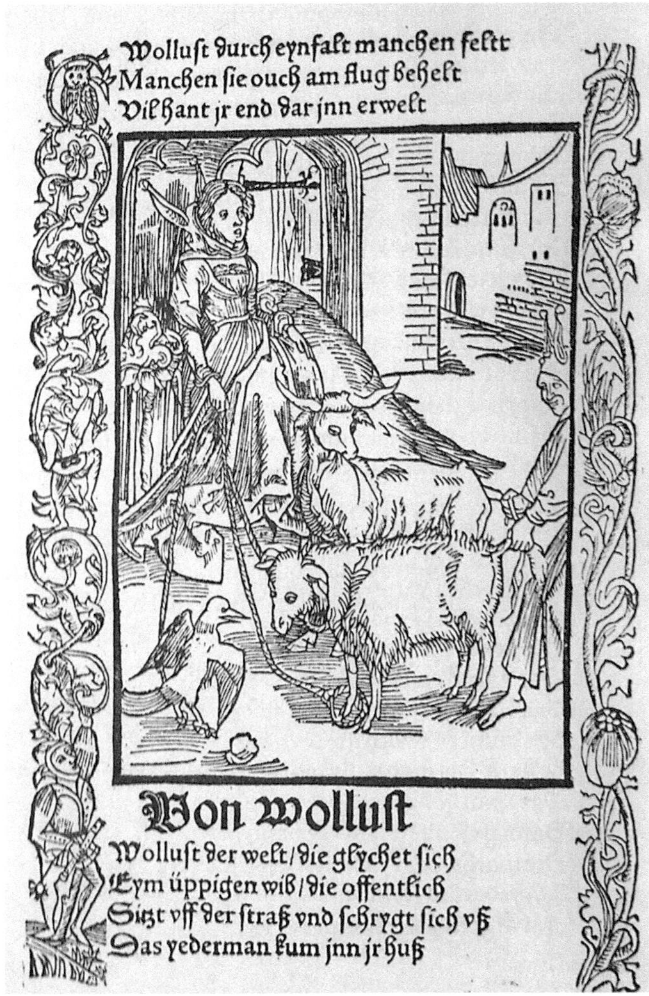
Wollust durch eynfalt manchen fellt
Manchen sie ouch am flug behelt
Vil hant jr end dar jnn erwelt
Von wollust
Wollust der welt / die glychet sich
Eym üppigen wiß / die offentlich
Sitzt vff der straß vnd schrygt sich vß
Das yederman kum jnn jr huß

8.4 "On Lust," from Sebastian Brant, *Ship of Fools*, 1494, anonymous woodcut illustration, octavo size (photo: Andersson)

the necks of two lovelorn fools (both wearing fools' caps) and other victims of love chosen for satirical effect: a tonsured monk, a monkey and a donkey. Behind Venus the foreboding skeleton of Death emerges, expressing a common moralistic message about sexual misconduct and reminding the viewer that earthly pleasures can lead to the death of the soul.[17] In the foreground, blindfolded Cupid readies his bow with which he is about to impale the next fool for love. Sebastian Brant's text above the woodcut image refers directly to the ropes shown in the image. Venus declares her intentions with the lovelorn fools she has captured: "I will pull on my rope many fools, monkeys, donkeys and cuckolds, and then seduce and betray them."[18] Brant's second text on this page, printed below the woodcut, emphasizes Venus' power over her fools. She says she will use her ropes to "pull" many fools toward her and turn each of them into a *Gouch*[19] or a cuckoo, a contemporary synonym for cuckolds.[20] Brant suggests that Venus and Cupid both create fools and cuckolds, potentially whenever a man falls in love. The emotional dependence and physical subjugation of the lovelorn as symbolized by the rope are, however, just the beginning of trouble between the sexes. It is what makes men vulnerable to the worst humiliation of all: becoming cuckolded.

Another chapter in Brant's *Ship of Fools*, entitled "On Lust" (*Von Wollust*), shows a similar allegorical female figure (Fig. 8.4), now without wings but wearing a fool's cap herself. She is a personification of Lust and Brant's text compares her to a sex worker in the street, procuring customers. The text states: "Worldly lust is like a voluptuous woman, who sits in the street and cries out for every man to come into her house."[21] She, too, holds various creatures snared by ropes: according to Brant these became her victims due to their own stupidity (*eynfalt*)—a cuckoo, a bull and a sheep. A fool amuses himself by pulling the latters' tails. Again, the ropes are the tangible sign of the power of lust over animals—and, by extension, of the prostitute over her clients—resulting in their physical and emotional enslavement.

The visual metaphor of the rope also appears in a number of 15th-century prints, such as the engraving by the Master of the Playing Cards (Fig. 8.5). An elegantly dressed lady riding on a donkey who appears to be embarking on a "hunting" expedition with a falcon is shown leading four monkeys on symbolic leashes. Instead of the falcon she would require during falconry, the printmaker has humorously illustrated a satirical cuckoo. At the right, four fools wearing fool's caps point to her; they are not bound with ropes like the monkeys, as they are already part of her entourage. Her comment about both her escorts is recorded in the inscription on the banderole.[22] She says: "I'll ride a donkey whenever I like; a cuckoo serves as my lure, with which I'll catch many fools and monkeys," and as the inscription points out, the cuckoo perched on her glove (here again called *Gauch,* the symbol of the cuckold) would seem to have already had a certain success as a lure. Both the three-part composition and the arches formed by the banderole suggest that the four fools and four monkeys are equally subservient to her. This allegorical engraving functions on two levels of meaning. What appears to be a hunting scene involving falconry expresses the power of women over lovelorn and potentially cuckolded men subjugated by their attraction to a beautiful woman. The engraver has drawn on the literary and visual traditions of the metaphorical hunt as an analogy of courtship, a familiar *topos* of the medieval imagery of courtly love. Perhaps the idea was derived from Ovid,[23] who metaphorically describes

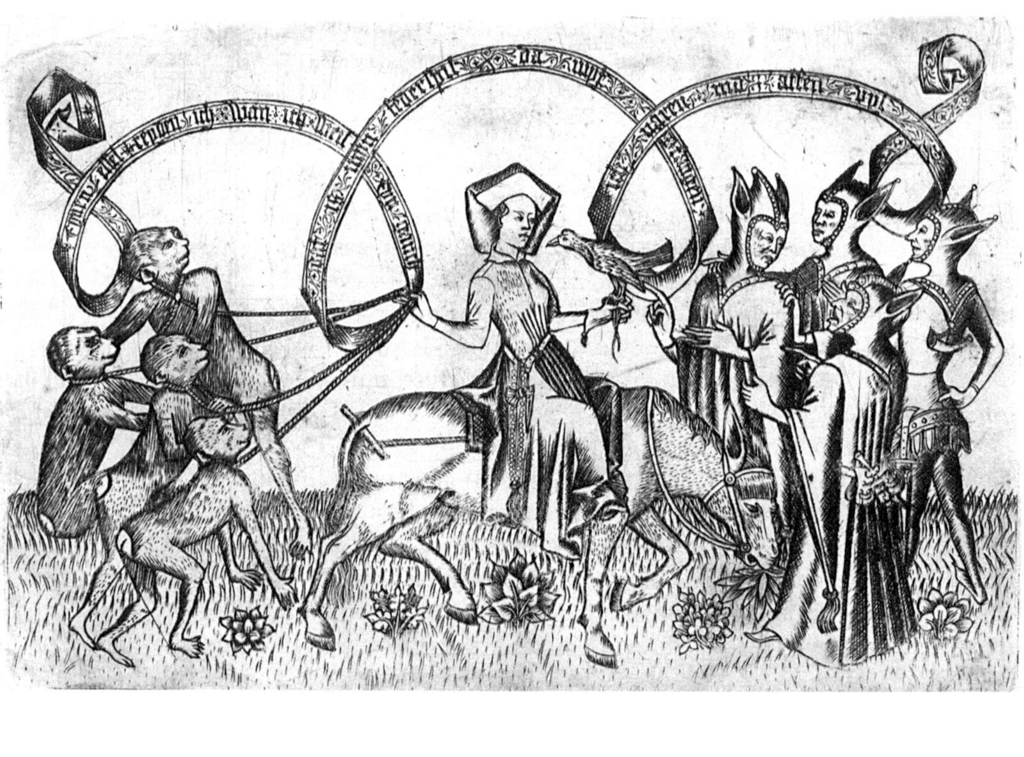

8.5 Master of the Playing Cards, *The Power of Women*, c. 1450, engraving, 11.3 × 17, 2 cm, Bayerische Staatsbibliothek Munich (Clm. 3941, fol. 139v)

women "hunting" and "catching" their mates like prey. The allusion was certainly common in 16th-century fool's literature: in Thomas Murner's *Geuchmat* of 1519, for example, women catch men with ropes in a chapter describing erotic seduction, appropriately entitled *Catching Fools*.[24]

Ropes are both the visual manifestation of an emotional bond and of a power relationship between the sexes; the battle of the sexes is in full swing, and falling in love can have dangerous consequences. In a carnival play of 1517 by the Nuremberg author Hans Sachs, entitled *The Courtiers of Venus* (*Das Hoffgesindt Veneris*), published in 1517, lovelorn fools are again ensnared, and Tannhäuser complains to Venus of being held as a prisoner on a rope.[25] Another literary text using this metaphor was a love song written by Niklaus Manuel's famous contemporary working in Basel, the artist Urs Graf, and published as a broadsheet about 1512.[26] In the second verse, the metaphorical bonds of Venus, here called *Venus strick*, describe the lover's captive state and emotional dependency on his sweetheart: "Alas my heart suffers such great pain because I cannot forget you and so I'm tightly bound with Venus' rope. Let me always be your lover." In the early 16th century, the rope analogy was also used in numerous satirical books belonging to the popular genre of fool's literature imitating Sebastian Brant's *Ship of Fools*. One of the most popular in northern Switzerland was Thomas Murner's treatise on folly, the *Narrenbeschwörung* of 1512.[27] Murner laments how love makes fools of even the strongest, wisest and noblest of men, such as the biblical Samson, robbed of his strength by Dalilah. Murner employs the metaphorical image of the rope to narrate the fates of wise kings, emperors and numerous famous men who were so foolish as to fall in love. In another passage, the author describes women less metaphorically and more realistically: they are actually leading their lovers around by ropes. Murner explains this practice with reference to the age-old idea that love is blind and thus these lovers literally cannot see, which makes them even more dependent on the women who lead them.

Niklaus Manuel himself was to use the metaphorical rope in a variety of works. In a drawing of Venus created about 1512 (Fig. 8.6 and Plate 11), Manuel depicts a female figure with large wings like Brant's Venus, balancing on a globe in mid-air and holding six ropes. Completely nude but for her necklace and headdress, she wears only a ribbon around one knee. She is unambiguously identified as Venus by the presence of Cupid, also shown with wings, who stands on her shoulders. The arrow in his drawn bow has a fool's cap affixed to it that he aims at his next victim, who will become an enamored fool, presumably wearing the cap. Here, the ropes Venus holds have nooses at the end and thus are a sort of lasso, one of which she holds aloft in her right hand, as if preparing to catch her next victim. Both Venus and Cupid occupy themselves with their prey, that is with the men—in the culture of this period, it's almost always men—who are about to be smitten with love. The victims are implied in the image, but not shown. The folly of love to which Cupid's victims are about to succumb is underscored by the

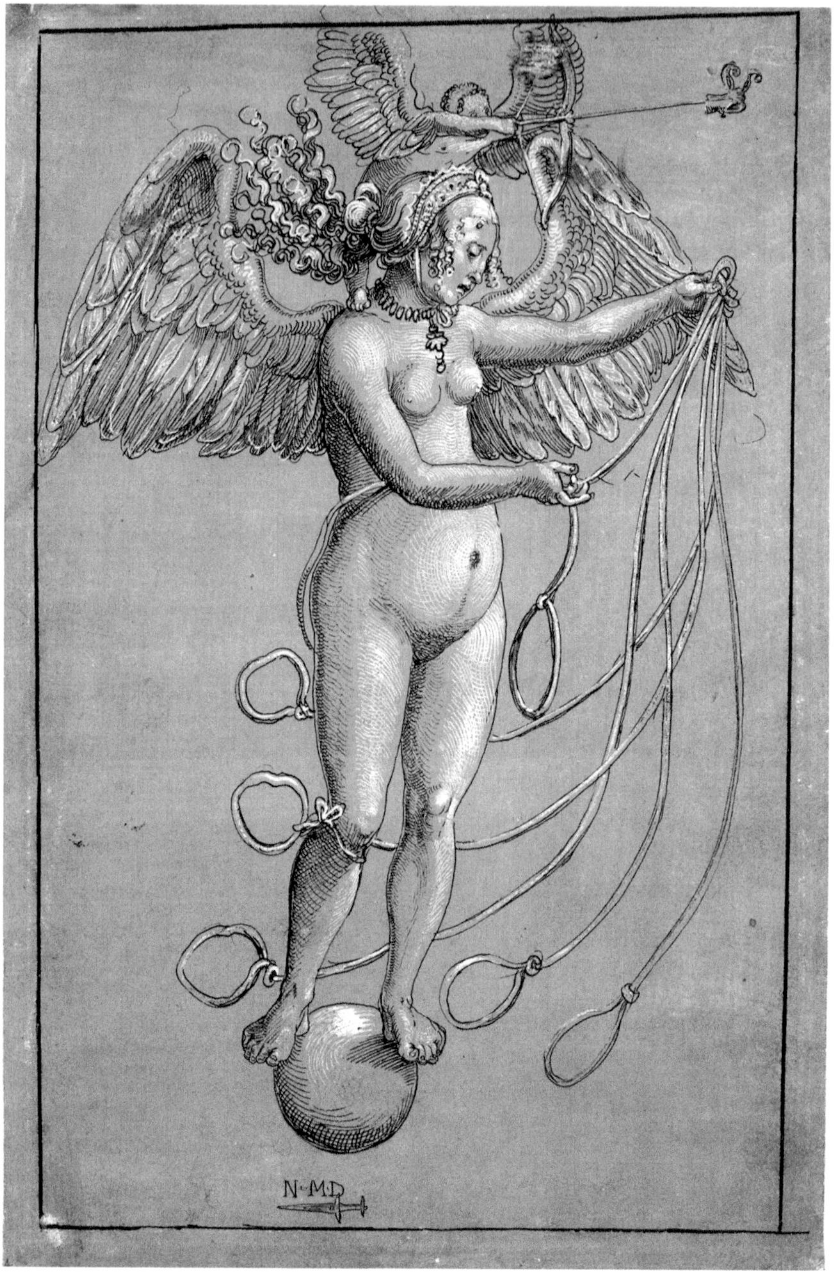

8.6 Niklaus Manuel Deutsch, *Venus*, c. 1512, chiaroscuro drawing, 31.4 × 21.7 cm, Kunstmuseum Basel, Kupferstichkabinett (photo: Martin P. Bühler)

fool's cap he shoots off on his arrow, offsetting the undeniably erotic nature of the drawing with a gentle moral satire.

Like Manuel's drawing of the cuckold, his drawing of Venus is quite large, with identical dimensions (31 × 21 cm), and is equally highly finished, although executed in different mediums. Here, Niklaus Manuel used pen and black ink on brownish-orange prepared paper, adding white highlights with a fine brush. He gave his composition a frame, a single black line applied with a quill pen and using a straight edge. The highlights showing where the light falls were executed in a white color that contains lead. It has oxidized in a few places, causing the white to turn greyish. Along the lower edge, the artist signed the drawing in his typical fashion with both his monogram, *NMD*, and the Swiss dagger. Like the artist's cuckold, the exceptional technical and artistic finesse suggests that it too was created as an independent work of art on a par with a small painting, and reveals the importance the artist evidently attached to the theme of Venus' power over men.

In another drawing by Niklaus Manuel, a pen and ink sketch he created about 1517 (Fig. 8.7), a young woman in contemporary dress holds a rope with a noose at the lower end. The degree of realistic detail in her clothes, expression and pose, as well as the absence of a banderole or other form of inscription, indicate that the artist has transposed the theme of amorous subjugation from the allegorical realm into that of a more personal reality. Placing a recognizable, functional object into the hand of an attractive, lavishly dressed young woman, Manuel has created a self-referential statement as he focuses the amorous allusion on himself. Manuel represents himself in this scene by placing conspicuously in the foreground his large and prominent monogram *NMD* alongside a Swiss dagger with the leather strap (by which it was worn on the body) laid out in the swirling shape of a love knot.[28] Manuel thus lays himself at her feet, both literally and metaphorically. The artist has also given this woman power over himself, as symbolized by her command of the lasso. She glances down at "him," present in the form of his monogram, seemingly fully cognizant of her power. The close proximity and the formal dialogue between the loops of the noose and of the intertwined love knot placed in the foreground eloquently express the artist's emotional entanglement.

A few years earlier, about 1512, Niklaus Manuel had created another drawing (Fig. 8.8) of an almost-nude man again wearing a pair of frilly pants, similar to those in his large drawing of a cuckold. In this earlier work, the artist even more emphatically shows the man as victim, leaning against a cross to which he is literally bound by ropes. Two more such bonds dangle from the crossbar above him to make the point more forcefully and more easily visible. While this drawing is a secular work, the cross surely alludes to Christ's Passion, although it has here been transformed into a locus for a different kind of suffering—that of the lovelorn man victimized by an amorous attachment. The artist shows us a martyr to love, a slave to the power of women, using a visual *topos* that was already in circulation in prints in this period.[29] Compared to the cuckold who exudes perplexity and helplessness, this figure inspires pity.

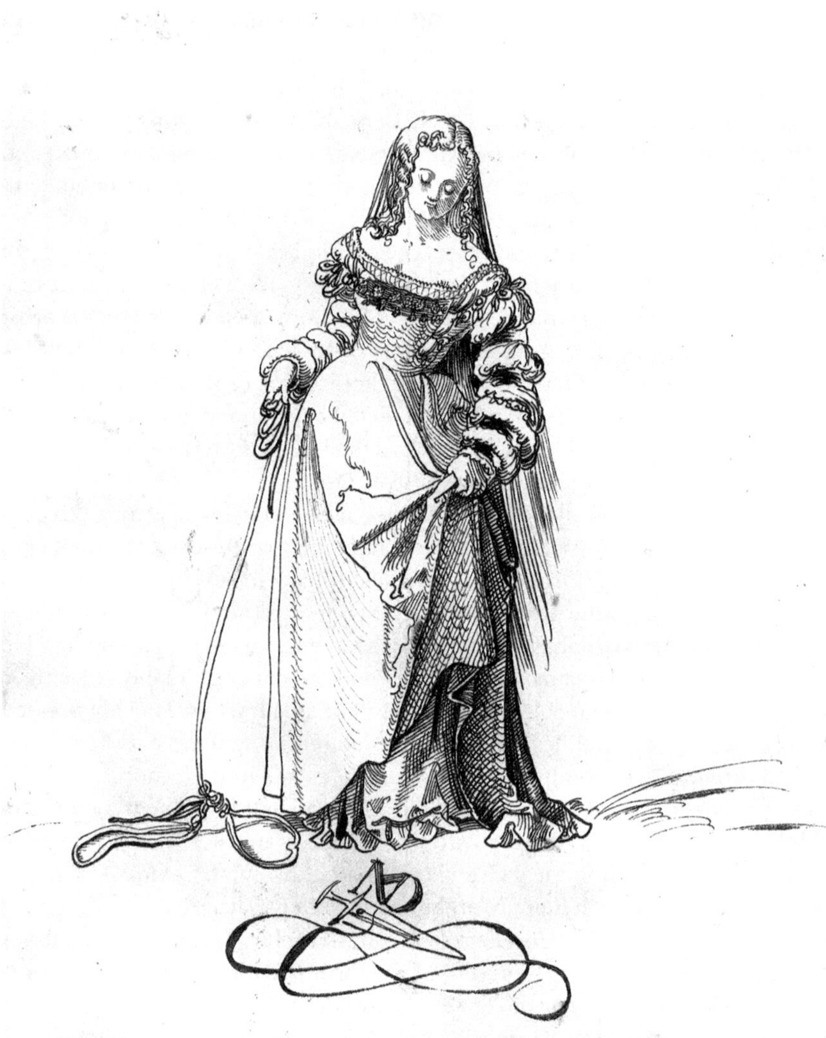

8.7 Niklaus Manuel Deutsch, *Woman holding a Lasso*, c. 1517, pen in black ink, 18.8 × 26.6 cm, Schweizerisches Landesmuseum Zurich (LM 25622)

An intriguing aspect of the symbolism of ropes during this period is found in practices of sympathetic magic. The tying of knots in ropes was believed to be an effective means of causing impotence, as noted by Bacon and Montaigne.[30] By tying three knots in a rope while repeating a spell, it was believed that a woman could sexually incapacitate a man who had abandoned her.[31] Magically-induced impotence was also believed to be a common affliction of newlyweds, where the string from a codpiece was the preferred instrument used to cast the spell.[32] In terms of the viewer's recognition of the symbolic significance of ropes, cords and other means of restraint, the metaphorical ropes depicted by Manuel would certainly have posed no problem in terms of the contemporary interpretation of his drawings.

Urs Graf

The other Swiss Renaissance artist from this time period whose work dealt with erotic subject matter of a satirical nature was Urs Graf.[33] The most original and innovative artist active in German-speaking Switzerland around 1508–1528, Urs Graf spent most of his life in Basel. Graf's most important body of work is composed of his approximately 150 drawings. This is the medium to which he made the most lasting contribution and to which he owes his place in Western art history. Most of these were created in pen and ink or in watercolor. His primary profession was that of a goldsmith, but almost none of his work in that medium is preserved. When not away from Basel participating in military campaigns as a Swiss mercenary, he also designed woodcuts, especially many book illustrations for local publishers, and made stained glass, a few paintings, engravings and a few etchings. Like Niklaus Manuel, Urs Graf used drawings in two different ways: as preparatory studies for works of art in other media, such as goldsmith's metalwork or stained glass, and as entirely independent works. In this latter category are to be found the most fascinating of his drawings, and many of these are humorous commentaries on the struggle between the sexes and satires on the German arch-rivals of the Swiss mercenaries, the *Landsknechte*.

One such drawing (Fig. 8.9) is closely related in theme to Manuel's suffering lover leaning against a cross (Fig. 8.8). While Graf's work is less extreme in the emotions it expresses, it is nonetheless more explicit regarding the erotic message. Graf's pen drawing, dated 1512, was created at the same time as Manuel's work in black chalk. It shows a male figure completely nude and attached to a tree by the metaphorical bonds of love, the ends fluttering in the breeze. Graf's figure is reminiscent of contemporary images of Saint Sebastian in which the saint is bound to a tree, column or post and riddled with arrows, but the "martyrdom" Graf sketched here is entirely secular. Graf's drawing was created about the time of his marriage to Sybilla von Brunn in Basel, and the lover metaphorically bound by an amorous attachment may reflect this circumstance in the artist's life.

There are other telling similarities between Niklaus Manuel's work and that of Urs Graf. Manuel's cuckold, for example, shares a number of details with a drawing by Graf of a semi-nude man holding a rope (Fig. 8.10), and thus raises the question of whether the latter might also represent a man afflicted with impotence. These two artists working in Bern and Basel knew each other's work well and the two similar drawings were probably created during the same year: Urs Graf dated his 1514 at the bottom left, while scholars have dated Niklaus Manuel's work to the same year. In Graf's drawing, the emphasis on the small proportions of the man's genitals (similar to Manuel's cuckold) appears to be intentional and meaningful, and both visually imply impotence. His condition does not, however, prevent his being in love. As in Manuel's drawing, Graf's figure glances down ruefully at a leash held in his hands, contemplating this conventional symbol of emotional and physical bondage. Yet Graf's image

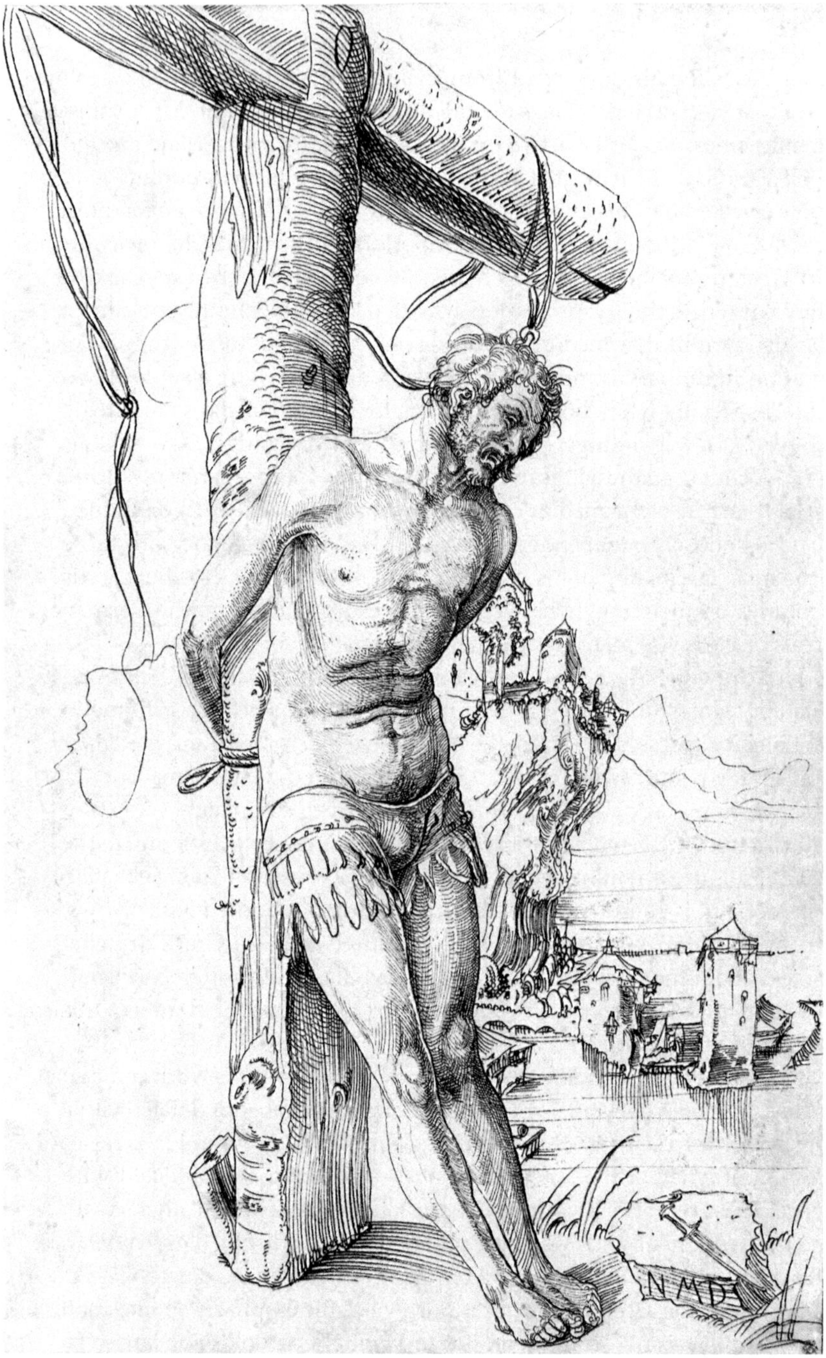

8.8 Niklaus Manuel Deutsch, *Victim of Love Tied to a Cross*, c. 1512, pen in black ink, 27.4 × 20.1 cm, Trustees of the British Museum, London (PD 1921.10.2.3)

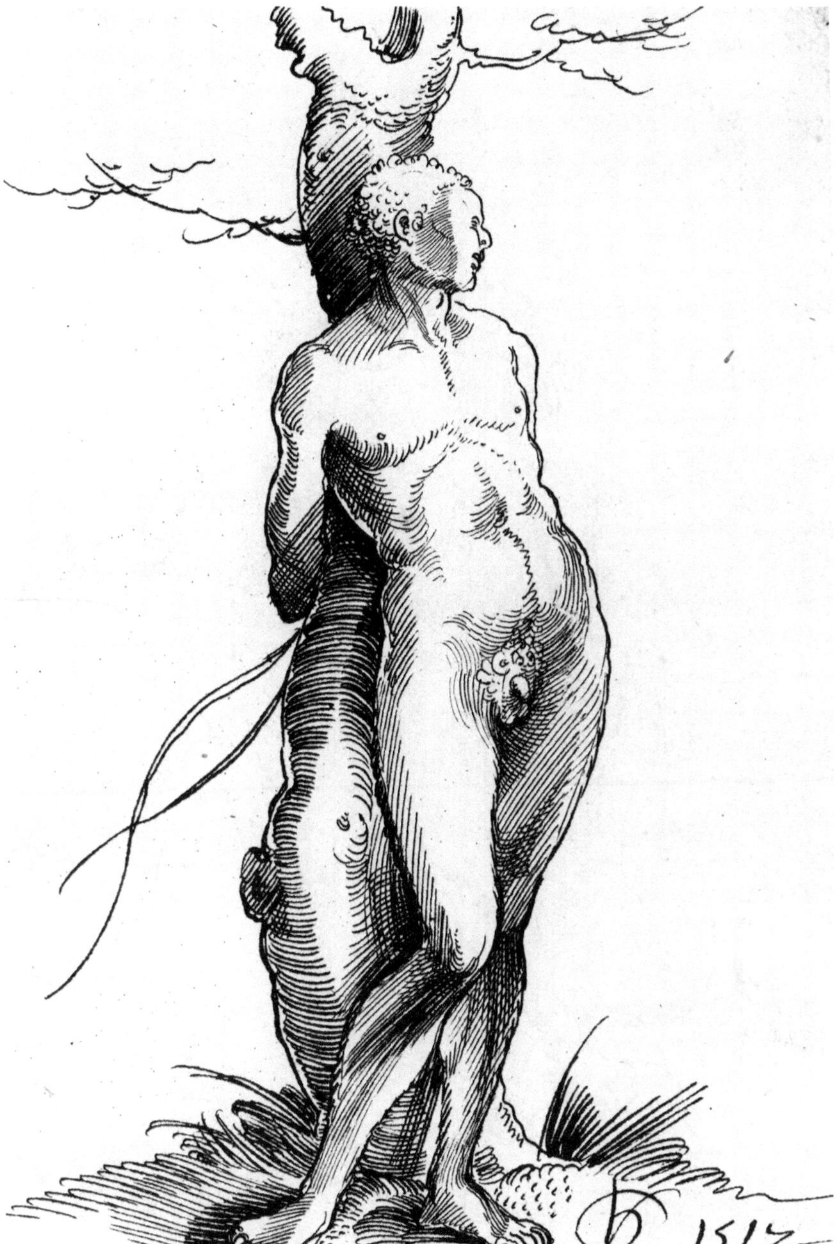

8.9 Urs Graf, *Nude Victim of Love tied to a Tree*, 1512, pen in black ink, 21.6 × 14.3 cm, Kunstmuseum Basel, Kupferstichkabinett (photo: Martin P. Bühler)

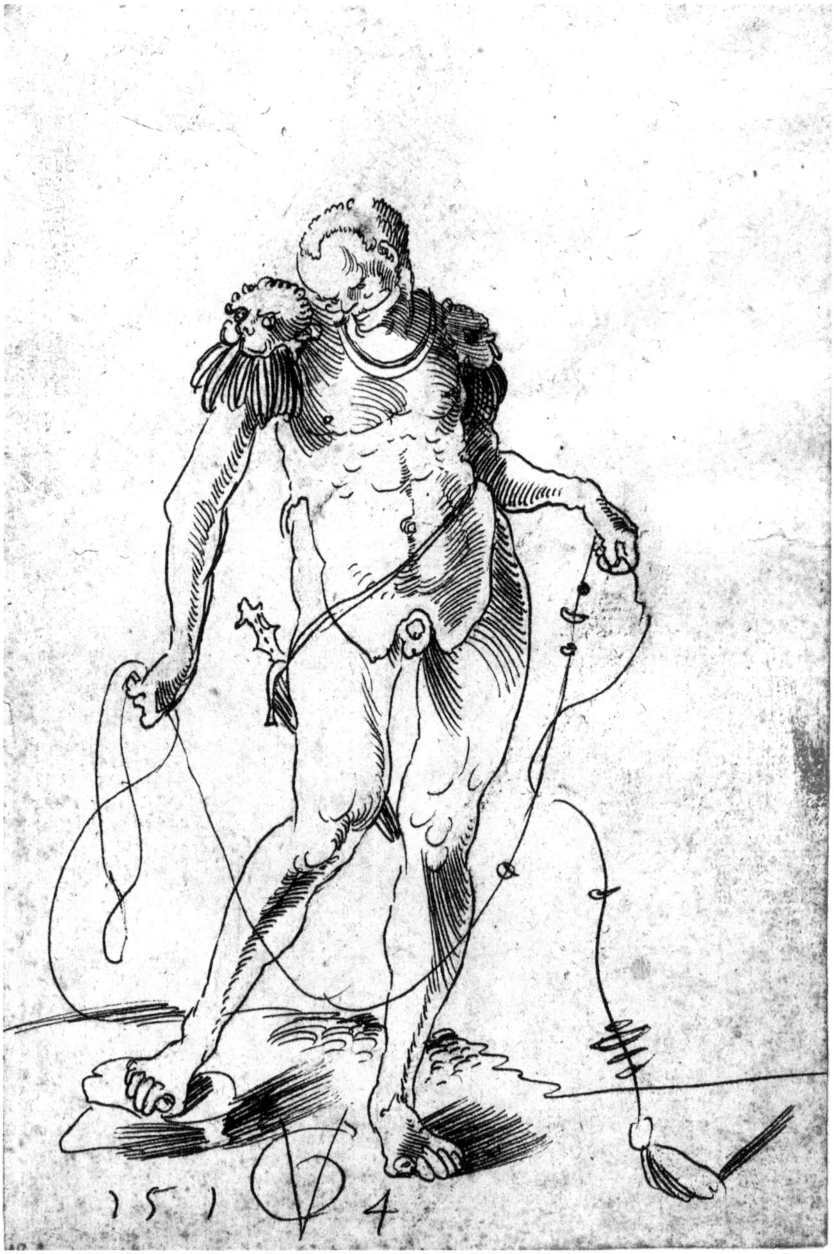

8.10 Urs Graf, *Half-Nude Man holding the Bonds of Love*, 1514, pen in black ink, 22.1 × 14.8 cm, Kunstmuseum Basel, Kupferstichkabinett (photo: Martin P. Bühler)

is somewhat more complex and multifaceted. The "macho" military garb of a cuirass with lion's heads at the shoulders and a sword slung around his waist offer a ludicrous contrast with his pitifully lacking "manhood." Since he is half nude, this man's cuirass would hardly have sufficed to protect him in battle. Moreover, a cuirass was never worn by mercenary soldiers, who needed to be fleet-footed rather than weighed down by a thick and heavy layer of leather. To Swiss mercenaries such as Urs Graf, such a cuirass would have looked outmoded and silly, which suggests that the artist has included it here for satirical effect. The man's weapon slung behind his thigh resembles in size and shape the short, wide swords used by the German *Landsknechte* rather than the much longer, slimmer Swiss variety. The moustache shown in the drawing was also typically worn by German *Landsknechte* rather than by the Swiss.[34] His being shown barefoot raises the question of whether he left his shoes on the battlefield; soldiers beating a hasty retreat were often reported to have lost their shoes while running to escape.[35] This detail would constitute yet another slur against his character: if this man fled the battlefield, the missing shoes are an accusation of cowardice. When interpreted in the context of contemporary military culture, the various details in the drawing suggest that Urs Graf meant to ridicule one of his favorite objects of scorn, the German *Landsknecht*. Graf ridicules him in personal, sexual and military terms, reviling his impotence and his amorous bondage at the same time as he suggests a lack of military readiness and cowardice in battle.

Such merging of sexual and military slurs also appears in an anonymous (and hitherto unpublished) Swiss drawing[36] of about 1510 (Fig. 8.11) that possesses similarities to Urs Graf's satire of a *Landsknecht* of 1514. It shows a partly nude man also wearing a cuirass with similar *épaulettes*, a sword slung across his torso and his lower limbs again undressed, and he, too, is barefoot. Whether he is a Swiss or a German soldier remains unclear, but the cock on his head unambiguously identifies him as a cuckold; it peers down at him while he seems to peer up at it, as if he did not know how it got there. His genitals are covered by a short tunic. Similar to Graf's impotent soldier, he, too, has lost his sexual and military prowess. There is, however, an additional detail meant to convey his incapacity: his injured left foot supported by a peg leg, a well-known satirical jab in Swiss art of this period since such a physical handicap would render him quite ineffectual as a soldier and create an additional source of impotence, both as a mercenary and as a man. He holds his bow in an awkward position behind his peg leg, a position that would make it useless as a weapon, and a sole arrow in his other hand. The reference to both bow and arrow would have also been recognized as having an amorous double meaning, one that is nonetheless qualified as being somewhat inadequate as he has no quiver, and thus has only one paltry shot left for his symbolic "bow." The outmoded cuirass, the feeble bow, the injured leg and the cockerel on his head all combine to make him look ludicrous, and extend the satirical intent to more than just impotence. This figure may in fact allude to contemporary misguided habits of military recruitment: despite their physical incapacity, the lame were sometimes signed up for battle, as happened in the case of a lame butcher conscripted in Bern in January, 1522.[37]

Urs Graf created some of the most vivid and harrowing narratives of early 16th-century warfare in his pen-and-ink drawings.[38] His images of war were based on personal experience, and he frequently interrupted his artistic career for months at a time to participate as a Swiss mercenary soldier in numerous

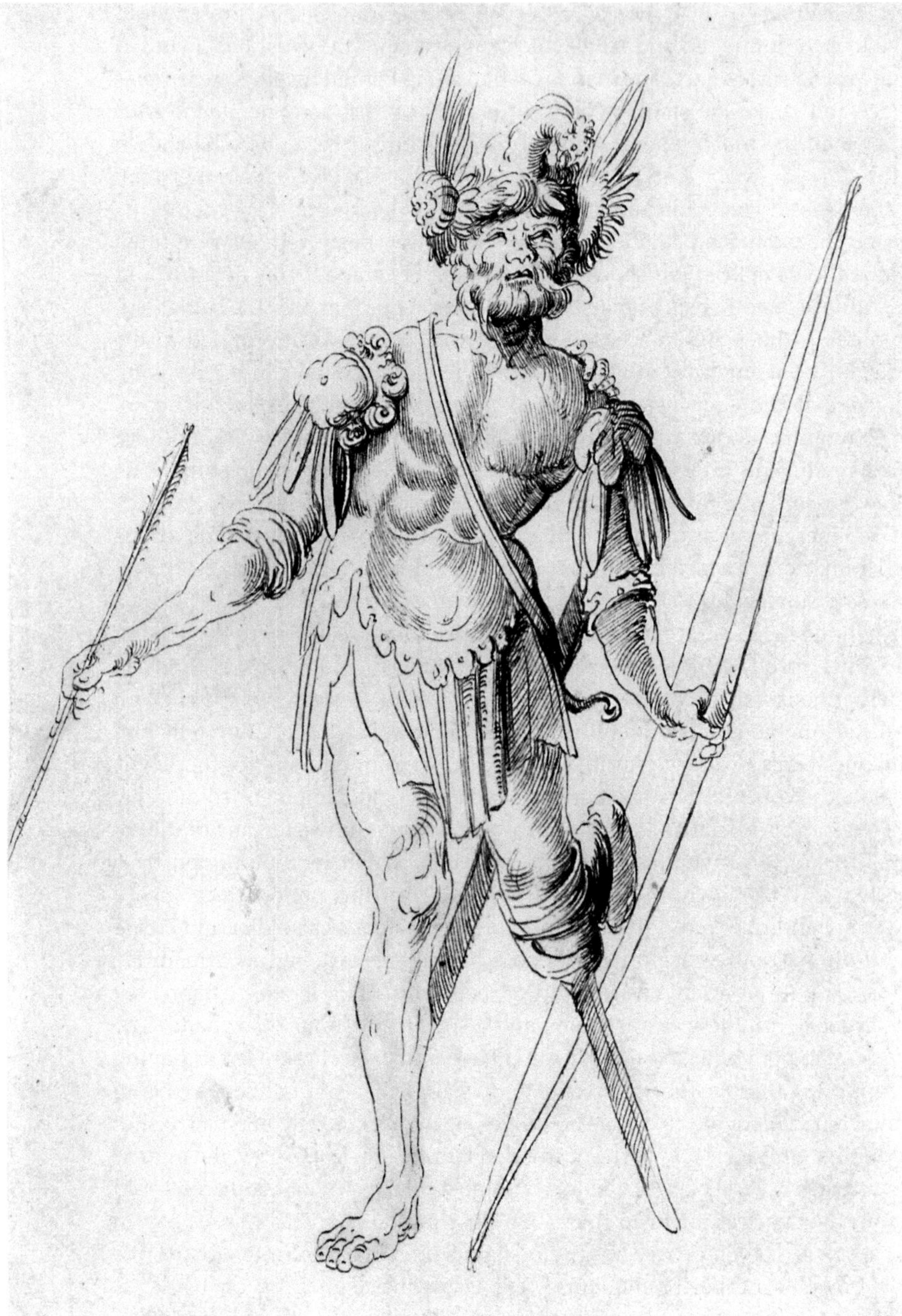

8.11 Anonymous Upper Rhenish artist, *Cuckold*, c. 1510, pen in black ink, 25.4 × 17.5 cm, Kunstmuseum Basel, Kupferstichkabinett (photo: Martin P. Bühler)

campaigns in northern Italy. Presumably he enjoyed the sense of adventure of the mercenary life and hoped to return home with wealth in the form of booty from a successful campaign. Graf is known to have participated in the mercenary campaigns of 1510, 1513, 1515, 1521 (and very likely in others that are undocumented), and his drawings powerfully capture the politics of mercenary warfare in the Swiss cantons. Initially, the mercenaries returning home with rich booty brought the cantons fame and fortune, but conflicts soon arose when Swiss soldiers signed up to serve different masters and wound up on opposing sides, battling each other.[39] Graf's earlier narrative treatment of soldiers in his drawings focuses on the excitement of the campaigns, the lure of ample booty, the pleasures of camp life out of doors and on the female camp followers who served the armies as cooks and sex workers. As in his drawing of 1514 (Fig. 8.10), he also created allegorical images and satires that reflect the bitter rivalry between the Swiss mercenaries and their arch-enemies, the German *Landsknechte,* in which the latters' sexual impotence serves to reiterate their inadequacy as soldiers.

One of Graf's most trenchant satires shows a soldier standing proudly erect with legs apart, balancing curious objects on his pike (Fig. 8.12). The diagonal cross of Saint Andrew, the German national emblem,[40] is slashed into his sleeve and breeches, identifying his nationality. The objects perched on or dangling from the pike symbolize the vices and impotence of the *Landsknecht.* The mouse, bird and spindle reveal his weakness for women; they are symbols of the female or of sexual activity. The mouse was a common metaphor for the female genitals,[41] and it reappears as such in Graf's humorous drawing of a prostitute taking her "mouse" for a walk.[42] The bird refers to sexual intercourse then as now; the verb *vögeln* is still common today in German slang.[43] The sexual meaning of the bird is evident for example in Cesare Ripa's *Iconologia,* in which the personification of lust is illustrated by a nude woman holding an *ucello* (bird), which was then—as still now—a euphemism for the male member. The spindle hanging from the soldier's pike is also a female symbol referring to spinning, women's most common type of work. In the 16th century, it also conveyed an erotic meaning; "having someone on one's spindle" meant having an illicit sexual relationship.[44] In Graf's drawing, the spindle hanging at the end of a leash (with the loop at the level of the soldier's head) suggests that the *Landsknecht* has fallen prey to the power of women. Like the mouse and the rat that holds a bayonet, the hedgehog creeping up the pike was considered to be a lowly, unclean creature. In this drawing, it symbolizes drunkenness, an idea reflected in the expression "drinking like a hedgehog."[45] Johann Fischart told the tale of a drunkard rationalizing his bad habit by explaining that he has a hedgehog in his stomach, which pricked if it was not kept afloat.[46] Due to this association, *The Hedgehog* became a common name for taverns in Germany. This custom continued well into the 19th century, judging by a caricature of Johannes Brahms making his way to the tavern *The Red Hedgehog,* followed by a small hedgehog symbolizing the portly

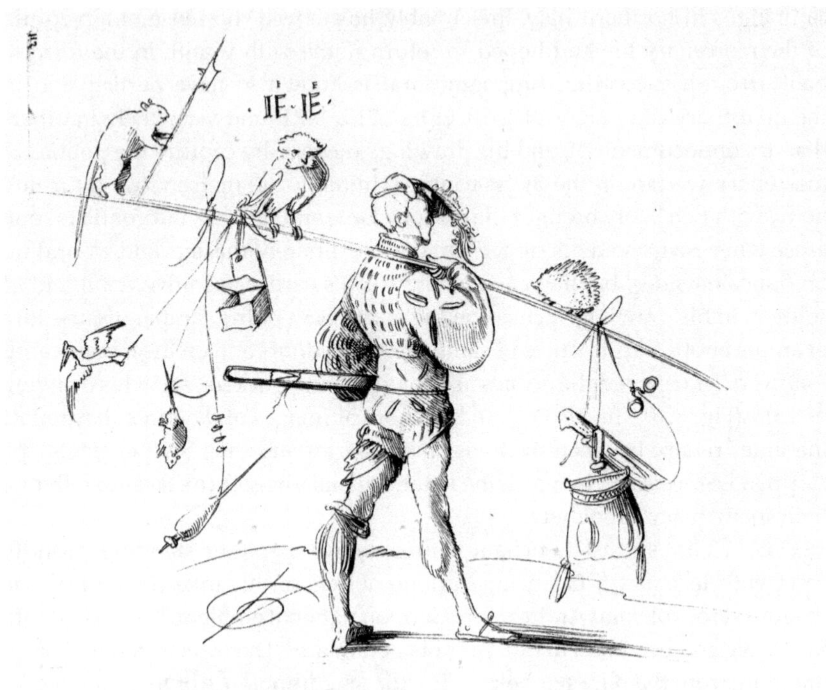

8.12 Urs Graf, Satire on the Vices of a German Landsknecht, c. 1514, pen in black ink, 21.2 × 25.4 cm, Kunstmuseum Basel, Kupferstichkabinett (photo: Martin P. Bühler)

composer's weakness for drink.[47] But Urs Graf may have intended a double entendre since the hedgehog was also used to symbolize female genitals. The expression "piercing the hedgehog," meaning to have sex, was common in the raucous language of 15th- and 16th-century carnival plays. In one such play, a man recounts his amorous adventures with his sweetheart, who "opened her garden" to him, while in her bed he "pierced her hedgehog."[48] Perhaps Graf intended to allude to both the vices of drunkenness and lust, since he frequently exploited the ambiguities of symbolism in his drawings. Finally, the *Landsknecht*'s lechery is also implied by the eyeglasses dangling near the hedgehog. They are the favorite tool of the voyeur, as Graf demonstrates in his drawing of about 1514 of an old fool lecherously peering through eyeglasses at a nude young woman.[49]

Hanging from the *Landsknecht's* pike are also a money purse and a dagger, widely used as the symbols of manliness and of the man's authority over his wife in the household, but these have here become separated from his person, suggesting that he is not quite "a man."[50] In the traditions of satirical imagery of this period, the money purse and dagger are often represented firmly in women's hands: in a drawing of an ill-assorted couple of 1502 attributed to Bernhard Strigel,[51] for example, a young woman has taken possession of an old man's purse and knife, while a demon hovering between them mocks his folly. In Hans Sachs's carnival play *Der bös Rauch*, a domineering wife declares that she will only allow her husband to return home to her if he himself will place his money bag and dagger around her waist and agree henceforth to let her always wear his symbols of domestic authority.[52]

Another symbolic item hanging from the German soldier's pike is a salt box, an additional reference to male sexual potency (or lack thereof). Its meaning is based on the superstitious custom of Graf's period that men carried salt in their pockets to guard against impotence.[53] Since the salt cellar hangs open and is empty, the German *Landsknecht* is presumably also impotent. In addition to such erotic slurs, the artist has drawn an owl (a conventional sign of doom and impending disaster) above the salt cellar,[54] with the letters *.IE.IE* in imitation of the owl's screech. A similar, onomatopoetic lament was frequently heard in Switzerland when bewailing a military defeat and its victims. In his *Bernese Chronicle*, Valerius Anshelm refers to a similar lament referring to the massacre of Swiss mercenaries near Milan in 1516.[55] Graf's drawing of a screeching owl would thus imply the *Landsknecht*'s imminent defeat.

Yet another satirical message is conveyed by the feather attached to the soldier's beret that hangs down so far in front of his face as to obstruct his vision. Again, the artist literally renders a popular expression, "hanging a feather in front of someone's nose,"[56] which meant to poke fun at him. That is certainly the artist's intention in this drawing. The proud stance of this German soldier belies his true situation. He lusts after women but is impotent. Rather than returning home from battle laden with booty carried on his pike, he carries instead the weight of his vices, his impotence and an impending military defeat. As in the previous drawings, Graf's German soldier is humiliated; he has lost both his sexual and military prowess, and is thus simultaneously deprived of his virility and social worth. Graf's satire vividly reflects the hatred and intense rivalry between Swiss and German mercenaries, expressed by the artist's apt manipulation of current erotic and military symbols, as well as his typically biting humor.

Mercenary Culture and Social Climate

The historical context of the works of art analyzed here played an essential role in their creation. In early 16th-century Switzerland, figures of authority, such as the clergy, were rapidly losing their honored status. In 1525, the Bernese town council instructed monks to stay in their monasteries and not loiter in town or run after prostitutes.[57] Marauding mercenaries of various nationalities, arriving in towns penniless from unsuccessful campaigns, became an ongoing social problem. In 1524, a type of anti-immigrant law decreed that foreign beggars, Germans and Italians that arrived destitute, should be banished from Bern or locked up.[58] To avoid paying for social services, city councils demanded that penniless Swiss mercenaries, now vagabonds and beggars, should not be given housing,[59] but should instead be made to return immediately to their home cantons.[60] It was above all the recently established culture of mercenary warfare in northern Switzerland, the sudden influx of wealth and the concomitant rapid social changes that came about within a few short years that had such a profound impact on Niklaus Manuel, Urs Graf and their generation. The pervasive sense of both vulnerability and opportunism that "speaks" from the artwork of this period is entirely new. To fully understand these images, a closer look at mercenary military history is necessary.

Swiss mercenaries had gained enormous military prestige from their resounding victories during the Burgundian wars of 1474–1477, especially at the battles of Grandson, Murten and Nancy. They defeated and later killed the Duke of Burgundy, Charles the Bold, who died on the battlefield in 1477. Henceforth, for over two generations, the Swiss mercenaries enjoyed the reputation of being unbeatable; they were called "invincible giants" (*unüberwintliche risen*).[61] Their military prowess was in enormous demand and highly paid during the subsequent wars in northern Italy between the Duke of Milan, the French king Louis XII, the Habsburg emperor Maximilian I and the pope. Both Niklaus Manuel and Urs Graf participated in the northern Italian campaigns between about 1510 and 1522.

The mercenaries from Switzerland were mostly young men in search of adventure and good pay. They were often unmarried apprentices, craftsmen from the towns or poor shepherds from the countryside. The Alsatian humanist Jakob Wimpfeling described the Swiss of this generation as defiant, arrogant and sinister men hailing from the wild Swiss forests, who were taught only how to handle weapons and to go to war.[62] His characterization is perceptive in so far as it highlights the single-minded focus of the Swiss population on mercenary warfare during the early 16th century. The mercenaries were either recruited by city officials, who received compensation from foreign powers, or volunteers. All were hoping to improve their economic situation. Many were cowherds from the Swiss mountains, which resulted in their German archenemies, the *Landsknechte,* inventing numerous derisive terms for them deriving from the word *Kuh* (cow): *Kuhmäuler* (cow-mouths), *Kuhbuben* (cow-boys) and *Kuhschwänze* (cow-tails). Soon, all Swiss mercenaries—whether shepherds, farmers, city dwellers, craftsmen, merchants or "nobles"—were called by the derogatory term "cow-Swiss" (*Kuhschweizer*).[63] It was obviously intended to suggest that they were uncouth, uneducated yokels who only understood the manual labor of dealing with large beasts but were unskilled in warfare. Yet the young cowherds brought from the mountainside to their new military occupation an extreme sense of male honor and conservative notions of personal conduct, which gave them an edge in terms of performance on the battlefield.[64] The mercenary campaigns were financially very attractive and the income, supplemented sometimes by a share of the booty, was critical for many during a period of steadily rising prices.[65] Typical of youth, few seem to have considered the inherent risks to life and limb in the hope for a better life. Monthly pay for a foot soldier was 4 ½ gulden, a good salary compared with what untrained day laborers could earn in the cities, if they could find work.[66]

As a member of the government of the city of Bern, Niklaus Manuel was directly involved in the politics of mercenary warfare. In principle, the state had a monopoly over military decisions when providing contingents of mercenaries from their towns to foreign leaders, who also paid the city leaders pensions in return for recruiting men. In practice, however, municipal authorities were unable to prevent scores of volunteers from enlisting independently with the highest bidder, so that (as mentioned above) the Swiss were in danger of fighting against each other on both sides of a conflict. Numerous city mandates outlawing such spontaneous enlistments and unregulated recruitment were ineffective and revealed the limits of state control.[67] In addition, problems arose from the lack of discipline among troops, not just guilty of pillaging and raping in the countryside, but also prone to desertions and unauthorized violence to gain booty. There was little hope for improvement in such a situation, especially due to the conflict of interest created by the pensions paid to Swiss political leaders by foreign powers desiring to hire mercenaries, and to the financial incentives available to individual volunteers. Most of the government leaders themselves were experienced captains of mercenary contingents and stood to gain large sums by maintaining the *status quo*.[68] Mercenary warfare and pensions were not outlawed until 1529 in Bern, following a similar decision in Zurich, as part of Reformation social regulations. The abolition and the draconian punishments for anyone countermanding these regulations, however, were relatively ineffective, and local observers commented that it would hardly be possible to stop all the young people from signing up, since one couldn't kill them all.[69]

The campaigns to recapture Milan[70] did in fact bring much money to Swiss cities but they also introduced new social problems and the detritus of war. Initially, euphoria reigned and greed silenced the skeptics. But soon, the high numbers of wounded and casualties took their toll on urban life. Cities had to deal with cripples, beggars, widows and orphans. Contemporary commentators blamed all the newly arisen social ills on mercenary warfare. Though the Swiss reformer Zwingli had consistently preached against mercenary war and the recipients of pensions who profited from the death of others, he nonetheless served as chaplain to mercenaries and died on the battlefield at Kappel in 1531. Zwingli considered mercenary warfare to be a "training ground for every vice imaginable" and an "inhuman, shameless and sinful practice."[71] He especially decried that mercenary habits were destroying the former unity of the cantons within the Swiss Confederacy.

In 1521, the chronicler of the city of Bern, Valerius Anshelm, likewise lamented the terrible social consequences of warfare in his city. In particular, he criticized changes in peoples' values and customs and especially the costliness and opulence of dress, blaming the latter on the new fashions mercenaries brought back from the campaigns.[72] He noted that all types of clothes for men and women had changed,[73] and was scandalized by the new slashed trousers and jerkins that often revealed naked skin underneath. Anshelm self-righteously records in 1521 that people wearing such scandalously erotic clothing had been fined five pounds in Bern.[74] Yet the vertical Swiss cross was often slashed onto jerkins, sleeves, backs or pants (as seen in Fig. 8.12) and became a national symbol to identify the nationality of the wearer. In battle, it was especially critical to distinguish the Swiss from their archrivals, the German *Landsknecht*, who wore the diagonal Saint Andrew's cross slashed into their clothes. Anshelm criticized other new fashions as well, especially the beret with ostrich feathers, and generally found all such innovations to be objectionable due to their expense. He reported that the sins of pride and vanity and peoples' desire for fun and entertainment were increasing daily, and complained that the new clothing's great expense lead to other ills, such as theft and fraud: "As opulent Pride increases and invents ever something new, so also expenses grow and more luxury is created. Just as expenses grow, so must fraud and dishonest ways of amassing money increase, too, so that the city is now full of useless and harmful shops [selling sumptuous goods]."[75] Predictably, he points out that yet another reprehensible consequence was the social leveling caused by the new clothes: different social classes were no longer easily distinguishable, as it was believed they should be, since everyone in the cities was now similarly dressed and sumptuary laws were ignored.[76]

The extreme contrasts between success and failure typical of mercenary warfare are vividly reflected in the drawings by Urs Graf and Niklaus Manuel. How suddenly a successful, prosperous soldier could lose everything and become a beggar is dramatically illustrated in a remarkable drawing of about 1514–1515 by Niklaus Manuel (Fig. 8.13, Plate 12). On the left side, a mercenary figure wears fine clothes of the latest fashion and a beret decorated with four very costly ostrich feathers. But his luck in war that presumably financed his lavish garb has already changed: three arrows pierce his face, hand and thigh. They are what Shakespeare called "the slings and arrows of outrageous fortune," the harbingers of a sudden reversal from riches to rags.[77] The right side of this allegorical figure shows a beggar beset by illness and war wounds, his Swiss sword broken, his bag containing only a useless rock, who supports himself on a beggar's staff. The handwritten text on the reverse of the sheet, possibly composed by Niklaus Manuel but not written in his own hand, emphasizes the moral: a woman will stay with a man as long as he's rich, but the moment his luck changes, she will abandon him precipitously. This luckless soldier thus reprimands the viewer: "I advise you, never rely on warfare" (*ich iedem raten will er buw vff kriegen nit zuo viel*).

Few men in northern Switzerland heeded the artist's sage advice. Niklaus Manuel himself returned to mercenary service in Lombardy in 1522, but the dramatic reversal between the glamorous versus the appalling nature of mercenary warfare was to remain a *leitmotiv* in his drawings, as in the poignant and ironic work of Urs Graf. The mercenary lifestyle can thus be understood as having conditioned, as much as any other social or cultural factor, the wistful and satirical drawings of these two Swiss artists in the tumultuous decades before the Protestant Reformation was to bring other concerns to the forefront of graphic art.

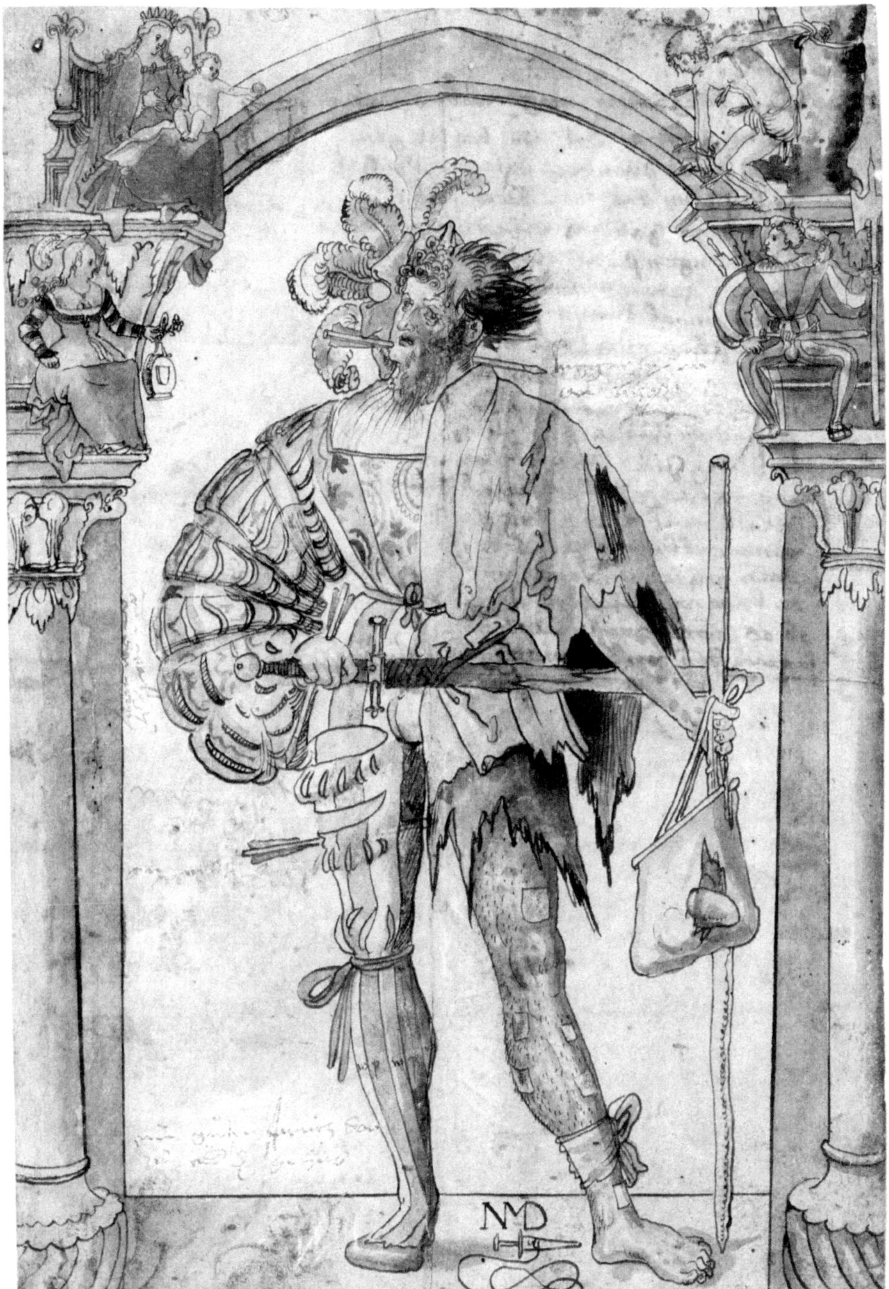

8.13 Niklaus Manuel Deutsch, Allegory on the Transitoriness of Luck in War, pen in black ink with watercolor on parchment, 31 × 21.3 cm, Kupferstichkabinett, Staatliche Museen zu Berlin (inv. 4287)

Works Cited

Early Printed Sources (pre-1900)

Geiler von Kaysersberg, Johannes, *Das buch Granatapfel, im latin genant Malogranatus: helt in ym gar vil vnd manig haylsam vnd susser vnderweysung vnd leer den anhebenden auffnemenden vnd volkommen menuschen mittsampt gaystlicher bedeütung des aussgannngs der kinder Israhel von Egipto : item ain merckliche Underrichtung der gaistlichen Spinnerin : item etlich Predigen von dem Hasen im Pfeffer und von siben Schwertern und Schayden nach gaistlicher ausslegung* (Augspurg: Hans Otmar, 1510). Schmid, Ruodolff, *Ein nüw wunderbarliche spilsüebung uß dem buoch Josuä fürnemlich zogen, wie die kinder Ißrael trockens fuoß durch den furt Jordans zogen und die zwey ersten küngrych Jericho und Aj yngnommen habind.* Nüwlich durch burger der statt Lenzburg gespil, Bern, 1580 (1579).

Wimpfeling, Jakob, *Soliloquium Jacobi Wimpfelingii pro pace Christianorum et pro Helvetiis ut resipiscant*, n.p. c. 1510.

Secondary Sources and Modern Editions

Amtliche Sammlung der ältern Eigenössischen Abschiede. Lucern: E. Schultze, 1856–1886.

Andersson, Christiane, "Jungfrau, Dirne, Fortuna: Das Bild der Frau in den Zeichnungen von Urs Graf," *Kritische Berichte* 16 (1988): 26–35.

Andersson, Christiane, "Martin Schongauers 'Kluge und Törichte Jungfrauen' und ihre Rezeption in der oberrheinischen Kunst," *Le Beau Martin: Etudes et Mises au Point, Actes du Colloque Martin Schongauer*, ed. Albert Châtelet. Colmar: Musée Unterlinden, 1994. 103–13.

Andersson, Christiane, "Urs Graf," *Biografisches Lexikon der schweizer Kunst*, vol. 1. Zurich: Schweizerisches Institut für Kunstwissenschaft, 1998. 423–4.

Andersson, Christiane, *Dirnen, Krieger, Narren: Ausgewählte Zeichnungen von Urs Graf.* Basel: Gute Schrift Verlag, 1978.

Andersson, Christiane, *Popular Lore and Imagery in the Drawings of Urs Graf*, Stanford University doctoral dissertation, Palo Alto, CA., 1977.

Anshelm, Valerius, *Die Berner Chronik des Valerius Anshelm*, hg. vom Historischen Verein des Kantons Bern, 6 vols. Bern: K.J. Wyss, 1884–1901.

Bächtiger, Franz, "Andreaskreuz und Schweizerkreuz: Zur Feindschaft zwischen Landsknechten und Eidgenossen," *Jahrbuch des Bernischen Historischen Museums* 51/52 (1975): 205–70.

Bächtold, Jakob, ed. *Niklaus Manuel. Bibliothek älterer Schriftwerke der deutschen Schweiz und ihres Grenzgebietes*, vol. 2. Frauenfeld: Huber, 1878.

De Quervain, Theophil, *Kirchliche und soziale Zustände in Bern unmittelbar nach der Einführung der Reformation (1528–1536).* Bern: G. Grunau, 1906.

Eisenbart, Liselotte Constanze, *Kleiderordnungen der deutschen Städte zwischen 1350 und 1700: Ein Beitrag zur Kulturgeschichte des deutschen Bürgertums, Göttinger Bausteine zur Geschichtswissenschaft*, 32. Göttingen: Musterschmidt, 1962.

Farner, Oskar, *Huldrych Zwingli: Der schweizerische Reformator.* Emmishofen: Blanke, 1917.

Feller, Richard, *Geschichte Berns, I. Von den Anfängen bis 1516*, 3rd revised edition. Bern: Lang, 1963.

Fischart, Johann, *Geschichtklitterung: Text der Ausgabe letzter Hand von 1590*. Düsseldorf: Rauch, 1964.

Friedländer, Max J. and Elfried Bock, *Staatliche Museen zu Berlin. Die Zeichnungen alter Meister im Kupferstichkabinett; Die deutschen Meister*. Berlin: Julius Bard, 1921.

Ganz, Paul, *Zwei Schreibbüchlein des Niklaus Manuel Deutsch von Bern*, Deutscher Verein für Kunstwissenschaft, Kommissionsverlag Julius Bard. Berlin, 1909.

Grieco, Allen J., "From Roosters to Cocks: Italian Renaissance Fowl and Sexuality," *Erotic Cultures of Renaissance Italy*, ed. Sara F. Matthews Grieco. Farnham, UK/ Burlington, VT: Ashgate, 2010. 89–140.

Grimm, Jakob and Wilhelm Grimm, *Deutsches Wörterbuch*. Leipzig: S. Hirzel, 1854–1962.

Keller, Adelbert von, *Fastnachtspiele aus dem fünfzehnten Jahrhundert, Bibliothek des literarischen Vereins in Stuttgart*. Stuttgart: Literarischer Verein, 1853.

Koegler, Hans, *Hundert Tafeln aus dem Gesamtwerk des Urs Graf*. Basel: Urs-Graf-Verlag, 1947.

Lehrs, Max, *Geschichte und kritischer Katalog des deutschen, niederländischen und französischen Kupferstichs im XV. Jahrhundert*, 1. Textband. Vienna: Gesellschaft für vervielfältigende Kunst, 1908.

Major, Emil and Erwin Gradmann, *Urs Graf*. Basel: Holbein-Verlag, 1942.

McLaren, Angus, *Impotence: A Cultural History*. Chicago/London, University of Chicago Press, 2007.

Müller, Christian, *Beschreibender Katalog der Zeichnungen, Offentliche Kunstsammlung Basel, Kupferstichkabinett, Die Zeichnungen des 15. Und 16. Jahrhunderts*, Teil 2B, Urs Graf. Basel: Schwabe, 2001.

Müller, Christian, *Sammeln in der Renaissance: das Amerbach-Kabinett, Zeichnungen alter Meister*, exhibition catalogue. Basel: Kupferstichkabinett der Öffentliche Kunstsammlung, 1991.

Murner, Thomas, *Die Geuchmat, Thomas Murners deutsche Schriften, Kritische Gesamtausgaben elsässischer Schriftsteller des Mittelalters und der Reformationszeit*, vol. 5, ed. Eduard Fuchs. Berlin: Walter de Gruyter, 1931.

Murner, Thomas, *Narrenbeschwörung, Thomas Murners deutsche Schriften, Kritische Gesamtausgaben elsässischer Schriftsteller des Mittelalters und der Reformationszeit*, vol. 2, ed. M. Spanier. Berlin: Walter de Gruyter, 1926.

Ovid, *Ars amatoria*, ed, Friedrich Maier. Bamberg: Buchner, 2001.

Posner, Donald, "An aspect of Watteau, peintre de la realité," *Etudes d'art français offertes à Charles Sterling*, ed. Albert Châtelet and Nicole Reynaud. Paris : Presses Universitaires de France, 1975.

Romer, Hermann, *Herrschaft, Reislauf und Verbotspolitik: Beobachtungen zum rechtlichen Alltag der Zürcher Solddienstbekämpfung im 16. Jahrhundert*. Zurich: Schulthess, 1995.

Sachs, Hans, *Sämtliche Fastnachtspiele in chronologischer Ordnung nach den Originalen, Neudrucke deutscher Literaturwerke des 16. und 17. Jahrhunderts*, ed. Edmund Goetze, Halle a.d. Saale, M. Niemeyer, 1880–1886.

Schaufelberger, Walter, "Zu einer Charakterologie des altschweizerischen Kriegertums," *Schweizerisches Archiv für Volkskunde* 54 (1958): 63f.

Schaufelberger, Walter, *Spätmittelalter: Handbuch der Schweizer Geschichte*. Zurich: Berichthaus, 1972.

Schwarz, Heinrich and Volker Plagemann, *Reallexikon zur deutschen Kunstgeschichte*. Munich: Beck, 1973.

Schweizerisches Idiotikon, Wörterbuch der schweizerdeutschen Sprache, hg. von der Antiquarischen Gesellschaft in Zürich. Frauenfeld: J. Huber, 1881ff.

Seligmann, Siegfried, *Der böse Blick und Verwandtes: Ein Beitrag zur Geschichte des Aberglaubens aller Zeiten und Völker*. Berlin: H. Barsdorf, 1910.

Simons, Patricia, *The Sex of Men in Premodern Europe: A Cultural History*. Cambridge: Cambridge University Press, 2011.

Aktensammlung zur Geschichte der Berner Reformation 1521–1532, ed. Steck, Rudolf and Gustav Tobler. Bern: K. J. Wyss Erben, 1923.

Storck, Karl, *Musik und Musiker in Karikatur und Satire, eine Kulturgeschichte der Musik aus dem Zerrspiegel*. Oldenburg: G. Stalling, 1910.

Talvacchia, Bette, "Il mercato dell'Eros: Rappresentazioni della sessualità femminile nei soggetti mitologici," *Monaca Moglie Serva Cortigiana: Vita e immagine delle donne tra Rinascimento e Controriforma*, ed. Sara F. Matthews-Grieco. Florence, Assessorato pubblica istruzione pari opportunita cultura delle differenze, progetto donne, 2001.

Varnhagen, Hermann, "Der Mailänder Feldzug vom Jahre 1522," *Mitteilungen der antiquarischen Gesellschaft in Zürich* 29 (1923): 101f.

von Tavel, Hans Christoph, "Niklaus Manuel Deutsch," *Neue Deutsche Biographie*, vol. 16. Berlin: Duncker und Humblot, 1990. 96–8.

von Tavel, Hans Christoph, *Niklaus Manuel: Zur Kunst eines Eidgenossen der Dürerzeit*. Bern: K. J. Wyss Erben, 1979.

Wackernagel, Hans Georg, *Kriegsbräuche in der mittelalterlichen Eidgenossenschaft*. Basel: K. Werner, 1934.

Wagner, Hugo, Cäsar Menz and Hans Christoph von Tavel, *Niklaus Manuel Deutsch: Maler, Dichter, Staatsmann*, exhibition catalogue. Kunstmuseum Bern, 1979.

Weisbach, Werner. "Ein Fuss beschuht, der andere nackt: Bemerkungen zu einigen Zeichnungen des Urs Graf," *Zeitschrift für schweizerische Archäologie und Kunstgeschichte* IV (1942): 108f.

Wermelinger, Hugo, "Lebensmittelteuerungen, ihre Bekämpfung und ihre politischen Rückwirkungen in Bern vom ausgehenden 15. Jahrhundert bis in die Zeit der Kappelerkriege," *Archiv des historischen Vereins des Kantons Bern* 55 (1971): 56f.

Wirth, Jean, *La jeune Fille et la Mort, Recherches sur les thèmes macabres dans l'art germanique de la Renaissance*. Geneva: Droz, 1979.

Das Narrenschiff: Faksimile der Erstausgabe von 1494, mit einem Anhang enthaltend die Holzschnitte der folgenden Originalausgaben, ed. Zarncke, Friedrich. Strassburg: K. J. Trübner, 1913.

Zischka, Ulrike, *Zur sakralen und profanen Anwendung des Knotenmotivs als magisches Mittel, Symbol oder Dekor, eine vergleichende volkskundliche Untersuchung, Tuduv-Studien* vol. 7. Munich: Tuduv-Verlagsgesellschaft, 1977.

Notes

1 This essay is dedicated to Kurt W. Forster with whom I first embarked on the study of Swiss Renaissance art.

2 Niklaus Manuel probably served as a mercenary at about age 23 in 1507 near Genoa, as his drawing of that year showing the siege of Castellazzo near Genoa implies (Wagner, Hugo, Cäsar Menz and Hans Christoph von Tavel, *Niklaus Manuel Deutsch: Maler, Dichter, Staatsmann*, exhibition catalogue, Kunstmuseum Bern, 1979, no. 139, pl. 75). He also served February to May, 1516, for the French king Francis I and again in 1522 at Bicocca and Novara. Urs Graf is documented as having served as a mercenary in 1510, 1513, 1515 and 1521.

3 For an overview see Wagner and von Tavel, *Niklaus Manuel Deutsch* and Hans Christoph von Tavel, "Niklaus Manuel Deutsch" in *Neue Deutsche Biographie* 16 (Berlin, 1990), 96–8.

4 Jakob Bächtold, ed. *Niklaus Manuel. Bibliothek älterer Schriftwerke der deutschen Schweiz,* Frauenfeld, 1978.

5 Bows at the shoulders of women's dresses are ubiquitous since they serve to attach the sleeves, as in Niklaus Manuel's drawing *Salome* (Wagner and von Tavel, *Niklaus Manuel Deutsch*, 90). Urs Graf's *Prostitute Walking her "Mouse"* wears a profusion of bows (Christiane Andersson, *Dirnen, Krieger, Narren: Ausgewählte Zeichnungen von Urs Graf* (Basel, 1978), Fig. 42. Graf's *Nude Fiddler* of 1523 and his *Allegory on the Transitoriness of Luck in War* are nude but for bows at the knees (Andersson, *Urs Graf*, figs. 51 and 34).

6 The motto NKAW appears in numerous drawings by Niklaus Manuel between c. 1510–1515 (Wagner and von Tavel, *Niklaus Manuel Deutsch*, 76, 77, 84, 85, 87 and 115).

7 Ibid., 76 and 87.

8 Paul Ganz, *Zwei Schreibbüchlein des Niklaus Manuel Deutsch von Bern*, Berlin, 1909, 1 and Wagner and von Tavel, *Niklaus Manuel Deutsch*, 123.

9 The drawing dates to c. 1510: Wagner and von Tavel, *Niklaus Manuel Deutsch*, no. 152, 87, and no. 147, 76 and cf. Christiane Andersson, *Popular Lore and Imagery in the Drawings of Urs Graf*, Stanford University doctoral dissertation, 1977, 171f.

10 Examples of his designs for stained glass and the glass panels made from these designs are illustrated in Wagner and von Tavel, *Niklaus Manuel Deutsch*, plates. 137, 139, 158, 166–7.

11 This seems a reasonable assumption though there is no contemporary documentation of such a practice. On artists sharing drawings with their friends for amusement, see also the essay in this volume on Baccio del Biano by Louise Rice, chapter 9.

12 Christian Müller, *Sammeln in der Renaissance: das Amerbach-Kabinett, Zeichnungen alter Meister,* exhibition catalogue, Kunstsammlung Basel, 1991.

13 Images of foolish virgins with and without the erotic allusions are common in northern art, see Christiane Andersson, "Martin Schongauers 'Kluge und Törichte Jungfrauen' und ihre Rezeption in der oberrheinischen Kunst," *Actes du Colloque Martin Schongauer*, ed. Albert Châtelet, Colmar, Musée Unterlinden, 1994, 103–13 and Christiane Andersson, "Jungfrau, Dirne, Fortuna: Das Bild der Frau in den Zeichnungen von Urs Graf," *Kritische Berichte*, vol. 16, 1988, 26–35. The sex worker in this drawing is clothed identically as the one Manuel clearly identified as a prostitute, calling her *Mätz* and *Diern*, in his *Dance of Death* frescoes (now destroyed but known from copies) in Bern of c. 1518 (Wagner and von Tavel, *Niklaus Manuel Deutsch*, 70). Manuel made several drawings of foolish virgins (ibid., 100–105) but no corresponding ones of wise virgins are known.

14 Niklaus Manuel's model book or *Schreibbüchlein* illustrates the camp followers cooking, hunting birds, giving directions and embracing men (ibid., 124 and 122).

15 Valerius Anshelm described these sandals among the new fashions brought from Italy, noting their costliness: *schuch, an zehen hangend, und doch zwifach türer, dan vornacher puntschuch. Die Berner Chronik des Valerius Anshelm, hg. vom Historischen Verein des Kantons Bern,* IV, 1893, 463.

16 *Das Narrenschiff: Faksimile der Erstausgabe von 1494, mit einem Anhang enthaltend die Holzschnitte der folgenden Originalausgaben,* ed. Friedrich Zarncke (Strassburg, 1913).

17 See for example Jean Wirth, *La jeune Fille et la Mort, Recherches sur les thèmes macabres dans l'art germanique de la Renaissance* (Geneva, 1979).

18 *An mynem seyl ich draffter yeich/ Vil narren, affen, esel, geüch / Die ich verfür betrüg vnd leych.*

19 See the term *Gauch* in *Grimms Deutsches Wörterbuch*, IV, col. 1525–1526.

20 *Frow Venus mit dem ströwen ars/ Byn nit die mynnst im narren fars / Ich züch zu mir der narren vil / Vnd mach ein gouch vss wem ich wil.*

21 *Wollust der welt / die glychet sich / Eym üppigen wib, die offentlich / Sitzt vff der strass vnd schrygt sich vss / Das yederman kum jnn jr huss.*

22 *Eynen essel reyden ich wan ich weil / Eyn gauch dat is myn federspil / Da myt fangen ich naren ind affen vyl.* Max Lehrs, *Geschichte und kritischer Katalog des deutschen, niederländischen und französischen Kupferstichs im XV. Jahrhundert, 1. Textband* (Vienna, 1908), 164.

23 Ovid, *Ars amatoria*, II, 427f and III, 669.

24 *Es ist eyn bsunderlicher list / Geuch zu fohen (fangen) syn gerist / Man foht ir glich so vill mit blicken / Alss mit iagen, garn, vnd stricken.* Thomas Murner's chapter entitled: *Den Gouch fohen (fangen), Die Geuchmat, Thomas Murners deutsche Schriften*, ed. Eduard Fuchs, V (Berlin, 1931), chapter 8, lines 904–7.

25 *Ir Pfeil hat mir mein hertz durch drungen / Darnach da hat sie mich gefangen / Und an ihr starckes seil gehangen, Hans Sachs: Sämtliche Fastnachtspiele in chronologischer Ordnung nach den Originalen, Neudrucke deutscher Literaturwerke des 16. und 17. Jahrhunderts*, ed. Edmund Goetze (Berlin, 1881), 13–14, lines 32–4.

26 *Allein min gertz [herz] / Das lydt gross schmerz / dass ich din nit vergessen kan / des wird ich dick / mit venus strick/gebunden hart / zu aller ffart ... Lass mich altzit dyn büelyn syn.* Emil Major and Erwin Gradmann, *Urs Graf* (Basel, 1942), illustrated on page 9.

27 *Venus strick vnd ire bandt / Manchen wysen gfangen handt; / Wen sy bindt/den bindt sy hart / Ir strick noch nie zerrissen wart. / Dalida sampson do mit fieng ... / Künig, keiser, fürsten, herren / Londt sich yrmetrütlin (woman's name) nerren, Narrenbeschwörung Thomas Murners deutsche Schriften*, ed. M. Spanier, 1512 (Berlin, 1926), chapter 47, lines 5–10.

28 Love knots appear often as part of Manuel's signature (seven examples dating between 1515 and 1527 are illustrated in Hans Christoph von Tavel, *Niklaus Manuel: Zur Kunst eines Eidgenossen der Dürerzeit* [Bern, 1979], 18). He also used love knots consistently as motifs in his drawings (Wagner and von Tavel, *Niklaus Manuel Deutsch*, 76, 77, 84, 85 and 87). See also Ulrike Zischka, *Das Knotenmotiv: Zur sakralen und profanen Anwendung des Knotenmotivs als magisches Mittel, Symbol oder Dekor, eine vergleichende volkskundliche Untersuchung*, vol. 7 (Munich: 1977).

29 See for example Bette Talvacchia, "Il mercato dell'Eros: Rappresentazioni della sessualità femminile nei soggetti mitologici," *Monaca Moglie Serva Cortigiana: Vita e immagine delle donne tra Rinascimento e Controriforma* (Florence, 2001).

30 Angus McLaren, *Impotence: A Cultural History* (Chicago and London, 2007), 45.

31 Ibid., xi.

32 On magical impotence see the essays in this volume by Bourne, Dune and Katritzky.

33 Christian Müller, *Öffentliche Kunstsammlung Basel, Kupferstichkabinett, Katalog der Zeichnungen, Teil 2B, Urs Graf* (Basel, 2001); Andersson, *Urs Graf*; Christiane Andersson, "Urs Graf," *Biografisches Lexikon der schweizer Kunst*, vol. 1 (Zurich, 1998), 423–4.

34 Graf shows a long moustache also in his other satires on the German enemy, such as *A Landsknecht in the Clutches of the Devil*, 1516 and *Al mein gelt verspilt (Landsknecht's money gambled away)*,1519, illustrated in Andersson, *Urs Graf*, Figs. 30 and 31 and in Hans Koegler, *Hundert Tafeln aus dem Gesamtwerk des Urs Graf* (Basel, 1947), 37 and 45.

35 Werner Weisbach, "Ein Fuss beschuht, der andere nackt: Bemerkungen zu einigen Zeichnungen des Urs Graf," *Zeitschrift für schweizerische Archäologie und Kunstgeschichte*, IV, 1942, 108f.

36 In this pen drawing the areas left unfinished along the figure's left side and a man's hand placed on his left shoulder reveal that the sketch is an incomplete copy after another drawing. Some details are reminiscent of Urs Graf's own drawings.

37 Valerius Anshelm reported on the recruitment of a lame baker for the French king: *An bestimpten orten in der Eidgnoschaft die erste mustrung und bezalung beschehen ... Claudo Hagelstein, ein mezger, an einem bein so lam, das er uf einem starken münch (castrated horse) mit siner büchs und gwer wolgerüst an die mustrung reit.* Anshelm, *Berner Chronik*, IV, 1893, 510.

38 Andersson, *Urs Graf*, 27–39.

39 This occurred for example in April 1500 at the Battle of Novara when Swiss pikemen fought both for Louis XII of France and for Ludovico Sforza, Duke of Milan. Richard Feller, *Geschichte Berns, I. Von den Anfängen bis 1516*, 3rd revised edition (Bern, 1963).

40 Franz Bächtiger, "Andreaskreuz und Schweizerkreuz: Zur Feindschaft zwischen Landsknechten und Eidgenossen," *Jahrbuch des Bernischen Historischen Museums*, 51/52, 1975, 205–70.

41 *Grimms Deutsches Wörterbuch*, vol. 12, col. 1819 defines *Maus* as a discreet term referring to the female sex organ (*das weibliche Geschlecht verhüllt)* and cites a ballad in which boys call a prostitute walking the streets at night "mouse": *"wenne si des obends uf der gassen loufen, so schrigent die knaben: ein mus, ein mus! Wil sie iemant koufen?"* In a Swiss play a fool calls an elaborately dressed sex worker *Müserin*, Ruodolff Schmid, *Ein nüw wunderbarliche Spilsüebung uss dem Buoch Josuä ... durch Burger der Statt Lenzburg gespilt*, n.p. 1579.

42 Andersson, *Urs Graf*, 60, Fig. 8.42.

43 For its usage in Switzerland in the 16th century, see *Schweizerisches Idiotikon*, I, col. 698. On the erotic meaning of birds in Italy see Allen J. Grieco, "From Roosters to Cocks: Italian Renaissance Fowl and Sexuality," *Erotic Cultures of Renaissance Italy*, ed. Sara F. Matthews-Grieco (Farnham, UK/Burlington, VT, 2010), 89–140.

44 The expression *jemanden an der Kunkel haben* was used by the Alsatian humanist Johann Geiler von Keisersberg in his "Die gaistlich spinnerin," in *Das Buch Granatapfel*, Augsburg, 1510, fol. O4d: *wenn es ... in unordentlicher liebe gefangen ... so spricht man es hat werk an der kunkel.* Elsewhere in the same text he says: *du hast villeicht den beichtvater selbs an der kunkel*, fol P6d. Cf. Donald Posner's article on the erotic significance of the spindle in a painting by Watteau, "An aspect of Watteau, peintre de la realité, *Etudes d'art français offertes à Charles Sterling*, ed. Albert Châtelet and Nicole Reynaud (Paris, 1975), 270–86.

45 *Wie ein Igel trinken.*

46 *Ich hab ein igel im bauch; der musz geschwummen haben*, Johann Fischart, *Geschichtklitterung: Text der Ausgabe letzter Hand von 1590* (Düsseldorf 1963), fol. 85v. Similarly in France: *il a un hérisson dans le ventre, s'il ne boit, il le pique*, Oudin, 210 cited in *Grimms Deutsches Wörterbuch*, IV, part 2, col. 2044.

47 Karl Storck, *Musik und Musiker in Karikatur und Satire, eine Kulturgeschichte der Musik aus dem Zerrspiegel* (Oldenburg, 1910), image inserted following p. 432.

48 *Mir öffnet ains mein puol ir gaden ,/ Und ward mich an ir pettlein laden, / Do solt ich ir ain igel stechen*, Adelbert von Keller, *Fastnachtspiele aus dem fünfzehnten Jahrhundert, Bibliothek des literarischen Vereins in Stuttgart* (Stuttgart, 1853), I, 338, lines 19–21. *Ich solt ir ein igel stechen*, ibid., 259, line 28.

49 Andersson, *Urs Graf*, 70, Fig. 50.

50 On the symbolism of purses as virile attributes, see Patricia Simons, *The Sex of Men in Premodern Europe: A Cultural History* (Cambridge, 2011).

51 Max J. Friedländer and Elfried Bock, *Staatliche Museen zu Berlin. Die Zeichnungen alter Meister im Kupferstichkabinett; Die deutschen Meister* (Berlin, 1921), accession no. 4256.

52 *Will mein Narr wider kummen ein / und mein genad wider erhaschen / So muss er darzu messr und taschen / mir selber guerten an mein seytten, / dass ich das trag zu aller zeytten, / dass ich im Haus sei Herr und man / Sonst will ich jn nicht nemen an. Hans Sachs, Sämtliche Fastnachtspiele, in chronologischer Ordnung nach den Originalen, Neudrucke deutscher Literaturwerke des 15. und 16. Jahrhunderts*, ed. Edmund Götze (Halle, 1883), III, 36–7, lines 242–9.

53 Siegfried Seligmann, *Der böse Blick und Verwandtes: Ein Beitrag zur Geschichte des Aberglaubens aller Zeiten und Völker* (Berlin, 1910), II, 38.

54 Heinrich Schwarz and Volker Plagemann, *Eule, Reallexikon zur deutschen Kunstgeschichte* (Munich, 1973), VI, col. 284f and col. 308–9.

55 *Ei, i, dass Got erbarm, das sind unsere doten von Meyland! Dass der Tuefel d'Franzosen und ir gelt haette! I, wo sind die alten, frommen Eidgenossen?* Anshelm *Berner Chronik*, IV, 173.

56 *Den das er nun die feder blass / Die er im hencket für die nass*, Murner, *Narrenbeschwörung*, chapter 12, *Fantasten beitzen*, lines 93–4.

57 *Fürhin die Münch inn iren klöstern beliben und nit also vagieren und den huren nachlouffen sollen*, in *Aktensammlung zur Geschichte der Berner Reformation 1521–1532*, ed. Rudolf Steck and Gustav Tobler (Bern 1923), I, 186, no. 596.

58 *Die frömbden starcken bättler und landstricher, tütsch und wälsch, allenthalb mit mercklichen scharen in unser landtschaft ziechen...damit wir ouch söllicher schädlicher lüt mögen abkomen, so wöllend die, so sich ungehorsam erzöugen und über gethane warnung under landtschaft nit würden rumen, väncklich annämen*, (1524) Steck and Tobler, *Aktensammlung*, I, 1923, 115, no. 397.

59 *Item geboten, die lands-, kriegs- und Jakobsbetler, husierer, heiden, frömden veldsiechen, und derglichen lüt hinweg zewisen und nit zuhusen*, a regulation (entitled *Einer stat Bern ernüwerte ordnung wider etliche miswesen*) recorded by Valerius Anshelm, *Berner Chronik*, V, 1896, 38.

60 *Die armen Kriegsleute, die bettelnd umherstreifen, sollen in jedem Ort schwören, sogleich in ihre Heimat zu ziehen. Eigenössische Abschiede*, vol. IV, Abteilung 1a (Brugg, 1873), 264, no. 124.

61 Anshelm, *Berner Chronik*, IV, 1893, 159.

62 *Soliloquium Jakobi Wimpfelingii pro pace Christianorum et pro Helvetiis*, n.p. 1510, chapter XI.

63 Walter Schaufelberger, "Zu einer Charakterologie des altschweizerischen Kriegertums," *Schweizerisches Archiv für Volkskunde* 54 (1958): 63f.

64 Hans G. Wackernagel, *Kriegsbräuche in der mittelalterlichen Eidgenossenschaft, Schriften der schweizerischen Gesellschaft für Volkskunde* 38 (1956): 306.

65 Hugo Wermelinger, "Lebensmittelteuerungen, ihre Bekämpfung und ihre politischen Rückwirkungen in Bern vom ausgehenden 15. Jahrhundert bis in die Zeit der Kappelerkriege." *Archiv des Historischen Vereins des Kantons Bern* 55 (1971): 56–7.

66 Hermann Varnhagen, "Der Mailänder Feldzug vom Jahre 1522," *Mitteilungen der antiquarischen Gesellschaft in Zürich*, 29 (1923), 101.

67 Hermann Romer, *Herrschaft, Reislauf und Verbotspolitik: Beobachtungen zum rechtlichen Alltag der Zürcher Solddienstbekämpfung im 16. Jahrhundert* (Zurich, 1995), 345 and 348.

68 Especially members of the patrician families: vom Stein, von Erlach, von Diesbach, von Wattenwyl and May. Walter Schaufelberger, *Spätmittelalter: Handbuch der Schweizer Geschichte* (Zurich, 1972), I, 365.

69 In 1533 Berchtold Haller wrote to the Reformer Martin Bucer: *Die unzempte jugent wirt louffen; wer wills weren? Wer will sy all köpfen?* Theophil De Quervain, *Kirchliche und soziale Zustände in Bern unmittelbar nach der Einführung der Reformation (1528–1536)* (Bern, 1906), 167.

70 Varnhagen, *Mailänder Feldzug*, 101.

71 *Krieg frömbder Herren vnd gelt ist ein schul aller lastren*, Oskar Farner, *Huldrych Zwingli: Der schweizerische Reformator* (Zürich, 1943), III, 299. *Das versöldet Kriegen ein unmenschlich, unverschampt sündtlich Ding ist*, Farner, II, 177.

72 *Wie dan vornacher bisshar alle übermass, üppikeit und ändrung der siten in ein schlechte, tapfere Eidgnoschaft uss frömden kriegen gebracht ist worden*, Valerius Anshelm, *Berner Chronik*, IV, 1893, 462–3.

73 *Alle kleidung an wib und man verändret worden*. Ibid., II, 1886, 389f. Anshelm objected to slashed clothes: *das ein grosse schand was gsin*.

74 Ibid., IV, 1893, 462–3.

75 *Wie nun die üppige hochfart zunimpt und stet nüws erdenkt, also nimpt ouch der unkosten zu und erdenkt kostbarkeit; und wie der unkosten zunimpt und kostbarkeit erdenkt, also muss ouch zunemen aller betrug und list, gelt zehaben, dahar die stät vol müessiger und schädlicher krämerien und gremplerien*, Ibid., IV, 1893, 462–3.

76 See Liselotte Constanze Eisenbart, *Kleiderordnungen der deutschen Städte zwischen 1350 und 1700, Göttinger Bausteine zur Geschichtswissenschaft*, 32 (Göttingen, 1962).

77 *Hamlet, Prince of Denmark*, Act 3, scene 1.

9

The Cuckoldries of Baccio del Bianco

Louise Rice

In the 1630s, the Florentine painter Baccio del Bianco (1604–1656) produced a series of comic drawings of daily life in the Tuscan capital, in which the citizens almost to a man sport the symbols of their wives' infidelities.[1] In a world gone horn-mad, the *cornuti* of Florence shop for the latest fashions in antlers, drop by the barbershop for a quick horn-trim, try on specialty hats at the milliner's, share their partners in a round dance, go on pilgrimage with their brother-sufferers, and take part in festivals celebrating the king of cuckolds, the great Becco himself. In Tuscan dialect, *becco* is both a billy goat and a cuckold; and this double sense plays an important part in Baccio's imagery. But goats have multiple associations, as we will see, and Baccio taps into all of them, complicating his cuckoldries with allusions to witchcraft and devilry on the one hand, fantasy and intellectual license on the other. In Baccio's hands, the comic trope of wifely infidelity becomes a template for invention, and the transgression of societal rules a metaphor for the free flight of fancy.

The drawings—there are nine of them in all, executed in black chalk and bearing consecutive inventory numbers in the Department of Prints and Drawings of the Uffizi Gallery in Florence—constitute an almost encyclopedic survey of the richly varied literary and visual gags associated with cuckoldry. They use a carnivalesque rhetoric of inversion to conjure up a topsy-turvy world, a world in which gender roles are reversed; in which all wives are by definition adulteresses and all married men cuckolds; a world furthermore full of contradictions and paradoxes, in which horns symbolize both virility and impotence, opposite ideas with a shared attribute.[2] The universality and at the same time the perversity of the cuckold's fate are the underlying fictions on which the drawings are based.

An obsessive preoccupation with female infidelity was, of course, nothing new.[3] *Chi non è morto, morirà; chi non è becco, diventerà,* so goes an age-old Tuscan proverb, which we might paraphrase: "Nothing is certain in this world, except death and horns." The saying appears on an anonymous Florentine print from around 1480, a fascinating precursor to Baccio's essays in horn lore, although markedly less genteel in its approach to the subject (Fig. 9.1).[4]

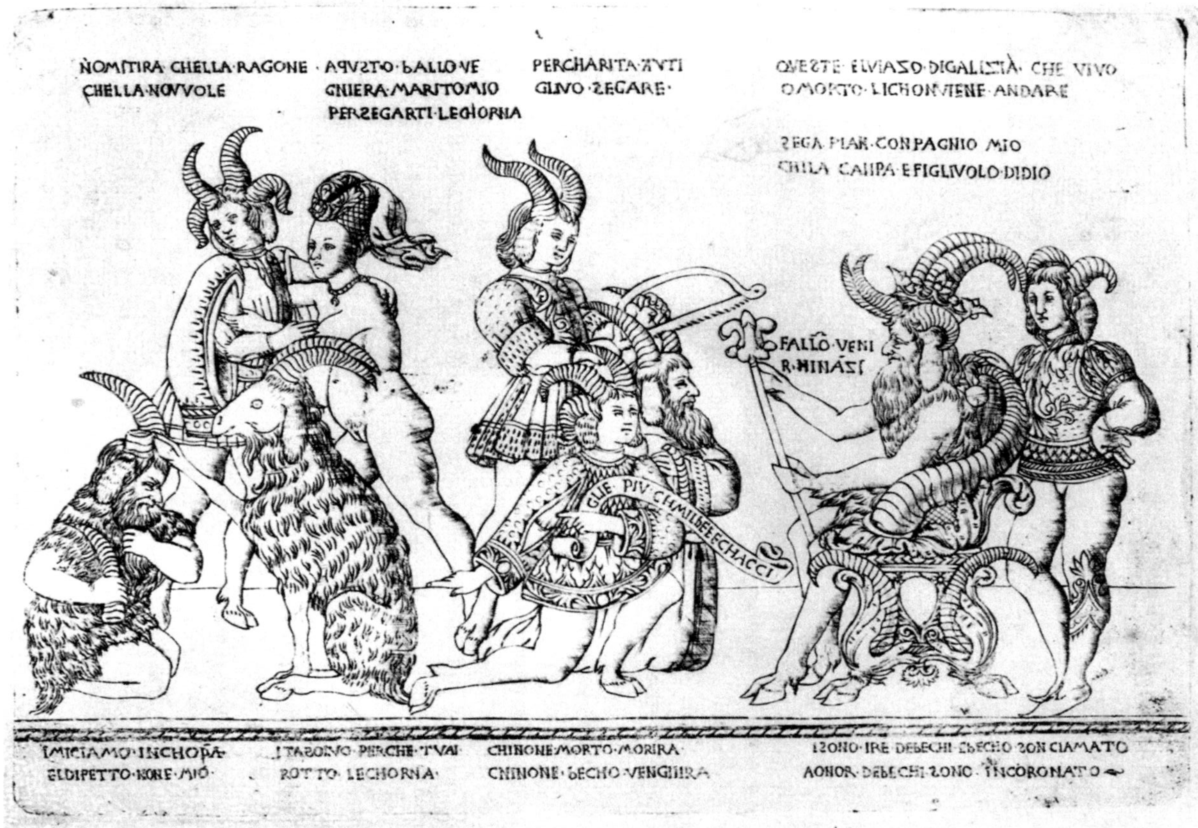

9.1 Anonymous Florentine, *Becco, King of Cuckolds, holds court*, c. 1480, engraving, 178 × 250 mm, Albertina, Vienna

Its depiction of the adulteress, in particular, is downright brutal. Naked, her pudenda exposed, the veil of her headdress falling in barely disguised labial folds, she is savage and sex-addled, out of control with desire. Meanwhile the cuckolds meekly approach Becco, king of the *becchi*, seated on a throne of horn on the right. He holds a scepter tipped with a Florentine *giglio* made of bundled phalluses. Note the punning caption next to the fleur-de-lis. *Fallo venir minanzi*, says the king, "Have him come before me." *Fallo*, in this context, means "have him," but we are surely meant to pick up on the fact that it also means "phallus." This kind of verbal and visual play was also dear to Baccio's heart and features in several of his cuckoldries.

Although of a type that was mass-produced for a popular market, this Quattrocento print is known today through a single surviving impression. We are reminded that compositions of this kind were terribly ephemeral; and the fact that we have relatively few drawings and prints of *cornuti* before Baccio's does not mean that they did not exist, nor even that they were particularly rare. The frequency with which the cuckold shows up in Renaissance literature suggests that he was similarly represented in the visual culture of the period. But whereas literary treatments have survived in large numbers, visual ones have been more subject to expurgation, censorship, and losses of various kinds. We must turn to the literary models, therefore, to establish a context for understanding the few visual ones that we have.

Among literary treatments, one of the best known and most entertaining is Giovanni Battista Modio's satirical dialogue on horns published in Rome in 1554 under the title *Il Convito* (literally "The Banquet," although given its decidedly Humanist flavor a better translation might be "The Symposium").[5] In it, Modio takes on the theme of the universality of the cuckold's condition, with one of his interlocutors bemoaning the fact that "while earlier eras are known as the age of gold, of silver, or of iron ... our own, by analogy, should be called the age of horn."[6] The world upside-down, the community of cuckolds, the age of horn: Modio's themes are the very ones that Baccio later elaborates in his nine Uffizi cuckoldries and related drawings.

Modio's *Convito* is set during Carnival.[7] While outside the streets teem with carriages full of men and women bent on merrymaking, a group of male friends—literati and academicians—gathers around a banqueting table in the *sala di Psiche* in Villa Farnesina. Perhaps Raphael's fresco overhead—his voluptuous celebration of marriage in paint—inspires the topic of conversation: for the diners agree to discourse on horns, and more specifically, "whence derives the general opinion, that when a husband has a lascivious wife he appears to the world to have horns on his head."[8] Each member of the party, in turn, offers his thoughts on the origins and meaning of the cuckold's horns. The tone is learned, witty and ludic, until the arrival of an unexpected guest who steals the privilege of speaking last and shifts the mood to one of seriousness, with his philosophical and rational defense of the married state. At the close of the dialogue, however, Carnival boisterously reasserts itself. Ten masked clowns (*mattacini*) dressed as satyrs (*cornuti animali*) tumble into the loggia and dance a round before the delighted guests. On this lighter note, the party disperses, leaving open and unresolved what moral, if any, the reader is to take away with him.

The backdrop of Carnival is crucial to understanding both Modio's dialogue and Baccio's drawings. Carnival was a time of exceptional license, when normal societal restrictions were relaxed.[9] Women were more on view than at other times of year, and in the parades, pantomimes and other comic enactments that were a regular feature of Carnival, the symbolism of sexual permissiveness was pervasive. A stock figure of fun at Carnival events was the cuckold. Mikhail Bakhtin posited that the cuckolded husband filled "the role of uncrowned old age, of the old year, and the receding winter" and his public humiliation—his crowning with horns—was thus central to the festival's subversive and anti-authoritarian impulse.[10] By the 17th century, in the cities at least, this kind of role-playing had largely been taken over by the clowns of the *Commedia dell'arte*, and cuckolds and cuckolding were constant themes in the street shows they staged during Carnival.[11] For Baccio and his contemporaries, then, the cuckold was almost synonymous with Carnival, and the cuckold's horns a symbol of all that Carnival stood for: the world turned upside-down (*il mondo alla rovescia*), authority upended, inhibitions unshackled and the imagination set free.

Baccio's cuckoldries have received surprisingly little attention in the literature. The series as a whole is occasionally cited, it is true, but until Massimiliano Rossi illustrated all nine of the sheets in the catalogue to an exhibition he co-curated in Corsica in 2011, fewer than half of them had been published.[12] The goal of this article, therefore, is to introduce Baccio's *mondo dei cornuti* to a wider audience and, through a close descriptive and iconographic reading of the drawings' rich imagery, to consider the broader historical circumstances and cultural assumptions that underlie their creation. Three general observations can be made at the outset. First, the drawings allude to many of the same themes touched on by the participants at Modio's symposium, which suggests either that Baccio knew and was thinking about Modio's text when he made them or (perhaps more likely) that he and Modio relied on a common repertory of humorous proverbs and conceits that had widespread currency at the time. Second, notwithstanding the existence of this common body of horn humor, the precise meaning of many of the scenes that Baccio represents is far from obvious, and in a few cases may involve private references impossible for us to parse. Third (and this is harder to put into words), the drawings have a sweetness of tone that is remarkable given their bawdy and misogynist subject matter. Baccio treats the fate of the married man as the lightest comedy of manners. Cuckoldom, for him, is a civilized place, populated by ladies and gentlemen of a certain class, whose passions are tempered by delicacy, and whose inconstancy is mitigated by tenderness. The drawings radiate erotic humor, but there is nothing boorish or savage about them. To quote George Rogers, whose 1660 treatise on cuckolds is similarly mild in tone: "Mirth and a good Conscience meet together, and I think they may as innocently kiss each other."[13]

Although the inventory numbers do not imply a fixed order of viewing, we may as well begin with the first in the sequence, Uffizi 3375 (Fig. 9.2). The *cornuti* of Florence go shopping for horns. Assisted by charming salesladies, they try on their horns for size, study the effect in a mirror, model hats custom-made to their specifications, and pay for their new appurtenances by the pound. Every sort of horn is on offer: goat, ram, bull, stag, even the timid snail. For snails, too, belong to the menagerie of cuckolds. Shakespeare refers to "the tender horns of cockl'd snails"[14] and jokes that the snail "brings his destiny [i.e. his horns] with him."[15] A rare example of a cuckoldry predating Baccio's, bearing an old attribution to Callot, represents a villainous-looking snail-eater, seated before a plate of snails, garlanded with the creatures, and making the sign of the horns with both hands (Fig. 9.3).[16] *Avere più corna di un cesto di lumache* (to have more horns than a basket of snails) is an Italian proverb, referring to husbands serially cuckolded by their wives.[17] (The idea that each act of adultery adds another pair of horns to the husband's head was widespread in the literature of the time and many of the cuckolds in Baccio's drawings wear multiple pairs of horns.[18]) Snails were clearly a favorite motif of Baccio's and are present, in one guise or another, in eight of the nine drawings in the series.

In this emporium for cuckolds, the wares are displayed on hangers, graduated by size and kind. The different types of horn imply different types of customer. For as we learn from Modio's *Convito*, not all *cornuti* are the same:

> From what has already been said, you will recognize that there are different kinds of cuckolds. Thus he who out of gluttony or drunkenness gives his wife freedom to pursue her own pleasures, may be called "goat;" he who cannot defend himself against either his wife or her lover because of the other's superior strength or power, may be called "sheep;" and he who, abandoning his wife and roaming elsewhere, does not fulfill his matrimonial duties but gives her reason to look outside for what she does not get at home, may be called "bull;" just as he who out of meanness of spirit and overwhelming jealousy, by suspecting everything and everyone, sparks desires in his wife that she might not otherwise have had, may, like Actaeon, be called "stag." But he who, by offering his wife to men of high rank, adds prestige and grandeur to his house, may be called, not without reason, "elephant." And because they are rarer than the others, it seems that these last, out of a certain respect that the world has for them as the favorites of lords and princes, are not called *cornuti*; and maybe it is also because it has not yet been resolved whether the elephant's tusk is horn or tooth. As for the others, one hears it said everyday, "he is a goat;" "he is a bull;" "he is a stag;" "he is a sheep." From which one may conclude, from the different appearances and natures of horned animals, likewise there are different kinds of cuckolds.[19]

On the right hand side of the drawing, beneath a row of horned trophies, shopkeepers polish, mend and sharpen horns as their clients anxiously look on. A lady-painter works on a half-length picture of a cuckold, her occupation recalling Benedick's boast, that if ever he were to marry, he would:

> … pluck off the bull's horns and set
> them in my forehead: and let me be vilely painted,
> and in such great letters as they write "Here is
> good horse to hire," let them signify under my sign
> "Here you may see Benedick the married man."[20]

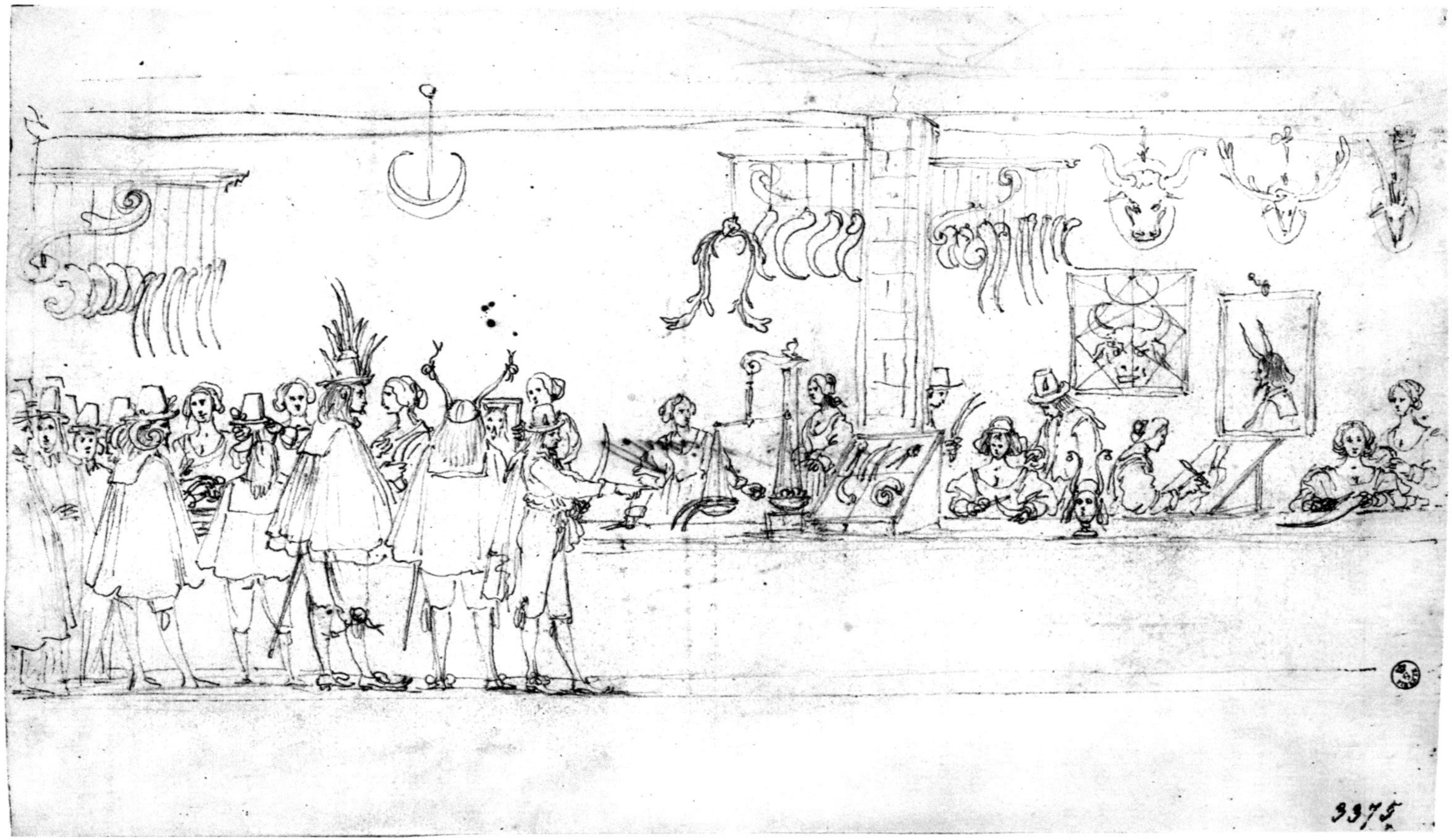

9.2 Baccio del Bianco, *The Horn Store*, c. 1638, black chalk, 252 × 418 mm, Uffizi (3375 F), Florence (permission: Ministero dei beni e delle attività culturali e del turismo)

The crescent, or horned, moon that hangs from the rafters on the left is yet another symbol of the cuckold's state that had wide currency in Baccio's day.[21]

The shoppers in Baccio's horn store seem almost proud of their shiny new accouterments, as though their vanity were enough to overcome their shame. In other drawings, too, we sense complicity and a willingness on the husbands' part to acquire the telltale sign. In Uffizi 3376, men crowd around a street vendor, buying horns as casually as they might *ciambelle*, or doughnuts (Fig. 9.7, far right). This little vignette parodies the kind of genre scene made popular by Callot in Florence and by the *bamboccianti* in Rome. Indeed, it so closely resembles Pieter van Laer's charming *Ciambella-seller* of c. 1630 (Galleria Nazionale, Rome) that one wonders if Baccio knew a version of it.

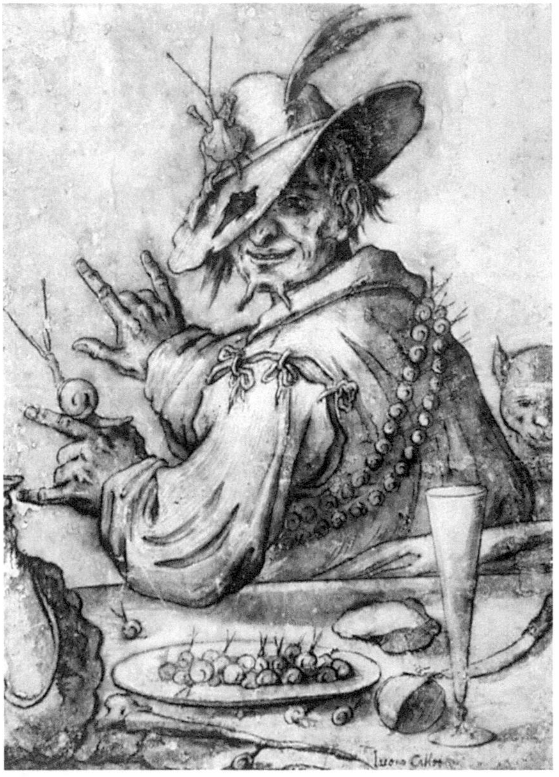

9.3 Attributed to Jacques Callot, *The Snail-Eater*, c. 1612–1617, pen and ink wash and white highlights, 470 × 370 mm, Uffizi (5803 S), Florence (permission: Ministero dei beni e delle attività culturali e del turismo)

In Uffizi 3383, a band of drums and cornetts strikes up a tune (Fig. 9.4).[22] To their rustic rhythm, five ladies and five gentlemen dance in a circle, each holding hands with two partners at once, a perfect metaphor for the spouse-swapping that makes cuckolds of husbands.[23] Dancing has always been thought to involve a dangerous kind of intimacy even under the most proper of circumstances, but in the fictional world of Cuckoldom it leads inevitably to adultery.[24] The ladies have come prepared and wear horns suspended on ribbons from their waistbands, ready to bestow on their mates. Those who are sitting out the dance are approached by handsome young gallants who offer themselves as partners. The husbands, meanwhile, commiserate with each other at the back of the queue, as they wait for a turn that never comes to dance with their own wives.

The horn store and the round dance are two of the easier drawings in the series. Others are more difficult to construe. This is due in part to the way Baccio composed them. A single sheet may feature multiple scenes and interpretation is complicated by the fact that it is not always clear where one scene ends and another begins, or what, if any, is the relationship between adjacent scenes. A case in point is Uffizi 3378, in which a man is sitting at a table gloating over a pile of coins, with bags and strongboxes full of money all around him (Fig. 9.5). A date on one of the moneybags—1638—is usually assumed to be that of the series as a whole. Through an open doorway, guarded by a servant, we glimpse a bed on which two pairs of feet are intimately intertwined. The brothel, it seems, is open to business. Who owns this house of ill repute?

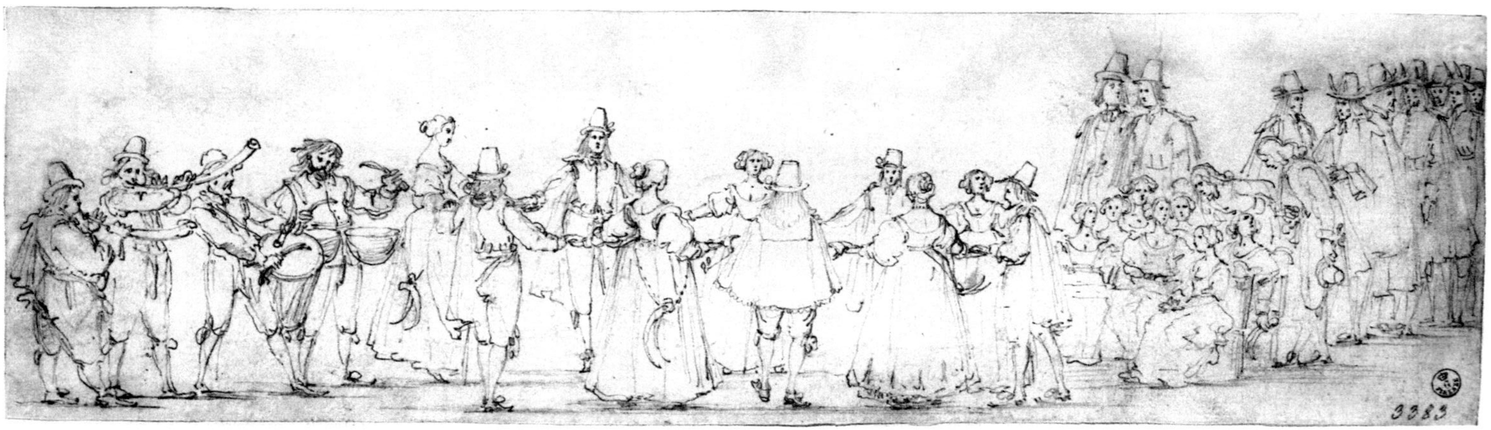

9.4 Baccio del Bianco, *The Round Dance*, c. 1638, black chalk, 122 × 420 mm, Uffizi (3383 F), Florence (permission: Ministero dei beni e delle attività culturali e del turismo)

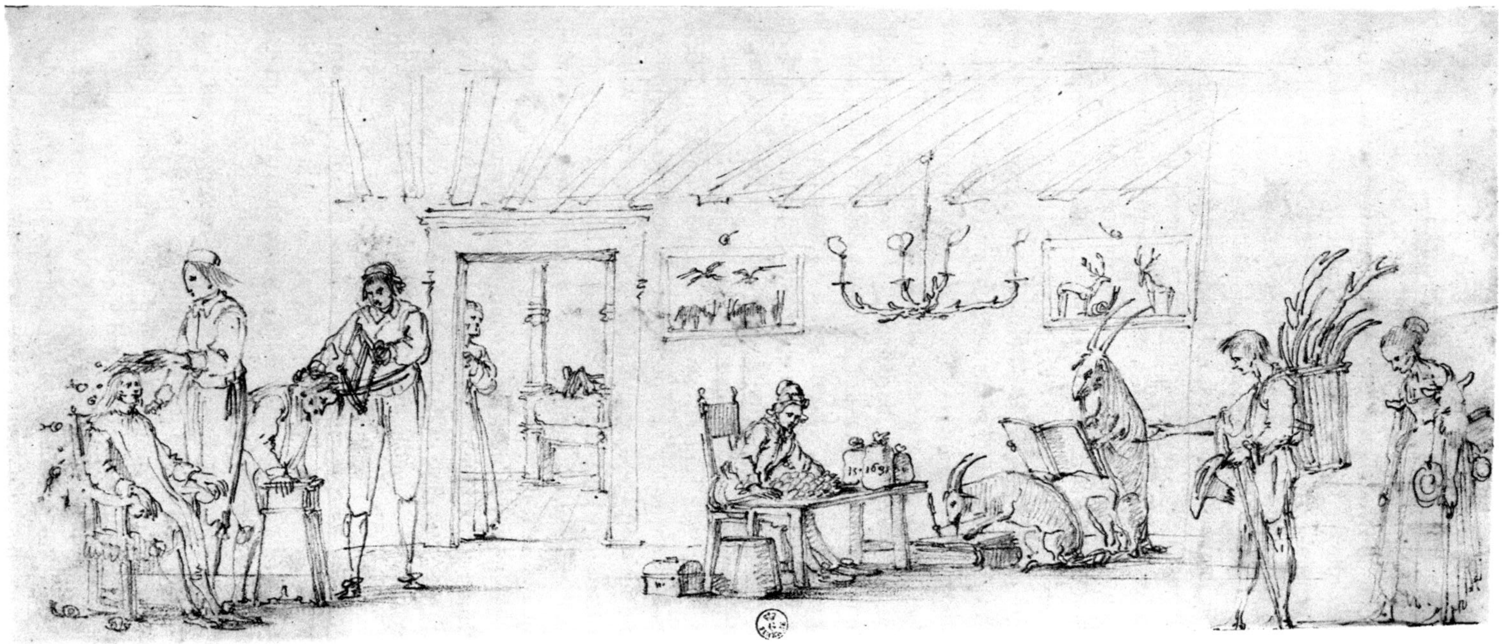

9.5 Baccio del Bianco, *The Wittol's Counting Room and other scenes*, c. 1638, black chalk, 175 × 395 mm, Uffizi (3378 F), Florence (permission: Ministero dei beni e delle attività culturali e del turismo)

It is the husband himself, for he is the kind of cuckold who profits from his wife's transgressions. He is what is referred to in Renaissance literature as a *cornuto volontario*, in English a contented cuckold, or wittol. Husbands come by their horns in all manner of ways and some, like this one, are complicit in prostituting their wives for money or other kinds of gain.[25] Pictures of horned animals decorate the wall of the wittol's counting room where, by the light of an antler chandelier, he pours over his ill-gotten gains, while beside him his two clerks—goats, the pair of them—keep the books.

In stark contrast, the couple on the right of the sheet are the poorest of the poor. The husband collects discarded horns for resale to others but wears none himself, because he has taken for his wife a woman too crippled and decrepit to tempt anyone to seduce her. He is safe from infidelity but on the other hand he cannot profit from his spouse like the man with the money. Here, the juxtaposition of the two scenes on the page is meant not so much to imply a continuity of action, as to emphasize the contrast between them. A thin vertical line indicating the corner of the wittol's room doubles as a kind of narrative boundary, even if the pauper's outstretched hand does accidentally cut across it.

On the left side of the sheet is a scene not directly related to the other two. Although at first glance we seem still to be in the wittol's counting room, we have in fact moved to a barbershop, where two married men are being treated for what ails them. One of them is having his horns sawn off. Shaving or sawing off the cuckold's horns was a commonplace trope in Renaissance Florence.[26] It is illustrated in the 15th-century print discussed above, where one of the cuckolds kneeling before King Becco's throne is having his horns cut off, while another holding his severed horn in his hand receives absolution from a goat (Fig. 9.1);[27] and it shows up also on painted majolica ware.[28] But what does it mean? Meek husbands who accept the infidelity of their wives quietly and let them get on with their adulterous affairs without resistance or remonstrance are said to have cut off their horns. This signifies, on the one hand, that they have rid themselves of the outward sign of their shame by keeping quiet about it; but, on the other hand, that they have undergone a kind of metaphorical castration, becoming docile eunuchs as a result. Here, as elsewhere in the parlance of cuckoldry, we encounter that curious confusion as to the precise meaning of horns, which seem to connote something phallic and anti-phallic at the same time. To saw off your horns (*segarti le corna*); to bury your horns; to keep your horns in your pocket, or to store them in your breast: all of these expressions seem to have roughly the same meaning—namely, to preserve your dignity and reputation by keeping silent about your wife's infidelity.[29] Vespasiano da Bisticci tells a story that perfectly illustrates the point. Approached by a citizen who wanted advice as to how to handle his wife's unfaithfulness, Cosimo de' Medici recommended that he take his horns and bury them in a ditch, so that no one would see them. "The man at once took Cosimo's meaning and, seeing that he had erred in talking about the business, kept silence afterwards and took the lady as an honest woman."[30] Yet at the same time, to be de-horned is to be emasculated, humiliated or more literally scorned (*scornato*). One of the speakers at Modio's banquet describes how shepherds treat an overly aggressive ram, who out a jealously and possessiveness prevents other males from mating with the ewes in his flock: they saw off his horns and this renders him submissive and mild.

> By the same token, those wretched men who unjustly and by force suffer the injuries committed against them by their wives, and who, unable to prevail against them, pretend not to notice, are likened to sheep; and some call them scorned/de-horned cuckolds, or say "I'll saw off your horns."[31]

The other of the barber's clients is having the snails combed out of his hair. This presumably means something similar to the sawing off of horns, and there is bound to be a corresponding expression or proverb, although I have not so far come across it. It is a motif that Baccio seems to have been particularly fond of, for it shows up again in another of the drawings, in which two snail-ridden husbands run their fingers through their hair in an effort to shake out the vermin (Fig. 9.8).

In Baccio's imaginary land of cuckolds, it is the women who have the upper hand, and who browbeat, cajole, lull, tempt or flatter their husbands into accepting their horns. A wife of a husband given to drinking too much encourages his dissipation, plying him with wine while surreptitiously placing the horns on his head (Fig. 9.6).[32] One woman wallops her submissive husband with an antler, dislodging a flurry of snails;[33] another taking advantage of her husband's slothfulness slips the horns on his head while he sleeps; yet another plays on her husband's vanity, encouraging him to admire his new look in the mirror (Fig. 9.7). And then there is the wife who steals up from behind while her husband is so immersed in his ledgers that he does not realize what has befallen him. Marriages, as everyone knows, are made in heaven; and as if to prove the point, Baccio includes a *deus ex machina* in the sky overhead: a platform of cloud whereon Venus crowns Vulcan with a coronet of horns, a celestial cuckolding attended by Taurus, Aires and Capricorn, the three horned members of the zodiacal menagerie.[34]

Uffizi 3382 consists of a string of four comic vignettes (Fig. 9.6). They are, from left to right:

1) A cuckold attempts to disguise his condition by hiding his horns under a floppy hat, but the telltale protuberances are spotted by an astonished bystander who also notices the snail rosettes on his breeches and shoes.
2) A street brawl erupts between two cuckolds, egged on by their women. Could it be that each man has cuckolded the other? One of the women, wielding an antler and horn, wears high pattens, a type of shoe sometimes (but not exclusively) worn by courtesans.
3) With the help of her maid, a wife befuddles her husband with drink and slips him the horns while he slumbers.
4) Young brides receive instruction in the housewifery of horns. In this school for wives, experienced "professors" demonstrate how to measure the thickness and straightness of horn using calipers and plumb lines. Elephant tusks contribute to the comedy, playing on the paradoxical meaning of horns as symbols of both virility and impotence.[35]

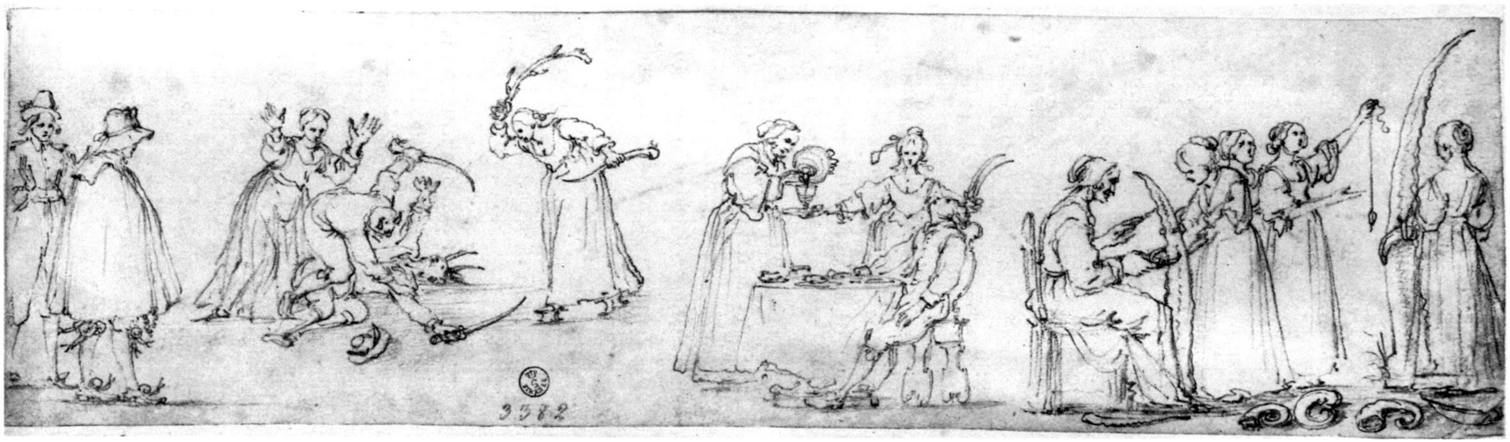

9.6 Baccio del Bianco, *The School for Wives and other scenes*, c. 1638, black chalk, 120 × 420 mm, Uffizi (3382 F), Florence (permission: Ministero dei beni e delle attività culturali e del turismo)

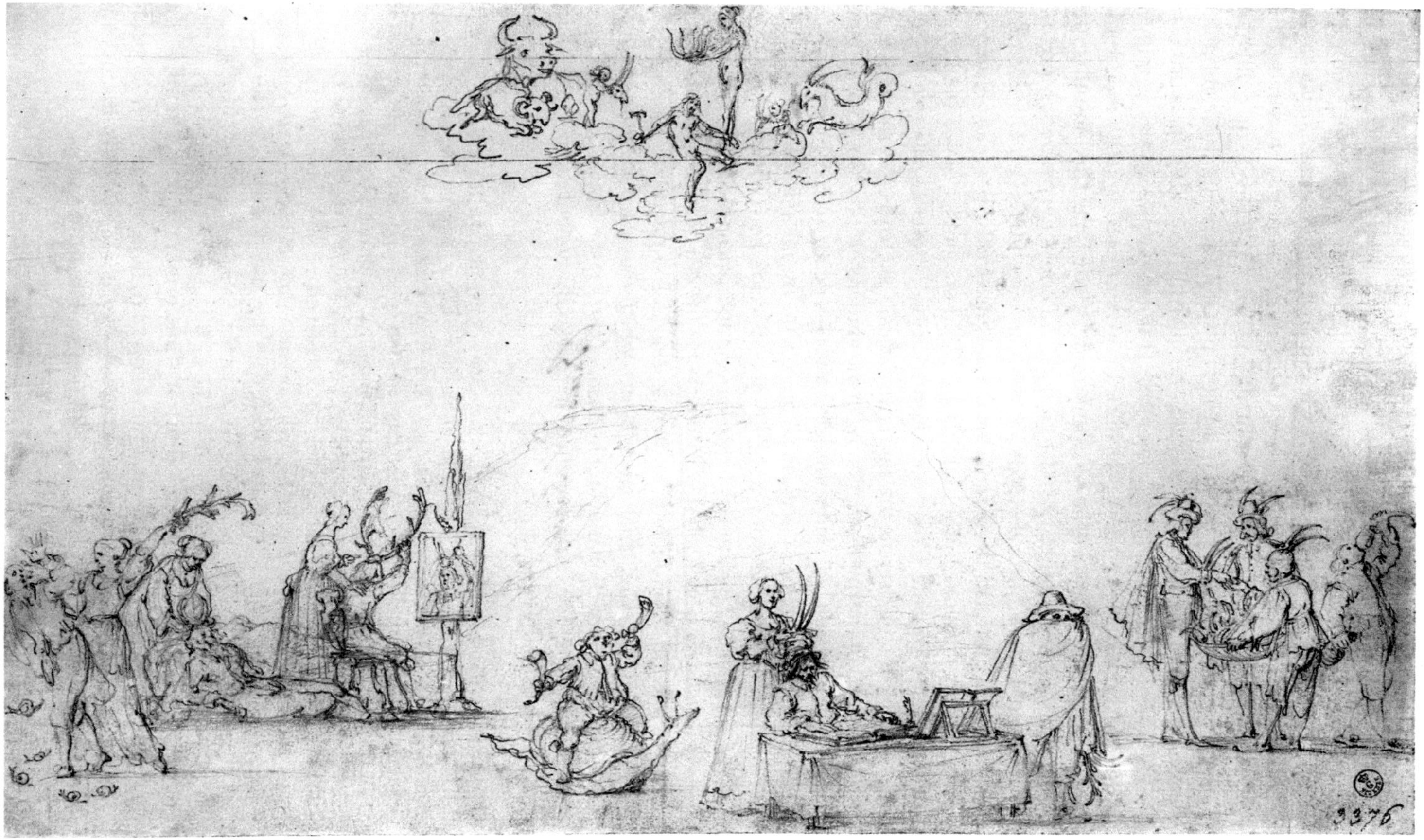

9.7 Baccio del Bianco, *A Marriage made in Heaven and other scenes*, c. 1638, black chalk, 252 × 410 mm, Uffizi (3376 F), Florence (permission: Ministero dei beni e delle attività culturali e del turismo)

This last scene is the only one in the series (apart from the bedroom scene in Uffizi 3378, which we barely glimpse) with overtly lewd subject matter. Its comico-pornographic treatment of the old bawd as school mistress and the young girls as pupils eager to learn the erotic arts (or what James Grantham Turner refers to as "the hard core curriculum") recalls Aretino's *Ragionamento* and other libertine texts in the pornodidascalian or School-of-Venus tradition.[36]

A more difficult drawing to disentangle is Uffizi 3376, made up of eight or nine separate scenes (Fig. 9.7). Particularly puzzling is the fat dwarf mounted on a slow-moving snail who heralds his arrival by tooting his horn. The figure has strong Florentine resonances. Is he one of the dwarfs employed at the Medici court? When we see him, are we supposed to recall the famous Nano Morgante, the favorite of Cosimo I de' Medici, depicted in numerous paintings and sculptures of the period? Valerio Cioli carved Morgante riding on a large tortoise (1560s; Boboli Gardens, Florence); Giambologna represented him astride a fantastical sea-slug (1580s; Bargello, Florence); and in a small bronze by Antonio Susini based on another of Giambologna's inventions, Morgante blows on a horn (1580s; Victoria & Albert Museum, London).[37] Even closer to the figure in Baccio's sketch is the marble dwarf mounted on an enormous snail, now in the gardens of Villa Medici at Careggi (begun by Valerio Cioli and completed after his death in 1599 by his nephew Simone Cioli).[38] Are these sculptural precedents meant to inform our reading of the figure in Baccio's drawing? Or does Baccio's horn blower have some other, unrelated significance? Is he, for example, meant to parody the town criers (*banditori*) whose job it was to traverse the city reading out the official notices and pronouncements known as *bandi*? The town criers went about mounted and carrying small silver horns, which they used to announce their arrival.[39] The connection may not be as tenuous as it sounds. According to one of Modio's symposiasts, the origin of the cuckold's symbol can be traced back to the horns of the *banditori*:

> Someone whose wife is giving him (as the saying goes) "the twisted spindles" [i.e. the horns] is only called "cuckold" if his shame is trumpeted in the piazzas, as they do with public announcements ... Therefore, since horns mean nothing in themselves, but only insofar as they represent the public opinion that the common man has of the husband's shame, and since, in former times, that shame was considered so great that it was quickly broadcast everywhere, as if it were big news, from this comes the cuckold's horn, based on the similarity to the *bandi* and other public pronouncements, which were made known to everyone by the sound of the trumpet or horn, since in those days they used to make trumpets out of horn.[40]

If the *nano* blowing his horn illustrates one origin myth, the youth at the far right drinking deeply from a horn cup may illustrate another. Boozing is one sure path to Cuckoldom, which is why one of Modio's discussants lays the blame for the cuckold's condition on his drunkenness.[41] That same speaker goes on to suggest that the cuckold's horns derive from the fact that the ancients drank their wine out of horn cups:

> Whereas today we drink out of glass or other material, in former times they used to drink out of animal horns ... Therefore when drunkenness has reduced a man to having an immodest wife, he is said to have horns on his forehead, either to show the world the occasion for his shame, or because the wine that he drank from the horn has raised a bump on his brow, because it's the property of wine, to hit you over the head.[42]

Thus the actions of the dwarfish *banditore* and the guzzling youth, as well as the objects they hold, may allude to variant accounts of the origins of the cuckold's horns.

Another perplexing character in this most crowded and complicated of the drawings in the series is the skulker with his cloak wrapped around his face who slinks away from center stage, carrying a partially concealed rack of antlers and another of horns. Is he a cuckold or a cuckold-maker? And is he connected to the oblivious businessman next to him on the sheet? Finally, what is the significance of the flat-topped hill in the background? This hill might not deserve notice were it not for the fact that a similar hill shows up in another of the drawings. The repetition would seem to suggest that a meaning of some sort attaches to it—like the cuckold's horns, its peak has been lopped off—but the precise signification remains obscure.

The other mountain serves as the backdrop to a scene of pilgrimage (Fig. 9.8, Uffizi 3379). A duo of elderly cuckolds ventures forth, perhaps on a votive mission to seek relief from their condition. Horns instead of scallop shells embellish their short pilgrim's capes, their broad-brimmed pilgrim's hats, and their pilgrim's staffs. A third gentleman watches them depart. A small horn dangles from the tip of his sword but there is otherwise no indication that he is either a cuckold or a pilgrim, and his relationship to the other two is ambiguous. Perhaps he is the cuckold-maker, just waiting for the husbands to be on their way before approaching their wives with an offer of consolation. The look—somewhere between distrustful and panic-stricken—that one of the pilgrims shoots in his direction seems to say it all.

A couple of the drawings hint at links between wifely infidelity and witchcraft. A convergence of iconographies contributes to this blurring of concepts. The goat is one common denominator. He is both the symbol of the cuckold and the witch's familiar, the devil in disguise.[43] Witches are often shown consorting with goats, or riding on them.[44] Horns are another shared motif. They are the attribute of the cuckold, but also of Satan, the cuckold-maker *par excellence*, who prefers to fornicate with married witches, since with his virgin devotees he cannot commit adultery.[45] Witches are reputed to have insatiable sexual appetites and this, too, implicates them in a web of related ideas about female rapaciousness and male inadequacy.[46] All of these themes come spectacularly together in an etching after a lost drawing by Parmigianino, which shows a witch mounted on a goat-phallus (that is, a phallus with its root and testicles transmogrified into the hind quarters of a goat), surrounded by horned creatures (a hybrid panther, a demon and a horned owl) and accompanied by a band of followers, prominent among whom is an elderly

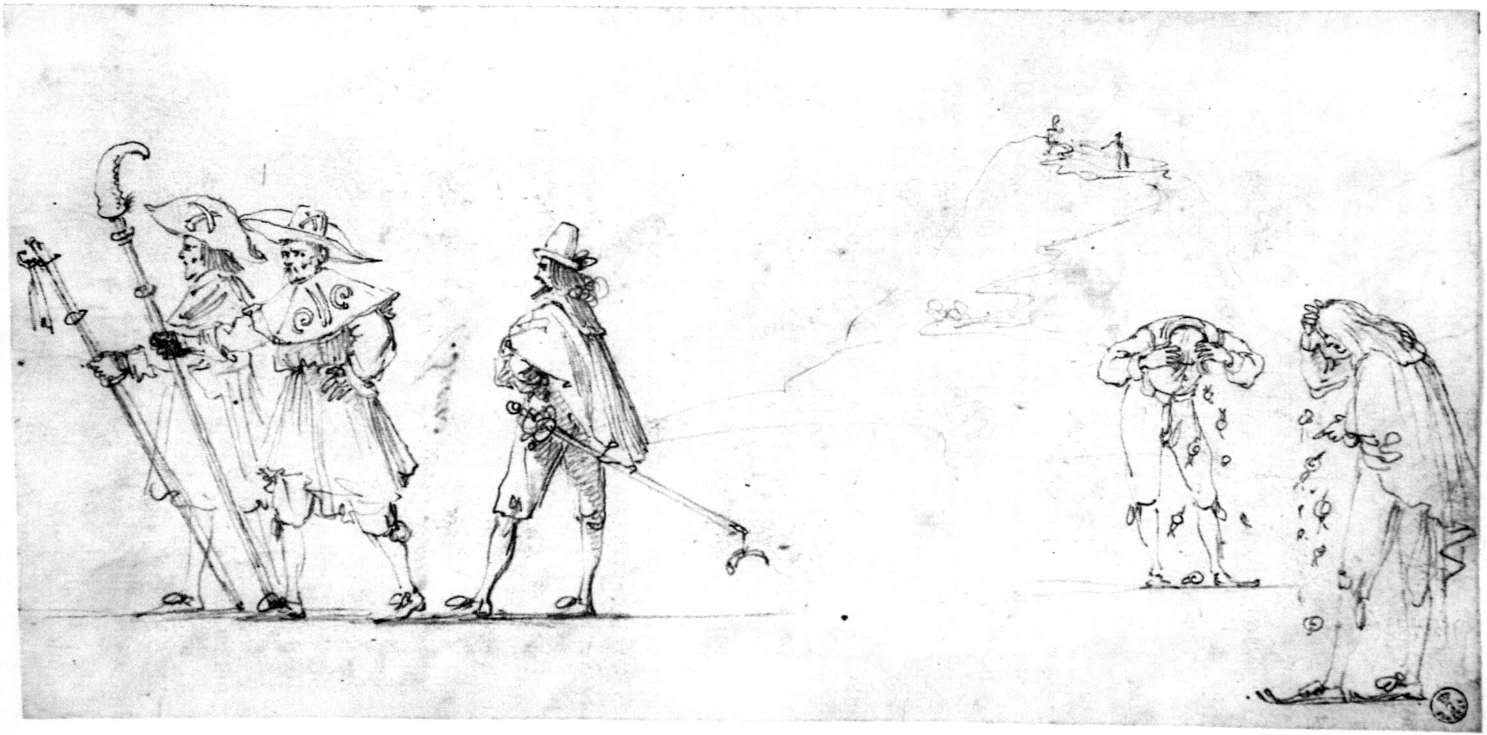

9.8 Baccio del Bianco, *The Pilgrim-Cuckolds and another scene*, c. 1638, black chalk, 175 × 340 mm, Uffizi (3379 F), Florence (permission: Ministero dei beni e delle attività culturali e del turismo)

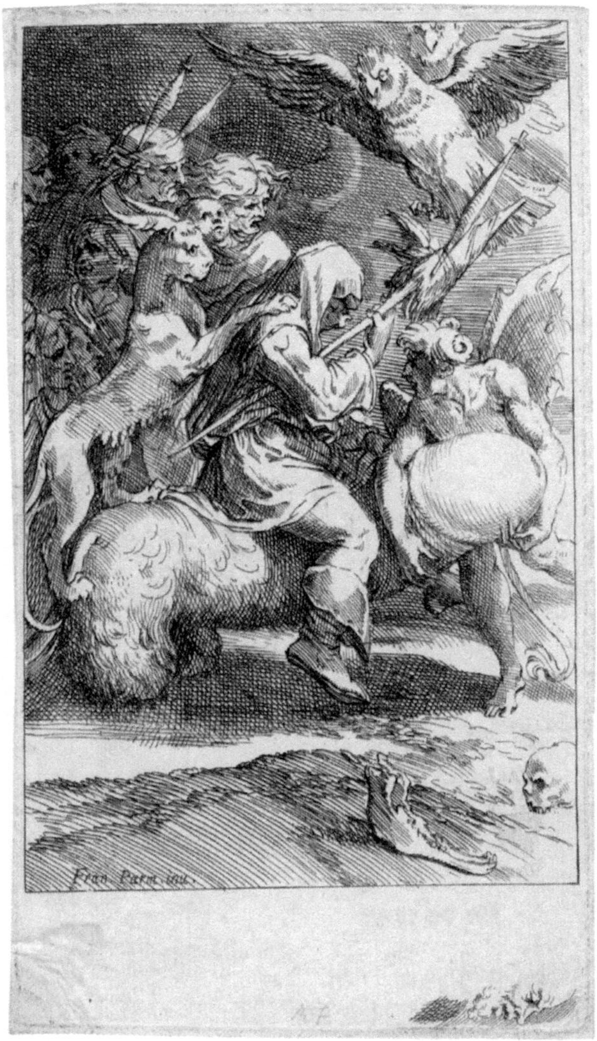

9.9 Bernard Picart, after a lost drawing by Parmigianino (1530s), *Witch riding a Phallus*, 1732, etching, 145 × 95 mm, British Museum, London

cuckold wearing the "twisted spindles" (Fig. 9.9).[47] A punning play on the word *becco* is, I suspect, the key to unlocking this image. For in addition to the two meanings already discussed (male goat and cuckold), *becco* has another significance. It is a bird's beak, and like the equivalent English word "pecker" it can be used in a bawdy sense to refer to the penis.[48] Parmigianino's goat-phallus is thus a *becco* times three, a licentious and paradoxical emblem of male sexual potency and impotence.

Nothing in Baccio's imagery is as hard core as this. But the association of women, goats and horns throughout the series strikes a faintly satanic chord, and the iconographic cross-referencing is nowhere more conspicuous than in Uffizi 3380, in which a coven of wives, gathered around a rustic sacrificial altar, seem bent on some diabolical ritual (Fig. 9.10). These ladies may not

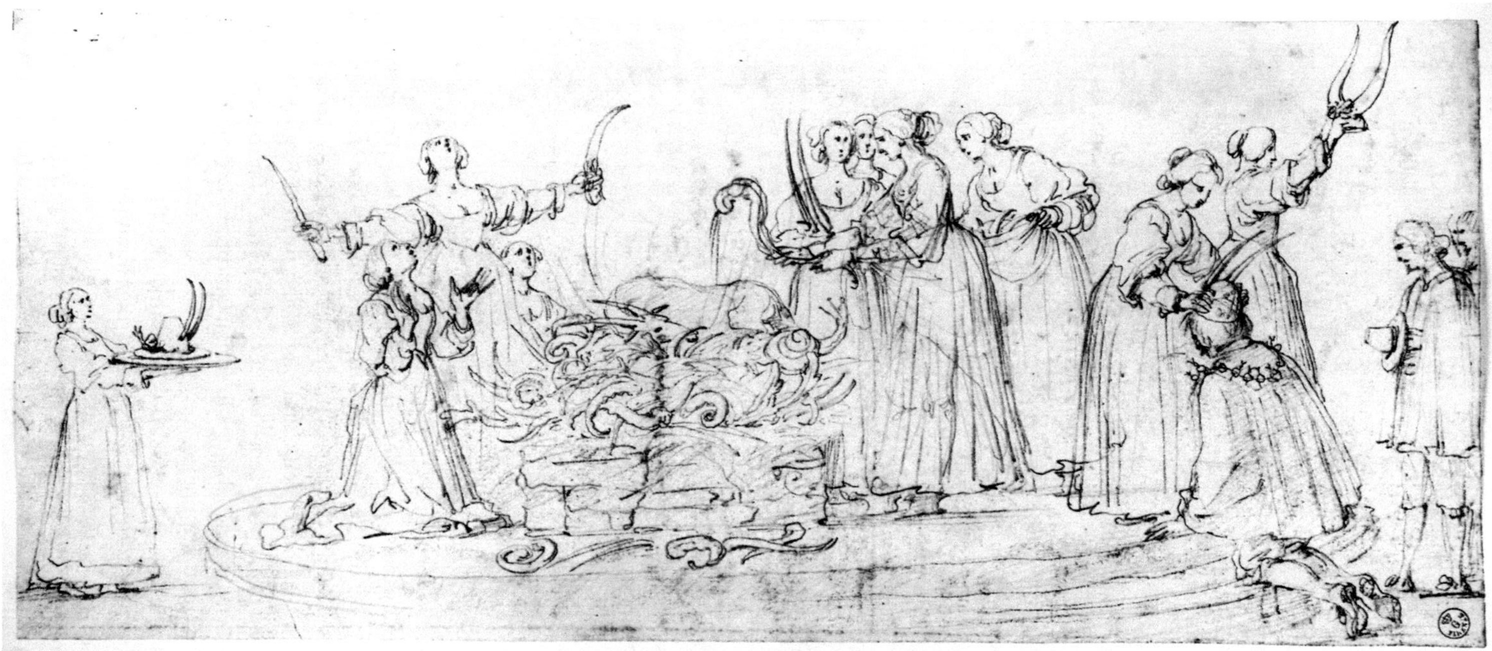

9.10 Baccio del Bianco, *Scene of Sacrifice and Ceremonial Induction into the Grand Order of Cuckolds*, c. 1638, black chalk, 175 × 390 mm, Uffizi (3380 F), Florence (permission: Ministero dei beni e delle attività culturali e del turismo)

look like witches but they certainly act like them, as they intone incantations and prayers while making offerings of horn. At the close of the ceremony, the wives induct their husbands into the Grand Order of Cuckolds, placing the chain of snails around their necks and crowning them with horns.[49]

An allusion to witchcraft may also be present in Uffizi 3377 (Fig. 9.11). Raised on a high table and enthroned on a recumbent goat, King Becco holds court. He is bedecked with the symbols of his rank: a hat sprouting multiple horns, a snail chain with horn pendent, snail rosettes at the cuffs of his breeches and on his shoes, and, in his left hand, a bell-tipped scepter of horn. Flanking him sit two wives on elaborate chairs of horn. They are the queens of his kingdom, while his courtiers are the two young gallants hovering off to the side, awaiting an opportunity to play their part. The prominence of the goat, together with the rigidly frontal and symmetrical position of the three principal figures, echoes a detail in the etching illustrating the witches' Sabbath in Pierre de Lancre's *Tableau de l'inconstance des mauvais anges et demons*, in which Satan in the guise of a multi-horned goat sits enthroned between twin consorts, the crowned Queen of the Sabbath to his right and another "less favored" to his left (Fig. 9.12).[50]

The triumph of King Cuckold ends the series on a high note (Fig. 9.13, Uffizi 3381). Holding a horn scepter and wearing a snail-shaped headdress sprouting multiple horns, he rides in a nautilus-shaped chariot pulled by a team of snails and preceded by a goat, with his entourage of husbands forming the vanguard. Becco's triumphal *carro* is immediately recognizable as the kind of fanciful carriage or float that wound through the city streets and took part in the great court spectacles staged during Carnival. It recalls similar animal-shaped Carnival *carri* in drawings and prints by Callot, Stefano della Bella and many others (Fig. 9.14). Of all Baccio's cuckoldries, this one is the most explicitly carnivalesque in its imagery and the one that most closely situates the series as a whole in a Carnival context.

The drawings are loose and sketchy in their handling, quite different from the highly polished drawings in pen and ink that Baccio produced when working on commission or in connection with more formal projects, and this may give us a hint as to the way they were created, and the way they were meant to be viewed. Baccio was admired by his contemporaries for his skill in inventing and rapidly jotting down funny little stories, dwarferies and caricatures, and we know from his 17th-century biographer Filippo Baldinucci that his lively wit made him popular at dinner parties (Baldinucci actually uses the word *conviti*), where he would entertain guests by sketching, causing them all "to die with laughter."[51] Perhaps the cuckold drawings were made in a similarly social context—at a dinner party or a gathering of friends. They have the feel of informal entertainments, sketched by a single hand, but perhaps collaboratively conceived and laughed over. The idea may, indeed, have been suggested by Modio's *Convito*, a treatise on cuckolds framed as a dinner table conversation among a group of male friends. We have seen the many parallels between the *Convito* and Baccio's cuckoldries. Perhaps the

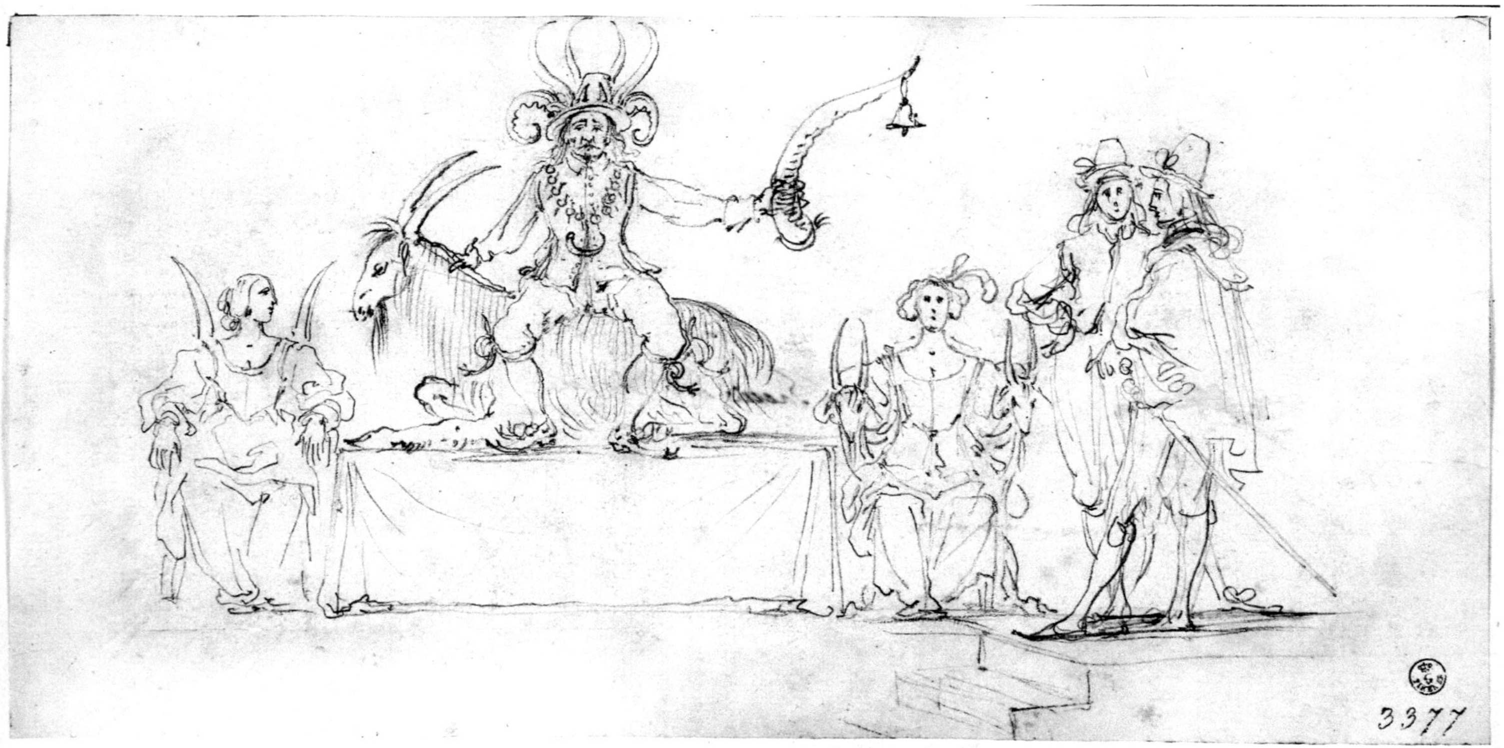

9.11 Baccio del Bianco, *Becco enthroned*, c. 1638, black chalk, 174 × 340 mm, Uffizi (3377 F), Florence (permission: Ministero dei beni e delle attività culturali e del turismo)

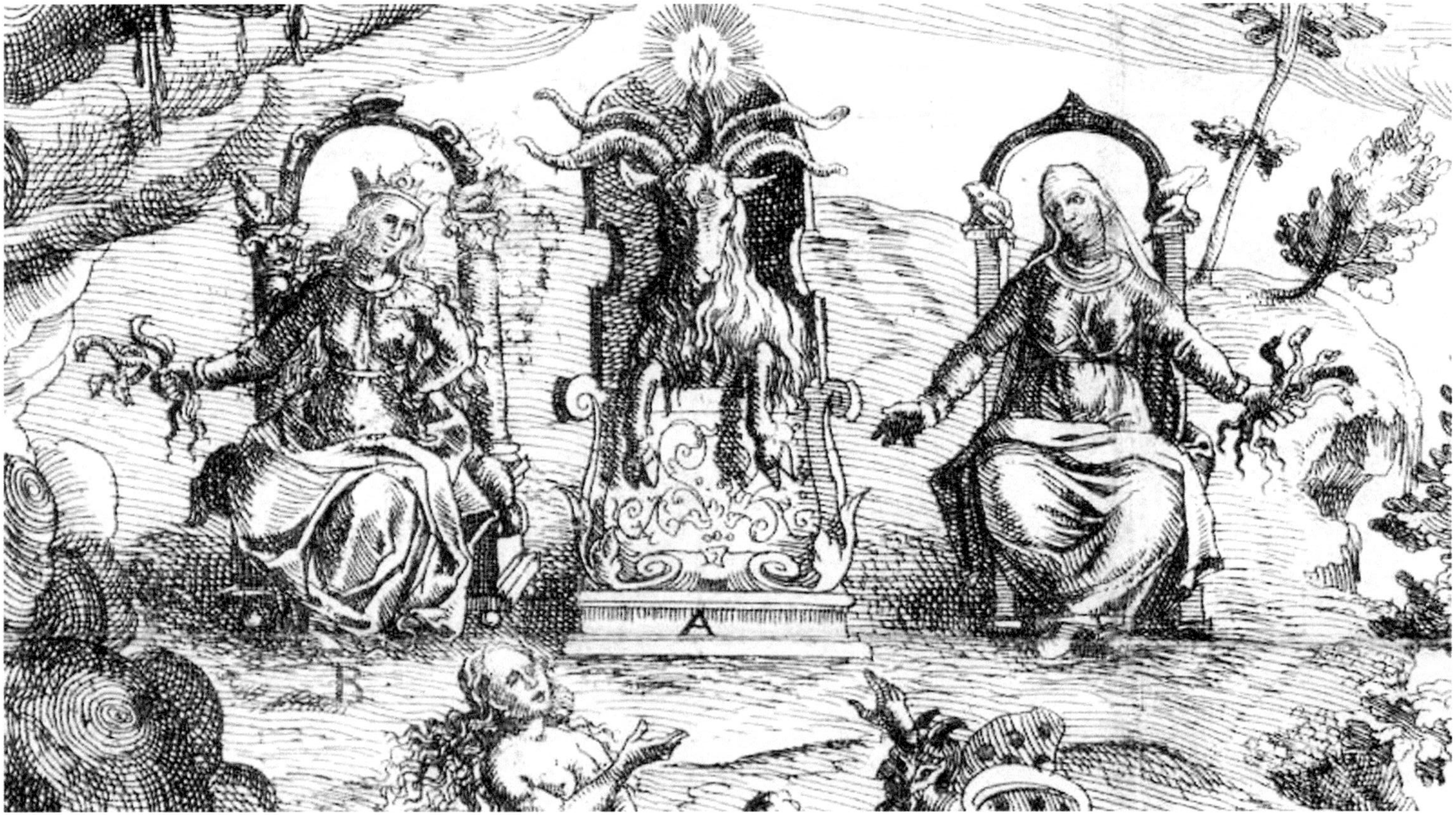

9.12 Anonymous, *Satan and his consorts*, detail from "Description et du Sabbat des Sorciers," in Pierre de Lancre's *Tableau de l'inconstance des mauvais anges et demons*, Paris, 1613, etching, Rare and Manuscript Collections, Cornell University Library, Ithaca, NY

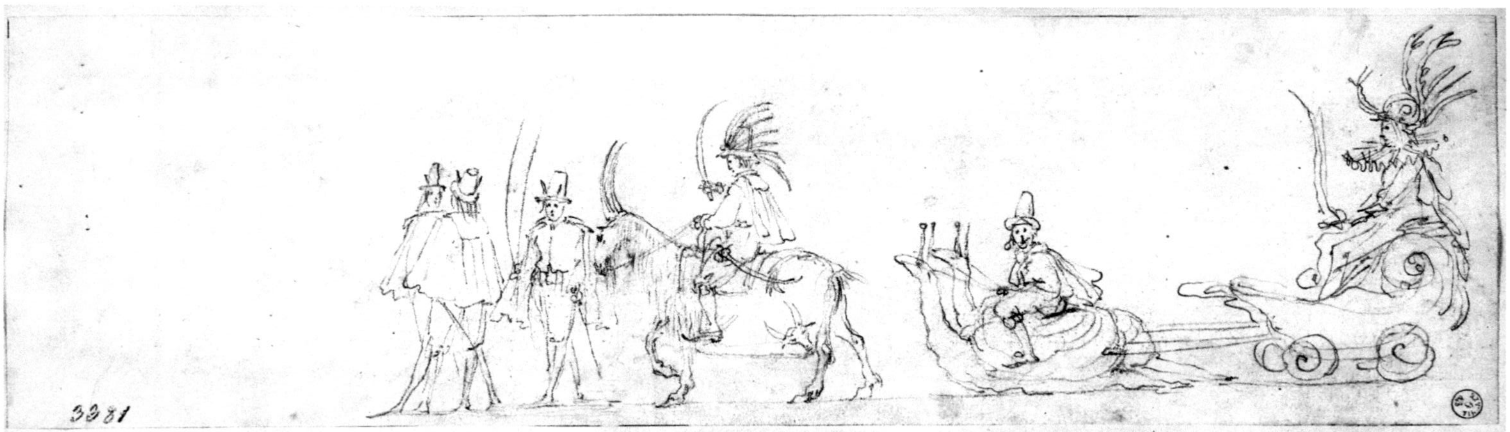

9.13 Baccio del Bianco, *The Triumph of King Cuckold*, c. 1638, black chalk, 120 × 420 mm, Uffizi (3381 F), Florence (permission: Ministero dei beni e delle attività culturali e del turismo)

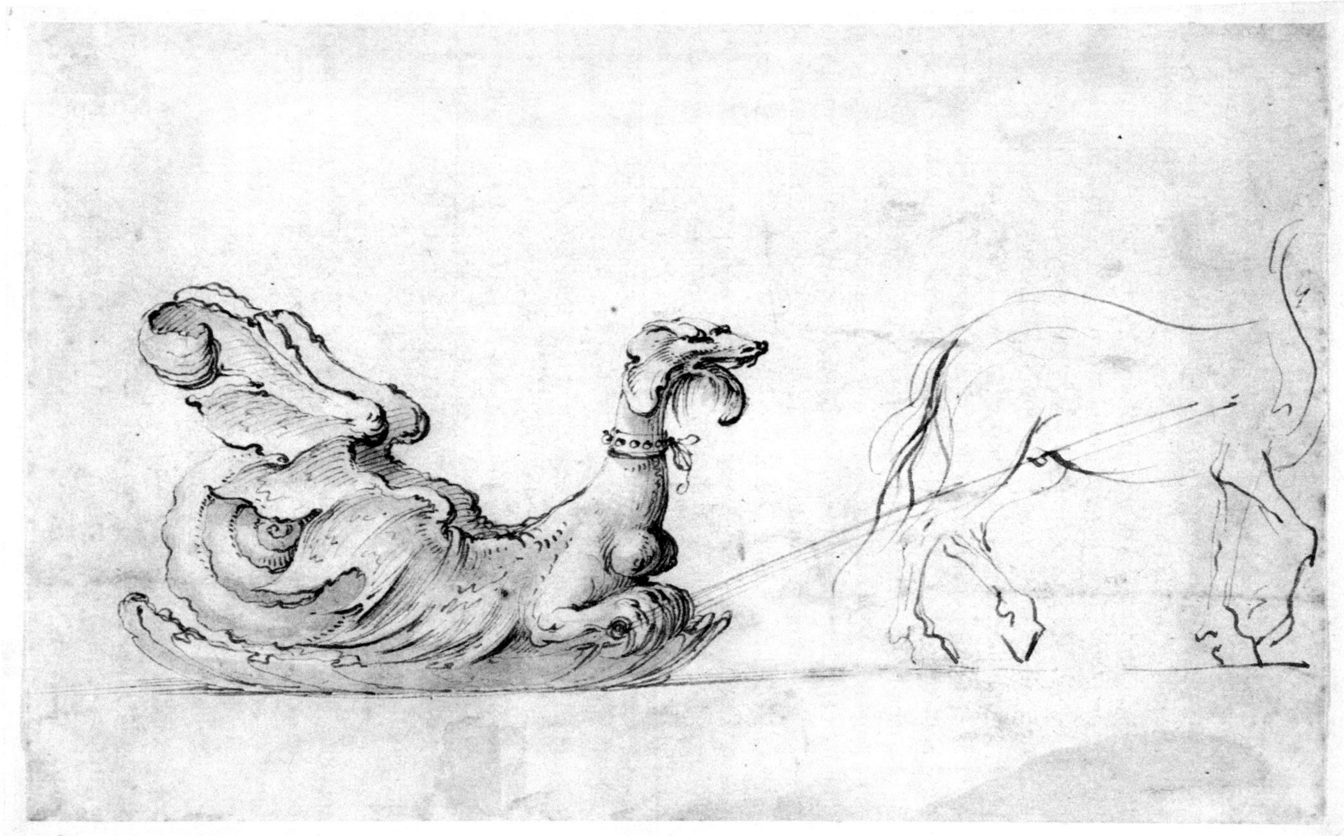

9.14 Stefano della Bella, *Design for a Carnival carro in the form of a hybrid snail*, pen and brown ink with gray-brown wash, 160 × 249 mm, Metropolitan Museum of Art, New York

fictional premise of the earlier work suggested to Baccio a similar form of amusement. Modio sets his dialogue during Carnival; and Baccio's drawings, too, have a distinctly Carnival flavor: comical, bawdy and transgressive—exactly the kind of thing he might have created to share among friends.

Much of the recent literature on cuckolds seeks to understand the obsession with female adultery in terms of specific political, religious or social anxieties. Could a similar case be made for Baccio's drawings? It might be relevant that, throughout much of the 1620s, Florence was ruled by women. When Ferdinando II de' Medici inherited the grand duchy from his father Cosimo in 1621, he was only ten years old. His mother Maria Maddalena of Austria and his grandmother Christina of Lorraine ruled as co-regents until he reached his majority in 1628. Even after that date, the two women continued to exert influence over the young grand duke and to play a prominent role in Florentine politics until their respective deaths in 1631 and 1637. Deeply religious and committed to supporting the policies of the papacy, the regents promoted a conservative agenda that an artist of liberal, not to say libertine, propensities like Baccio must have found unappealing.[52] In their effort to validate and make more palatable the concept of female rule, they sponsored a cultural program that dramatized the heroic virtue and nobility of women and commissioned treatises presenting the equality of the sexes "as both an absolute value and a necessary condition for the well-ordered state."[53] Needless to say, not everyone was convinced by this pro-woman propaganda. Although the Uffizi drawings date from 1638, 10 years after the official end of the regency, it may not be too far-fetched to see in them a satirical commentary on the perniciousness of female government, echoing a kind of political misogyny left over from that period.

Another event at the Medici court that may have influenced Baccio's series was the marriage of the grand duke to his first cousin Vittoria della Rovere, arranged in 1633 by their grandmother Christina of Lorraine and celebrated in 1637, shortly before the drawings were made. This was a dynastic union and by all accounts a deeply unhappy one. At some point during the marriage, the pious Vittoria discovered her husband in bed with one of his pages, a spectacle that so shocked and disgusted her that she ceased to have spousal relations with him for a number of years.[54] The episode almost certainly occurred after the drawings were made and has no direct bearing on them. But those who, like Baccio, frequented the court were probably aware of the grand duke's homosexual predilections even before the marriage and, if so, the drawings may reflect a sardonic response to the absurdly hyped allegorical representations of joyous matrimony that accompanied the wedding celebrations in 1637. Baccio himself played a leading part in concocting a mythology of happy marriage around the grand ducal couple. A skilled scenographer and designer of costumes and stage machines, he collaborated with Alfonso Parigi in preparing the principal entertainment at the festivities, a lavish spectacle entitled *Le Nozze degli Dei* ("The Marriage of the Gods"), held in the courtyard of Palazzo Pitti in June of that year.[55] The mythological *deus ex machina* in Uffizi 3376 is so strikingly similar in design (if not in tone) to the stage machinery in *Le Nozze degli Dei* that it does suggest a certain convergence of the two projects in Baccio's imagination (Fig. 9.7).[56] If in the months following that bombastic production he made drawings for his own private pleasure and the enjoyment of his friends that depict a very different and less idealized view of marriage, it would hardly be surprising. He would not have been the only one to seize on the celebrations as an opportunity for satire. Massimiliano Rossi has noted parallels between Baccio's cuckoldries and certain passages in the mock-heroic *poemetta Lo Sconcio sposalizio* ("The Indecent Nuptials") by his close friend, the painter Francesco Furini.[57] Just as Raphael's *Marriage of Cupid and Psyche* sets the stage for Modio's dialogue on horns, the *Nozze degli Dei* provides a backdrop against which both Baccio's drawings and Furini's verses can be viewed.

In the end, though, Baccio's cuckoldries probably have less to do with Medici politics than with society in general, and in particular that branch of society with which the artist was most familiar, the *cavalieri suoi amici* and their ladies, the well-to-do gentry of Florence. In other words, they satirize the very audience they were meant to amuse. It is worth remembering that Florentine men of the patrician class married extraordinarily late in life. In fact, throughout the seventeenth century, the typical Florentine bridegroom had fully 15 years seniority over his bride.[58] Where the age disparity between husbands and wives was so extreme, it is hardly surprising that certain anxieties—however couched in comedy—surrounded the married state. The theme was explored by another of Baccio's friends, the poet and playwright Giancinto Andrea Cicognini,[59] whose literary production included a farce entitled *Il Cornuto nella propria opinione*, as well as satirical verses on the immoral behavior of Florentine noblewomen, which in their burlesque tone are strikingly similar to Baccio's drawings.[60] It was with friends like Furini and Cicognini, then, and in the circles they frequented, that Baccio's cuckoldries found their intended audience.[61]

Whatever the circumstances of their creation—whether they were sketched in the artist's studio or in some more social setting, whether they were made during Carnival or at some leaner time of year—the drawings are the record of a virtuoso performance, one in which Baccio took the starring role, contriving clever conceits and eliciting the laughter and admiration of his viewers with his lively invention, flickering speed and sureness of touch. Ultimately they are best understood as *capricci*. The term refers to an exercise in free and spontaneous invention and/or improvisational form.[62] It implies a degree of license, an easing of the rules. But the word has many shades of meaning, and if in an intellectual and artistic context it suggests originality, genre-bending and experimentation, in a bawdy or libertine context it connotes freedoms of a very different kind. Thus Modio describes a wife's extramarital adventure as a *capriccio*;[63] and Aretino inserts the word into the title of his pornographic dialogue on the adulterous conduct of wives (*La seconda giornata del capriccio aretino nella quale la Nanna narra alla Antonia la vita delle maritate*).[64] The Uffizi cuckoldries perfectly embody both meanings of the word. *Capriccio* has a goatish ring to it and was popularly believed to derive from *capro*, the nimble goat whose lightness of foot and sprightly bounding seemed to symbolize creative experimentation.[65] In Baccio's *becco* we find an earthier manifestation of that same capricious goat: for he is the comic catalyst that liberates the artist's imagination, unleashes his improvisational genius, and gives free rein to his licentious and carnivalesque sense of fun.

Works Cited

Manuscripts and Early Printed Sources (pre-1900)

Capaccio, Giulio Cesare. *Gli Apologi di Giulio Cesare Capaccio, secretario della fedelissima città di Napoli, con la giunta delle Dicerie Morali*, Naples: Gio. Iacomo Carlino, 1602.

Cicognini, Giacinto Andrea. *Le Scappinate sopra le dame di Fiorenza*. Florence: Biblioteca Riccardiana, MS. Cod. 3146, ff. 199–217; MS. Cod. 3160, ff. 1–20.

Coppola, Giovanni Carlo. *Le Nozze degli dei, favola dell Abbate Gio. Carlo Coppola rappresentata in musica in Firenze nelle reali nozze de Serenissimi Gran Duchi di Toschana Ferdinando II e Vittoria Principessa d'Urbino.* Florence: Amadore Massi e Lorenzo Landi, 1637.

Doni, Anton Francesco. *La Zucca del Doni fiorentino*. Venice: Girolamo Polo, 1551, 1589.

Rogers, George. *The Horn Exalted, or Roome for Cuckolds, Being a Treatise concerning the Reason and Origin of the Word Cuckold, and why Such are said to wear Horns.* London: J. Cadwel, 1660.

Select Proverbs, Italian, Spanish, French, English, Scotish, British, etc., Chiefly Moral. London: Philip Monckton, 1707.

Tassoni, Alessandro. *De' pensieri diversi di Alessandro Tassoni libri dieci*. Venice: Barezzi, 1646.

Vespasiano da Bisticci, *Vite di uomini illustri del secolo XV*, ed. Adolfo Bartoli. Florence: Barbera, Bianchi e comp., 1859.

Secondary Sources and Modern Editions

Angiolillo, M. *Sv* "Bianco, Baccio del," *Allgemeines Künstlerlexikon*. Munich: Saur, 1995, X. 439–40.

Aretino, Pietro. *Ragionamento de la Nanna et de la Antonia fatto in Roma sotto una ficaia*, Venice, 1534, in *Sei giornate*, ed. Angelo Romano. Milan: Mursia, 1991.

Aretino, Pietro. *The Secret Life of Wives*, ed. Paul Bailey, trans. Andrew Brown. London: Hesperus Press, 2006.

Bacci, Mina. "Lettere inedite di Baccio del Bianco," *Paragone* XIV (1963): 68–77.

Bakhtin, Mikhail. *Rabelais and his World*, trans. Hélène Iswolsky. Bloomington: Indiana University Press, 1968, 1984.

Baldinucci, Filippo. *Notizie de' professori del disegno da Cimabue in qua, 6 voll., Santi Franchi, Firenze 1681–1728*, ed. Ferdinando Ranalli, 5 vols. Florence: V. Batelli e Compagni, 1845–1847.

Bernardi, Walter. *Il paggio e l'anatomista. Scienza, sangue e sesso alla corte del Granduca di Toscana*. Florence: Le Lettere, 2008.

Boggione, Valter and Giovanni Casalegno. *Dizionario storico del lessico erotico italiano. Metafore, eufemismi, oscentità, doppi sensi, parole dotte e parole basse in otto secoli di letteratura italiana*. Milan: Longanesi & C., 1996.

Bolzoni, Lina. "Il mondo utopico e il mondo dei cornuti: plagio e paradosso nelle traduzioni di Gabriel Chappuys," *I Tatti Studies* VIII (1999): 171–96.

Broedel, Hans Peter. *The* Malleus Maleficarum *and the Construction of Witchcraft. Theology and Popular Belief*. Manchester: Manchester University Press, 2003.

Bruster, Douglas. "The Horn of Plenty: Cuckoldry and Capital in the Drama of the Age of Shakespeare," *Studies in English Literature, 1500–1900*, XXX (1990), 195–215.

Burke, Peter. *Popular Culture in Early Modern Europe*. London: Ashgate, 1978, 3rd ed., 2009.

Cancedda, Flavia and Silvia Castelli. *Per una bibliografia di Giacinto Andrea Cicognini. Successo teatrale e fortuna editoriale di un drammaturgo del Seicento*. Florence: Alinea, 2001.

Cheng, Sandra. "Parodies of Life: Baccio del Bianco's Comic Drawings of Dwarfs," in *Parody and Festivity in Early Modern Art. Essays on Comedy as Social Vision*, ed. David Smith. Farnham, UK/Burlington, VT: Ashgate, 2012, 127–41.

Cusick, Suzanne. *Francesca Caccini at the Medici Court. Music and the Circulation of Power*. Chicago: University of Chicago Press, 2009.

Daumas, Maurice. *Au bonheur des mâles. Adultère et cocuage à la Renaissance 1400–1650*. Paris: Armand Colin, 2007.

Ekserdjian, David. *Parmigianino*. New Haven/London: Yale University Press, 2006.

Fumagalli, Elena and Massimiliano Rossi, eds. *Florence au grand siècle entre peinture et littérature*, exhib. cat. Ajaccio: Palais Fesch-Musée des Beaux-Arts, 2011.

Gilbert, Allan. "The Prosperous Wittol in Giovanni Battista Modio and Thomas Middleton," *Studies in Philology* XLI (1944): 235–7.

Gregori, Mina. "Baccio del Bianco tra Firenze e Madrid," *Paragone* LX (2009): 15–90.

Gualtieri, Luigi (attributed to). "Storia della nobile e reale famiglia de' Medici," in Luca Ombrosi, *Vita dei Medici sodomiti*. Rome: Canesi, 1965.

Harness, Kelley. *Echoes of Women's Voices. Music, Art and Female Patronage in Early Modern Florence*. Chicago: University of Chicago Press, 2006.

Hartmann, Lucrezia. *Capriccio: Bild und Begriff*. Nürnberg: Druckschnelldienst Nürnberg, 1973.

Heikamp, Detlef. "Il Nano Morgante: tentative di un ritratto," in *Giambologna. Gli dei, gli eroi*, ed. Beatrice Paolozzi Strozzi, exhib. cat. Florence: Giunti, 2006. 286–301.

Henke, James. *Courtesans and Cuckolds. A Glossary of Renaissance Dramatic Bawdy (Exclusive of Shakespeare)*. New York/London: Garland, 1979.

Hind, Arthur. *Early Italian Engravings. A Critical Catalogue with Complete Reproduction of All the Prints Described, Part I. Florentine Engraving and Anonymous Prints of the Other Schools*, 2 vols. New York: B. Quaritch, 1938.

Hoppe, Ilaria. "Maria Magdalena von Österreich (1589–1631) die vergessene Regentin," in *Die Frauen des Hauses Medici*, ed. Christina Strunk. Petersberg: Imhof, 2011, 107–15.

Hults, Linda. *The witch as muse: art, gender, and power in early modern Europe*. Philadelphia: University of Pennsylvania Press, 2005.

Kahn-Rossi, Manuela. *Ritratti in barocco. La festa nella caricatura toscana del Seicento*. Locarno: R. Rezzonico, 1985.

Kanz, Roland. *Die Kunst des Capriccio. Kreativer Eigensinn in Renaissance und Barock*. Munich: Deutscher Kunstverlag, 2002.

Lancre, Pierre de. *On the Inconstancy of Witches. Pierre de Lancre's Tableau de l'inconstance des mauvais anges et demons, (1612)*, ed. Gerhild Scholz Williams. Tempe: Arizona Center for Medieval and Renaissance Studies, 2006.

Lea, K. M. *Italian Popular Comedy. A Study in the Commedia dell'arte, 1560–1620, with Special Reference to the English Stage*, 2 vols. New York: Russell & Russell, 1962.

Litchfield, R. Burr. "Demographic Characteristics of Florentine Patrician Families, Sixteenth to Nineteenth Centuries," *Journal of Economic History* XXIX (1969): 191–205.

Lorenzi, Lorenzo. *Witches: Exploring the Iconography of the Sorceress and Enchantress*, trans. Ursula Creagh. Florence: Centro Di, 2005.

Massar, Phyllis Dearborn. "Scenes for a Calderon Play by Baccio del Bianco," *Master Drawings* XV (1977): 365–75.

Modio, Giovanni Battista. *Il Convito, overo del peso della moglie, dove ragionando si conchiude, che non può la donna dishonesta far vergogna a l'huomo*, Rome, 1554, in *Trattati del Cinquecento sulla donna*, ed. Giuseppe Zonta. Bari: G. Laterza & figli, 1913, 309–70.

Muir, Edward. *Ritual in Early Modern Europe*. Cambridge: Cambridge University Press, 1997, 2nd ed., 2005.

O'Bryan, Robin. "Groteque Bodies, Princely Delight: Dwarfs in Italian Renaissance Court Imagery," *Preternature: Critical and Historical Studies on the Preternatural* I (2012): 263–80.

Panek, Jennifer. "'A Wittall Cannot be a Cookold': Reading the Contented Cuckold in Modern English Drama and Culture," *Journal for Early Modern Cultural Studies* I (2001): 66–92.

Rathe, Alice. "Le Capriccio dans les lettres italiennes," *Les Lettres Romanes* XXXIV (1980) : 207–45 and 321–51.

Rice, Louise. "Cardinal Rapaccioli and the Turnip-sellers of Rome: A Satire on the War of Castro by Baccio del Bianco," *Master Drawings* XLVII (2009): 53–69.

Rossi, Massimiliano. "Furini poeta," in *Un'altra bellezza. Francesco Furini*, ed. Mina Gregori and Rodolfo Maffeis, exhib. cat. Florence: Mandragora, 2007, 107–19.

Stephens, Walter. *Demon Lovers: Witchcraft, Sex, and the Crisis of Belief*. Chicago: University of Chicago Press, 2002.

Strunk, Christina. "Christiane von Lothringen Großherzogin der Toskana (1565–1636) ein 'weiblicher Herkules,'" in *Die Frauen des Hauses Medici*, ed. Christina Strunk. Petersberg: Imhof, 2011, 75–93.

Strunk, Christina, ed. *Medici Women as Cultural Mediators (1533–1743)*. Milan: Silvana, 2011.

Tal, Guy. *Witches on Top: Magic, Power, and Imagination in the Art of Early Modern Italy*, PhD dissertation, Indiana University, 2006.

Ternois, Daniel. *Jacques Callot. Catalogue complet de son oeuvre dessiné*. Paris: F. de Nobele, 1962.

Thiem, Christel. *Florentiner Zeichner des Frühbarock*. Munich: Bruckmann, 1977.

Turner, James Grantham. *Schooling Sex. Libertine Literature and Erotic Education in Italy, France, and England, 1534–1685*. Oxford: Oxford University Press, 2003.

Turrini, Giovanna, ed., et al. *Capire l'antifona: dizionario dei modi di dire con esempi d'autore*. Bologna: Zanichelli, 1995.

Vespasiano, da Bisticci. *The Vespasiano Memoirs. Lives of Illustrious Men of the XVth Century*, trans. William George and Emily Waters. London: G. Routledge & Sons, 1926.

Waldman, Louis. "A Satiric Image on a Maiolica Pharmacy Jar," *Burlington Magazine* CXXXIV (1992): 375–8.

White, Veronica. "Serio Ludere: Baroque Invenzione and the Development of the Capriccio," PhD dissertation, Columbia University, 2009.

Zika, Charles. *Exorcising our Demons: Magic, Witchcraft, and Visual Culture in Early Modern Europe*. Leiden: Brill, 2003.

Notes

1 On Baccio del Bianco, see Filippo Baldinucci, *Notizie dei professori del disegno da Cimabue in qua*, ed. Ferdinando Ranalli, Florence, 1847 (1974), V, 16–51; Angiolillo, M. *sv* "Bianco, Baccio del,"*Allgemeines Künstlerlexikon*, X (Munich, 1995), 439–40; Mina Gregori, "Baccio del Bianco tra Firenze e Madrid," *Paragone*, LX, 2009, 15–90. The more recent literature on Baccio as a satirist is summarized in Louise Rice, "Cardinal Rapaccioli and the Turnip-sellers of Rome: A Satire on the War of Castro by Baccio del Bianco," *Master Drawings*, XLVII (2009), 53–69; and Sandra Cheng, "Parodies of Life: Baccio del Bianco's Comic Drawings of Dwarfs," in *Parody and Festivity in Early Modern Art. Essays on Comedy as Social Vision*, ed. David Smith, Farnham, UK/Burlington, VT, 2012, 127–41. On Baccio's cuckoldries in particular, see Christel Thiem, *Florentiner Zeichner des Frühbarock* (Munich, 1977), 383–4; Manuela Kahn-Rossi, *Ritratti in barocco. La festa nella caricatura toscana del Seicento*, Locarno, 1985, 63; *Florence au grand siècle entre peinture et littérature*, eds. Elena Fumagalli and Massimiliano Rossi, exhib. cat., Ajaccio, 2011, 252–7.

2 On the paradoxical symbolism of horns, see James Henke, *Courtesans and Cuckolds. A Glossary of Renaissance Dramatic Bawdy (Exclusive of Shakespeare)* (New York & London, 1979), 129–30, with numerous relevant citations, including this one from George Chapman, Ben Jonson & John Marston, *Eastward Ho*, 1605 (IV. 1): "Farewell, thou horn of pleasure, the ensign of the huntsman! Farewell, thou horn of destiny, th'ensign of the married man!" See also Valter Boggione and Giovanni Casalegno, *Dizionario storico del lessico erotico italiano. Metafore, eufemismi, oscentità, doppi sensi, parole dotte e parole basse in otto secoli di letteratura italiana* (Milan, 1996), 285.

3 Maurice Daumas, *Au bonheur des mâles. Adultère et cocuage à la Renaissance 1400–1650* (Paris, 2007).

4 Bartsch, XIII, 112, no. 9; Arthur Hind, *Early Italian Engravings. A Critical Catalogue with Complete Reproduction of All the Prints Described, Part I. Florentine Engraving and Anonymous Prints of the Other Schools* (New York, 1938), I, 73–4; II, plate 108. Hind helpfully transcribes and translates all of the textual tags, but the precise meaning of the print remains obscure.

5 The full title of Modio's dialogue is *Il Convito, overo del peso della moglie, dove ragionando si conchiude, che non può la donna dishonesta far vergogna a l'huomo* (Rome, 1554). The edition used here appears in *Trattati del Cinquecento sulla donna*, ed. Giuseppe Zonta (Bari, 1913), 309–70. Many other 16th and 17th-century texts treat the theme of the cuckold, including Anton Francesco Doni, *La Zucca del Doni fiorentino* (Venice, 1589), 41–7; Giulio Cesare Capaccio, *Gli Apologi di Giulio Cesare Capaccio … con la giunta delle Dicerie Morali* (Naples, 1602), 168–9; Alessandro Tassoni, *De' pensieri diversi di Alessandro*

Tassoni libri dieci (Venice, 1646), 364–8; and in England, George Rogers, *The Horn Exalted, or Roome for Cuckolds, Being a Treatise concerning the Reason and Origin of the Word Cuckold, and why Such are said to wear Horns*, London, 1660, which includes a partial paraphrase of Modio (8–17). On the adulterous conduct of wives, the classic text is Pietro Aretino's *Ragionamento de la Nanna et de la Antonia fatto in Roma sotto una ficaia* (Venice, 1534), in *Sei giornate*, ed. Angelo Romano, Milan, 1991; translated into English as *The Secret Life of Wives*, ed. Paul Bailey, trans. Andrew Brown (London, 2006).

6 Modio, op. cit., 344: "… si come dell'altre età è stato detto che altra fu d'oro, altra d'argento, et altra di ferro, così la nostra, per la cattiva opinione che ha di se stessa, si può per similitudine chiamar di corno …" The conceit is picked up by later imitators; see, for example, George Chapman, *All Fools*, 1605 (V. 2): "… so the World into the Golden age, the Siluer, the Brasse, the Iron, the Leaden, the Wooden; / and now into this present age, which wee tearme the Horned age."

7 For an excellent summary and analysis of Modio's text, see Lina Bolzoni, "Il mondo utopico e il mondo dei cornuti: plagio e paradosso nelle traduzioni di Gabriel Chappuys," *I Tatti Studies*, VIII, (1999), esp. 182–8.

8 Modio, op. cit. at note 5, p. 318: "… se farete a mio modo, ragionaremo oggi delle corna, e donde è venuta questa generale opinione, che quando un marito ha la moglie lasciva, par al mondo ch'egli abbi le corna in testa."

9 Peter Burke, *Popular Culture in Early Modern Europe*, 3rd ed. (London, 2009), 255–86; Edward Muir, *Ritual in Early Modern Europe*, 2nd ed. (Cambridge, 2005), 93–124.

10 *Rabelais and his World*, trans. Hélène Iswolsky (Bloomington, IN, 1968, 1984), 241–3.

11 See, for example, the anonymous *commedia dell'arte* scenario, *Li Tre Becchi* (transcribed and translated in K. M. Lea, *Italian Popular Comedy. A Study in the Commedia dell'arte, 1560–1620, with Special Reference to the English Stage*, 2 vols. (New York, 1962), II, 580–84). On Carnival as the feast of cuckolds, see Daumas, op. cit. at note 3, esp. 136–46. See also Johannes Lingelbach's *Carnival in Rome* (c. 1650–1655; Kunsthistorisches Museum, Vienna), in which, at the very center of the composition, a masker in costume is handed the horns by a figure on horseback.

12 *Florence au grand siècle*, op. cit. at note 1, 252–7.

13 Rogers, op. cit. at note 5 above, preface.

14 *Love's Labour's Lost*, IV. 3.

15 *As You Like It*, IV. 1. See also Henke, op. cit. at note 2, 245.

16 Uffizi 5803 S; see Daniel Ternois, *Jacques Callot. Catalogue complet de son oeuvre dessiné* (Paris, 1962), 53–4. I am grateful to Sara Matthews-Grieco for bringing this extraordinary drawing to my attention and providing the photograph illustrated here.

17 *Capire l'antifona: dizionario dei modi di dire con esempi d'autore*, ed. Giovanna Turrini et al. (Bologna, 1995), 53.

18 For example, Nicholas Breton, *I Pray You Be Not Angry*, 1605 (II. 8): a promiscuous wife will "set more hornes then haires on my head."

19 Modio, op. cit. at note 5, 346–7: "Percioche chiunque per ingordigia o per ebbrezza da il largo a la moglie di far i suoi piaceri, può esser chiamato 'becco'; chi per altrui potenza o forza, senza ch'egli o della moglie o dell'adultero possa vendicarsi, si può chiamar 'montone'; e chi, per abbandonar la moglie et andar vagabondo, non compie al natural uso del matrimonio, ma da materia di cercar di fuori quel che non trova in casa, si potrà dir 'toro'; si come chi per viltà d'animo e per soverchia gelosia, porgendo gli occhi pertutto, accende nella mente della sua donna quei desideri, che forse da se stessa avuti non averebbe, a guisa d'Atteone, si potrà chiamar 'cervo.' Ma chi, compiacendo della sua moglie a gran maestri e valentuomini, da principio a la casa sua di riputazione e grandezza, non senza ragione potrà chiamarsi 'elefanto.' A questi ultimi dunque, perche sono in minor numero degli altri, pare che per un certo rispetto che ha loro il mondo, come favoriti de' signori e de' principi, non si da il nome di 'cornuto': e forse anco per non essersi ancora esso risoluto se questo animale ha corna o denti. Dove degli altri tutto il giorno si sente dire, 'egli è un becco,' 'egli è un bue,' 'egli è un cervo,' 'egli è un montone.' Per che si può conchiudere che, da diverse similitudini e nature d'animali di corno, sieno anche diverse spezie di cornuti." On the equivocal sense of the elephant's tusk, see note 35 below.

20 *Much ado about nothing*, I. 1.

21 See, for example, Shakespeare's *Midsummer Night's Dream*, V.1. Baccio used the crescent moon in a similarly equivocal sense in a satirical drawing he produced a few years later, in which he took cruel aim at the bungling Cardinal Rapaccioli, commissioner general and special legate to the army of Pope Urban VIII during the first war of Castro. The crescent moon incised like a maker's mark on the blade of the cardinal's oversized, misshapen sword is one more emasculating gibe in a scene already permeated with sexual innuendo. The drawing, in the Morgan Library, is illustrated and discussed in Rice, op. cit. at note 1, 53–69.

22 The cornett (*cornetto*, or little horn, in Italian) is a curved wooden wind instrument that resembles a hollowed-out animal horn, and both its name and its shape make it an obvious symbol of the cuckold. I know of no examples, outside Baccio's drawing, where the instrument is specifically so identified, but they are bound to exist. In Renaissance literature, hunting horns, post horns, bugles of one sort or another regularly allude to the cuckold's fate; and Mozart taps into this same tradition when he uses French horns (in Italian, *corni*) to accompany Figaro, who, believing that he has been cuckolded by his bride Susanna, chastises all women for their universal infidelity (in the closing measures of "Aprite un po' quegl'occhi," *Le Nozze di Figaro*, act IV). I am indebted to my brother John Rice for suggesting this last comparison.

23 From Boccaccio to Ophuls, the round dance or circle dance (in Italian, *ballo tondo* or *ridda*; in French, *la ronde*) has suggested itself as a metaphor for erotic exchange. It appears, for example, in one of Callot's *capricci* (c. 1617), where youthful Columbina dances a round dance with eight elderly cuckolds. See also Boggione and Casalegno, op. cit. at note 2, 162–3; and note 50 below.

24 In the language of innuendo, any sort of dance or dancing can refer to the sexual act, as in (to cite another passage in Mozart's *Nozze di Figaro*) Figaro's angry response to the count's efforts to claim his *droit de seigneur*: "Se vuol ballare, signor contino, il chitarrino le suonerò." For numerous earlier examples, see Boggione and Casalegno, op. cit. at note 2, 161–5.

25 Modio, op. cit. at note 5, 320–21; Allan Gilbert, "The Prosperous Wittol in Giovanni Battista Modio and Thomas Middleton," *Studies in Philology* XLI (1944): 235–7; Douglas Bruster, "The Horn of Plenty: Cuckoldry and Capital in the Drama of the Age of Shakespeare," *Studies in English Literature, 1500–1900* XXX (1990): 195–215; Jennifer Panek, "'A Wittall Cannot be a Cookold:' Reading the Contented Cuckold in Modern English Drama and Culture," *Journal for Early Modern Cultural Studies* I (2001): 66–92. On the theme of the contented cuckold, see also the essays in this volume by Musacchio, Giannetti, Katritzky, and Matthews-Grieco.

26 See the essays in this volume by Musacchio and Bourne.

27 The relevant captions read: PERCHARITA AVTI GLIVO SEGARE (For pity's sake, help him saw); SEGA PIAN CONPAGNIO MIO CHILA CANPA E FIGLIVOLO DI DIO (Saw gently, my comrade, whoso escapes it is a child of God); ITASOLVO PERCHE TVAI ROTTO LECHORNA (I absolve you, as you have broken your horns) and, above the woman, A QV[E]STO BALLO VEGNIERA MARITO MIO PER SEGARTI LE CHORNA (I would come to this dance, my husband, to saw off your horns). Hind, op. cit. at note 4, p. 73.

28 Louis Waldman, "A Satiric Image on a Maiolica Pharmacy Jar," *Burlington Magazine*, CXXXIV (1992), 375–8.

29 See, for example, *Select Proverbs, Italian, Spanish, French, English, Scotish, British, etc., Chiefly Moral*, London, 1707, 05: "He who hath horns in his Bosom, needs not put them on his Head." Or, from Rogers's *Horn Exalted* (op. cit. at note 5, prefatory poem): "Surely those hornes are far the best, / That quiet lye within the brest." Foolish husbands make a fuss, "When wiser Cuckolds chew the cud, / And hide their hornes within their hood, / Or at least pare them when they bud." On the virtues of discretion, see also the essay in this volume by Matthews-Grieco.

30 Vespasiano da Bisticci, *Vite di uomini illustri del secolo XV*, ed. Adolfo Bartoli, Florence, 1859, 262: "Costui subito intese Cosimo, e parvegli avere errato a publicare questo caso; e per questo seguitò il consiglio di Cosimo, di non ne parlare più; e tolsesi questa sua donna per buona, come si doveva istimare ch'ella fusse." The translation is taken from *The Vespasiano Memoirs. Lives of Illustrious Men of the XVth Century*, trans. William George and Emily Waters (London, 1926), 226; cited by Hind, op. cit. at note 4, p. 73.

31 Modio, op. cit. at note 5, p. 323: "Dalla qual similitudine queste meschine genti, che ingiustamente e per forza patiscono cotale ingiuria delle mogli, e, non potendosene prevalere fanno vista di non s'accorgere, si sono poi assomigliati ai montoni; e, a comparazione di quegli, ad altri si dice cornuto scornato, overo 'ti segherò le corna.'" Later in the same dialogue, the derivation of the word *scornato* is again referred to (341–2): "Eran dunque le corna segno di potenza e d'onore, la qual cosa si può giudicare, essendo anco insin ad ora tra noi un cotal modo di dire pervenuto; che, quando uno ha patito qualche ingiuria o in parole o in fatti, ne se n'ha potuto prevalere, gli si dice: 'Egli è rimasto scornato,' cioè senza difensione e senza honore."

32 The scene exactly parallels a passage in Modio (op. cit. at note 5, p. 326), where one of the participants draws a connection between Becco (cuckold) and Bacco (god of wine), observing that: "… quando la moglie d'un di costoro vuol per avventura trarsi un capriccio e star la notte presso ad altro huomo che al marito, l'empie tanto di vino per addormentarlo, che il fa parer Bacco istesso."

33 The browbeaten cuckold, not only betrayed but physically abused by his wife, is a stock figure in the comedy of the time. See, for example, English Broadside Ballad Archive, Pepys 4.134 (http://ebba.english.ucsb.edu/ballad/21798/image).

34 Rogers, op. cit. at note 5, p. 23: "No doubt man is the sport of the stars … Luna horn'd, Aries horn'd, Taurus horn'd, besides Capricorn and other beasts, which Astrology puts in heaven, have their operations upon us; and 'tis said that marriages are made their also."

35 For the elephant's tusk as phallic symbol, see Aretino, op. cit. at note 5, p. 92: "Rimandati gli altri a casa, si ritenne il successore del cavaliere: che, col suo dente di liofante, la racconsolò di maniera che, posta da canto la vergogna, deliberò di torlo per marito." The fact that, in Italian, the tusk is often referred to as the elephant's tooth (*dente*) leaves the door to equivocation wide open, since in Italian bawdy *dente* is a common synonym for penis. See Boggione and Casalegno, 308, as well as the passage in Modio quoted in note 19 above.

36 See James Grantham Turner, *Schooling Sex. Libertine Literature and Erotic Education in Italy, France, and England, 1534–1685* (Oxford, 2003), especially the Introduction and Part I: "Erotic Education and the (Hard) Core Curriculum."

37 Detlef Heikamp, "Il Nano Morgante: tentative di un ritratto," in *Giambologna. Gli dei, gli eroi*, ed. Beatrice Paolozzi Strozzi, exhib. cat. (Florence, 2006), 286–301; Robin O'Bryan, "Groteque Bodies, Princely Delight: Dwarfs in Italian Renaissance Court Imagery," *Preternature: Critical and Historical Studies on the Preternatural* I (2012): 263–80.

38 O'Bryan, op. cit., 269–72 and figs. 14–15. A small bronze version is in the Louvre Museum; http://www.louvre.fr/en/oeuvre-notices/dwarf-snail. In all these representations, the dwarf is naked and the humor is clearly sexually inflected. His mounts—tortoises, slugs, and snails—are funny not only because they are slow rather than fast, and large when they should be small, but because their ability to extend and retract their heads gives them phallic connotations; cf. Boggione and Casalegno, op. cit. at note 2, p. 282; Henke, op. cit. at note 2, p. 245. Baccio delighted in similar imagery. He made numerous comic drawings of dwarfs (*caramogi*), and among them is at least one in which two dwarfs—one mounted on a snail, the other on a tortoise—face off against each other in single combat; illustrated in Cheng, op. cit. at note 1, p. 133, Fig. 10.3.

39 Stephen Milner, "*Fanno bandire, notificare et expressamente comandare: the Information Economy of Renaissance Florence*," lecture delivered in the Department of Italian Studies, New York University, March 26, 2012.

40 Modio, op. cit. at note 5, p. 336: "… non per altro uno, a cui la moglie faccia, si come si dice, 'le fusa torte,' è detto 'cornuto,' se non perche della sua infamia, come dell'altre cose publiche, si suonano i corni per le piazza. … Essendo dunque le corna non cosa essenziale in se, ma piu tosto una publica opinione, che il volgo communemente ha dell'infamia d'un marito, ed essendo questa infamia in quel tempo tanto enorme, che, si come suole essere dell'altre cose grandi, si spargeva prestamente pertutto, ne venne poi il nome delle corna, togliendo la similitudine dai bandi e dall'altre cose pubbliche, le quali si fanno sapere a tutti a suono di tromba o di corno; poiche insin a quel tempo usavan farsi le trombe di questa materia." For the expression "far le fusa torte," the *Vocabolario della Crusca* offers the somewhat prudish definition, "è il romper di fede, che si fanno marito, e moglie, e anche si dice degli amanti." In fact, it means "to give the horns," as is unambiguously illustrated by Fig. 9.9, in which an elderly *cornuto* wears a pair of spindles tied to his temples with a headband.

41 See note 32 above.

42 Modio, op. cit. at note 5, 326–7: "Percioche, dove noi ora beviamo in vetro o in altra materia, essi solean già bere nelle corna degli animali … Poscia dunque che l'ebbreza ha ridotto costui ad aver la moglie impudica, s'è detto aver le corna in fronte , o per mostrar al mondo la cagione della sua vergogna, o perche il vino, ch'egli bebbe nel corno, gli ha la fronte percossa, poiche la proprietà del vino è di tentar la testa."

43 See, for instance, Pierre de Lancre, *On the Inconstancy of Witches. Pierre de Lancre's Tableau de l'inconstance des mauvais anges et demons, (1612)*, ed. Gerhild Scholz Williams, Tempe, Arizona, 2006, 96: "… the Devil emerges in the form of a billy-goat. … Others say that he seems to be a big billy-goat, with two horns in front and two in back."

44 See Linda Hults, *The witch as muse: art, gender, and power in early modern Europe* (Philadelphia, 2005), passim; Lorenzo Lorenzi, *Witches: Exploring the Iconography of the Sorceress and Enchantress*, trans. Ursula Creagh (Florence, 2005), passim.

45 Pierre de Lancre, op. cit. at note 43, 234–5.

46 Hans Peter Broedel, *The* Malleus Maleficarum *and the Construction of Witchcraft. Theology and Popular Belief* (Manchester/New York, 2003), 167–88. See also Walter Stephens, *Demon Lovers: Witchcraft, Sex, and the Crisis of Belief* (Chicago, 2002). On the association of witchcraft with impotence—often considered a primary cause of cuckoldry—see the essay by Matteo Duni in this volume.

47 David Ekserdjian, *Parmigianino*, New Haven and London, 2006, 116–17; see also Charles Zika, *Exorcising our Demons: Magic, Witchcraft, and Visual Culture in Early Modern Europe* (Leiden, 2003), 303–4; Guy Tal, "Witches on Top: Magic, Power, and Imagination in the Art of Early Modern Italy," PhD dissertation, Indiana University, 2006, ch. 2. For the motif of the "twisted spindles," see note 40 above.

48 For numerous examples from Renaissance literature, see Boggione and Casalegno, op. cit. at note 2, 174–5, 283.

49 On companies and brotherhoods (confraternities) of cuckolded husbands, see Matthews-Grieco in this volume.

50 The etching, entitled, "Description et figure du sabbat des sorciers," appears in the second edition of Pierre de Lancre, *Tableau de l'inconstance des mauvais anges et demons*, Paris, 1613, between pages 118 and 119. The print shares other motifs with Baccio's series. The round dance is represented twice, once with witches alone, and once with witches and devils holding hands and dancing in a circle. Another vignette shows a group of ladies and gentlemen wearing Carnival masks, with the caption: "Ce sont les grands Seigneurs & Dames, & autres gens riches & puissans, qui traictent les grands affaires du Sabbat, où ils paroissent voilez, & les femmes avec des masques, pour se tenir tousiours a couvert & incognues." A good reproduction of the whole composition is available at: http://library24.library.cornell.edu:8280/luna/servlet/detail/CORNELL~10~1~51499~101124:Description-et-figure-du-sabbat-des.

51 Baldinucci, op. cit. at note 1, 31–2: "Quello però, in che Baccio del Bianco fu eccellente, e forse anche singolare, in materia di finire, fu l'inventare e toccar di penna storiette piacevoli, caramogi, e ritratti di persone con disegno caricato; in genere di che gli sovvenivano cose da fare altrui morir dalle risa. Si trovò più volte in casa di cavalieri suoi amici in occasione di conviti, ove bene spesso era chiamato, a cagione del suo bello e piacevolissimo spirito, a rappresentare in carta il convito, e le persone, caricando i volti di ciascuno de' cavalieri, e delle dame in modo, che tutti si rendevano ridicolosi quanto mai dir si potesse, e contuttociò si riconoscevano per quei ch'egli erano."

52 Harold Acton, *The Last Medici* (London, 1932 [1980]), 30, 111, 192.

53 Suzanne Cusick. *Francesca Caccini at the Medici Court. Music and the Circulation of Power*, Chicago, 2009, 195. On the cultural politics of the regents, see also Kelley Harness, *Echoes of Women's Voices. Music, Art and Female Patronage in Early Modern Florence* (Chicago, 2006); Christina Strunk, "Christiane von Lothringen Großherzogin der Toskana (1565–1636) ein 'weiblicher Herkules,'" in *Die Frauen des Hauses Medici*, ed. Christina Strunk (Petersberg, 2011), 75–93; Ilaria Hoppe, "Maria Magdalena von Österreich (1589–1631) die vergessene Regentin," in ibid., 107–15; and the several relevant articles in *Medici Women as Cultural Mediators (1533–1743)*, ed. Christina Strunk (Milan, 2011).

54 Attributed to Luigi Gualtieri, *Storia della nobile e reale famiglia de' Medici*; published as Luca Ombrosi, *Vita dei Medici sodomiti* (Milan, 1965), 33. The manuscript does not state when the episode is supposed to have occurred, although it does specify that it resulted in an estrangement that lasted 18 years. Since Vittoria had three children in the first five years of her marriage, between 1637 and 1642, and none thereafter until 1659, it would stand to reason that the period of the estrangement began sometime in the early 1640s. However, given that the page named in the manuscript, a certain Bruto della Molara, was born only in 1639, the chronology remains problematic. See Walter Bernardi, *Il paggio e l'anatomista. Scienza, sangue e sesso alla corte del Granduca di Toscana* (Florence, 2008), 76–8.

55 *Le Nozze degli dei, favola dell Abbate Gio. Carlo Coppola rappresentata in musica in Firenze nelle reali nozze de Serenissimi Gran Duchi di Toschana Ferdinando II e Vittoria Principessa d'Urbino*, Florence, 1637, illustrated with etchings by Stefano della Bella recording all of the stage sets. The book is available online at: http://www.archive.org/stream/lenozzedeglideif00copp#page/n1/mode/2up. For Baccio's activities as a stage and costume designer, see Mina Bacci, "Lettere inedite di Baccio del Bianco," *Paragone* XIV (1963), 68–77; Thiem, op. cit. at note 1, 183; Phyllis Dearborn Massar, "Scenes for a Calderon Play by Baccio del Bianco," *Master Drawings*, XV, 1977, 365–75; Gregori, op. cit. at note 1.

56 A connection between Baccio's *cornuti* and the 1637 wedding extravaganza was first proposed by Massimiliano Rossi ("Furini poeta," in *Un'altra bellezza. Francesco Furnini*, ed. Mina Gregori and Rodolfo Maffeis, exhib. cat. (Florence, 2007), 113; *Florence au grand siècle*, op. cit. at note 1, 252).

57 Ibid.

58 R. Burr Litchfield. "Demographic Characteristics of Florentine Patrician Families, Sixteenth to average age at which aristocratic Nineteenth Centuries," *Journal of Economic History* XXIX (1969), 199. On average, patrician men were around 35 when they married for the first time, patrician women around 20.

59 On Cicognini's connection with Baccio, see *Florence au grand siècle*, op. cit. at note 1, 264–5, cat. 62; citing Flavia Cancedda and Silvia Castelli, *Per una bibliografia di Giacinto Andrea Cicognini* (Florence, 2001), 52–4, n. 91.

60 "Le Scappinate sopra le dame di Fiorenza" (Florence: Biblioteca Riccardiana, MS. Cod. 3146, ff. 199–217; MS. Cod. 3160, ff. 1–20). The term *scappinata* refers to the Commedia dell'arte character Scappino (Scapin), thus situating Cicognini's satirical verses in the same Carnival context as Baccio's cuckoldries.

61 Baccio often returned to the theme of the cuckold in his drawings. See, for example, Uffizi 17659 F, in which a lover takes leave of his mistress, while her husband (or possibly her father) emerges from the cellar where he gone to fetch a barrel of wine. In a drawing for a frontispiece with *caramogi*, a cuckold tries to hide behind a mask but his companions expose his unhappy state, two of them making the sign of the horns while a third blasts loudly on a horn and points (Florence, Biblioteca Nazionale Centrale, MS. Magliabechiano,cl. XVIIII, 6; illustrated in *Florence au grand siècle*, op. cit. at note 1, 258–9, cat. 61 and Cheng, op. cit. at note 1, 131, Fig. 10.2).

62 The word was first used in this sense in connection with literary and musical compositions; Callot may have been the first to apply it to the visual arts, when he dedicated to Lorenzo de' Medici, uncle of Grand Duke Ferdinando II, a set of 50 small etchings of miscellaneous subjects, which he entitled *Capricci di varie figure* (c. 1617).

63 See note 32 above.

64 See note 5 above.

65 Callot hints at the goatish origins of the word in the title plate to the *Capricci*, which he frames between two goat-legged satyrs. The word may, in fact, have an entirely different and non-caprine root, but the popular view that goats were somehow involved had wide currency, and is reflected in the many goats, fauns, and satyrs in *capricci* by Tiepolo, Goya, Fragonard, and others. See Lucrezia Hartmann, *Capriccio: Bild und Begriff* Nürnberg, 1973), 7–9; Alice Rathe, "Le Capriccio dans les lettres italiennes," *Les Lettres Romanes* XXXIV (1980): 207–45, 321–51; Roland Kanz, *Die Kunst des Capriccio. Kreativer Eigensinn in Renaissance und Barock*, Munich, 2002. I am grateful to Veronica White for sharing with me the relevant pages of her PhD dissertation, "Serio Ludere: Baroque Invenzione and the Development of the Capriccio" (Columbia University, 2009) in which she ably summarizes the complex literature on this question.

Picart's Browbeaten Husbands in 17th-Century France: Cuckoldry in Context[1]

Sara F. Matthews-Grieco

Prints can be used as a kind of weather vane with respect to social climate, especially when specific issues gather critical mass in visual media. In the case of printed pictures produced for the open market, the subject of cuckoldry seems to have reached a high level of social and commercial pertinence in images produced at the middle level of the print trade in 17th-century Paris, roughly between 1630 and the mid-1660s. The topicality of cuckoldry is also borne out by other areas of cultural production, such as theatre and satirical literature,[2] but the first question that comes to mind regarding the abundance of surviving images on this topic is whether this critical mass might be entirely serendipitous. Is it due to the eclectic collecting habits of art amateurs at the time? The images bound in volumes by collectors have not always survived as single sheets, and thus the preservation of many documents from the lower levels of the print market is solely due to the whims of early modern print enthusiasts.[3] For example, the bound volumes of *facéties* (drolleries) collected by the Abbé de Marolles (1600–1681), who had a particular interest in humorous images and "popular" prints, ended up in the Bibliothèque Royale in 1667 and are still preserved in the Cabinet des Estampes of the Bibliothèque de France in Paris.[4] Print collecting was already a gentleman's hobby all over Europe by the mid-16th century, yet there certainly seem to be fewer surviving engravings dealing with cuckoldry, impotence and adultery in Cromwell's England and Counter-Reformation Italy.[5] What explanation can be given for what appears to be a quantitative surge of Parisian print production on cuckoldry, and why was there a market demand for such images at this point in time?

This essay will address three questions. The first has to do with visual discourse: what were the causes and the consequences of cuckoldry as implied by prints? In other words, what are the domestic, social and economic concerns translated by such images? The second question has to do with the contemporary environment in which these prints were produced: what do we know about adultery in 17th-century France? What can court cases and current legislation reveal about the social climate, and in particular the reasons for which female adultery and male cuckoldry are so widely portrayed in popular engravings? Finally, the middle level of the Parisian print market was influenced by current events, popular spectacles, urban gossip and local politics. Given the multiplication of theatres and the vogue for plays featuring cuckolds (real and imaginary) in mid-17th-century Paris, the relationship of these prints to contemporary comedy cannot be neglected, especially as the public that filled the *parterre* of the city's theatres—made up of artisans, merchants and lower bourgeoisie—was also the target audience of "popular" prints.[6]

Parisian printmakers were, like printmakers throughout Europe, rather opportunistic with regard to the market opportunities provided by current events.[7] For example, the Protestant engraver Abraham Bosse produced an image representing *David and Goliath* (1651), which prominently features the slingshot that permitted a mere boy to overcome a fearsome giant. The image is commented by a text that assigns divine agency to the weapon that killed the tyrant. Cleverly disguised as an episode from the Old Testament, this print provided a bi-medial form of visual and textual propaganda in support of the revolt known as the *Fronde* (literally, slingshot) by suggesting both biblical precedent and celestial legitimation for the current political upheaval.[8] At the same time, on an equally fraught register, Bosse—like many of his contemporaries—produced numerous series of prints about marriage and domestic life. These multi-sheet narrative "dramas" (the same sort of dramas that were simultaneously being acted out in Parisian theatres) engaged in the current debates on conjugal mores and the relationship between the sexes.[9] Finally, many engravers also issued prints representing recent theatrical successes, for such souvenirs provided an opportunity to make a quick profit on a print run. Surviving examples of this sort of ephemera are Bosse's engraving of actors on stage at the Hôtel de Bourgogne (c. 1633–1634), Molière in the role of Sganarelle in a print by Claude Simonin (1661), and a frontispiece to *LEscole des Maris* engraved by François Chaveau (Paris, 1661).[10]

The primary objective of this essay is thus to draw renewed attention to the importance of printed pictures as a primary source.[11] Prints played a role as both a symptom and an agent of change in the early modern world, and can thereby shed light on the society that produced them. Printed pictures also reveal some of the essential presuppositions of early modern sexual culture, such as a commonly shared attitude towards the body where the private is also public, and belongs less to its owner than to an institution (such as the social institution of marriage) and thus to the larger community. Above all, prints were a commercial product, and responded to market conditions: notably curiosity and novelty, taste and expectations, supply and demand. By examining mid-level prints on cuckoldry/adultery in terms of their contemporary context, it is possible to reach a number of conclusions about the role played by this specific product in relation to current events.

This essay will explore in particular the explicit and implicit agendas that were being addressed by French engravings on cuckoldry in terms of the wider social and political climate of mid-17th-century France.

Lagniet's *Illustrated Proverbs*

The series of prints that constitutes the focus of this study belongs to a large and heterogeneous collection of engravings published in Paris. Generally thought to have been printed between 1657 and 1666, they are bound under the collective title: *Receuil des plus illustres proverbes divisé en trois livres*, more commonly known as the *Illustres Proverbes* of Jacques Lagniet.[12] Very little is known about Lagniet (c. 1600–1675). The title page of the *Illustres Proverbes* points out that his print shop was located on the Quay de la Mégisserie, at Fort l'Evêque (located about halfway between the Louvre and Châtelet). The art enthusiast and print collector Michel de Marolles, Abbé de Villeloin, lists Lagniet in his *Book of Painters and Engravers* only to specify that he was a "mediocre engraver" (*médiocre graveur*).[13] Other art critics and gazetteers of the time do not seem to have considered this engraver–printer worthy of attention, which implies that this sole mention was probably due to the fact that Marolles had a special interest in facetious and satirical subjects that were not considered of any particular value, either artistic or monetary.[14]

The compilation used for this investigation is currently held at the Bibliothèque Nationale de France and contains 294 prints that were bound together in the first half of the 18th century.[15] This is not the only collection of *Illustrated Proverbs* attributed to Lagniet. There is a compilation of 404 plates now at the Getty Research Library, while other volumes (some now lost) have been said to contain over 500 prints.[16] In these various compilations, the Lagniet proverbs are usually bound with a number of extraneous allegorical or facetious images that may have been engraved, printed or sold by the Lagniet workshop, as well as other miscellaneous engravings, most of which can be ascribed to Parisian print production in the middle decades of the 17th century.[17]

The Lagniet volumes are generally divided into three books: the first is introduced by a collective title page which lists all three—the "Moral Proverbs," the "Joyous and Pleasant Proverbs" and the "Life of Beggars in Proverbs" (*RECEUIL DES PLUS ILLUSTRES PROVERBES DIVISES EN TROIS LIVRES, LE PREMIER Contient les proverbes moraux LE SECOND Les proverbes joyeux et plaisans LE TROISIEME Represente la vie des Gueux en proverbes, mis en lumiere par Iacques Lagniet a PARIS* (Fig. 10.1).[18] Within the collection, the second and third "books" each have their own title page, while subsidiary series ranging between 6 and 30 prints are announced with yet other title pages. In the Paris volume there is, for example, a series inspired by the topsy-turvy world called "Asinine situations" (*Anneries*), another sub-series entitled the "Exemplary Life of Two Friends" (*Le tableau et la vie exemplaire de ces deux amys*) with a rather scatological title page,[19] and a long sub-series of

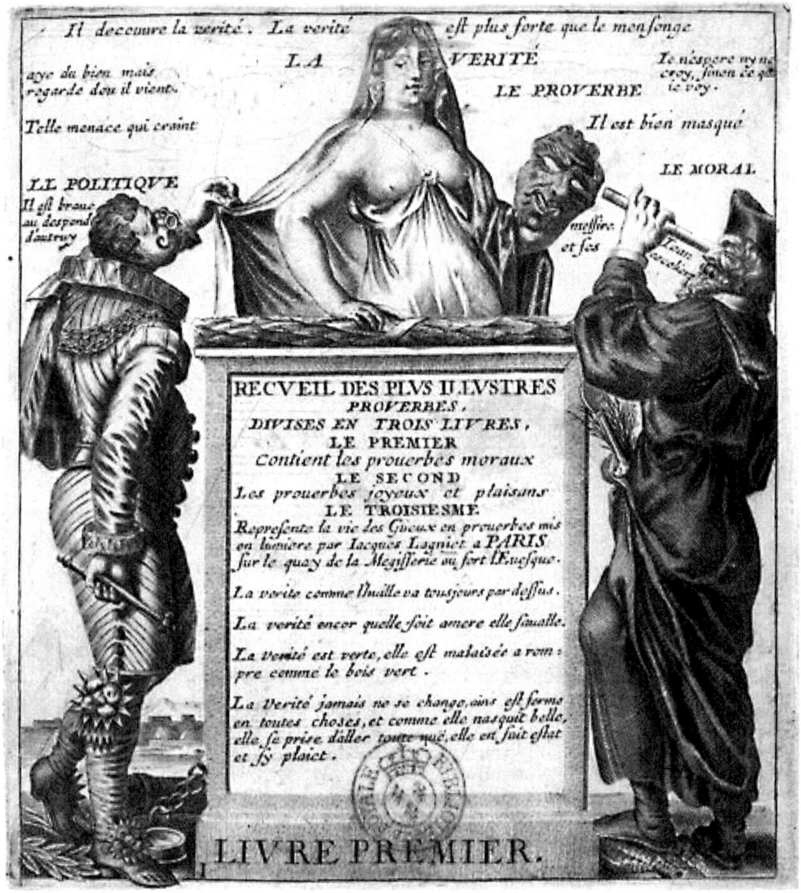

Il decouure la verité. La verité est plus forte que le mensonge
LA VERITÉ
LE PROVERBE
aye du bien mais regarde dou il vient.
Telle menace qui craint
Il est bien masqué
LE MORAL
LE POLITIQVE
Il est braue au despend d'autruy
RECVEIL DES PLVS ILLVSTRES PROVERBES.
DIVISES EN TROIS LIVRES,
LE PREMIER
Contient les prouerbes moraux
LE SECOND
Les prouerbes joyeux et plaisans
LE TROISIESME
La verité encor quelle soit amere elle saualle.
La verité est verte, elle est malaisée a rom:pre comme le bois vert.
LIVRE PREMIER.

10.1 Jacques Laginet, *Recueil des plus illustres proverbes divisés en trois livres: le premier contient les proverbes moraux, le second les proverbes joyeux et plaisans, le troisiesme représente la vie des gueux en proverbes*, Paris, c. 1660, title page, engraving, Rés. Z-1746 in 8°, Bibliothèque Nationale de France, Paris

over 30 engravings dedicated to a current comic favorite: *Till Eulenspiegle*.[20] Curiously, the Paris volume also contains a series of prints on costumes, and a considerable number of odd prints with no apparent thematic connection to the others if not for the fact that they illustrate proverbs, or topics which contemporaries seem to have found rather hilarious (such as drunkenness and defecation). Sometimes these odd prints feature numbers, suggesting that they were originally part of a larger series, but their place in the Paris volume does not seem to follow a particular logic.

The eclectic contents and seemingly serendipitous order of all Lagniet compilations is due to the nature of print retailing at this time. Engravings could be bought singly, in shorter or longer series, and many circulated in the second-hand market until they were compiled and bound in volumes by 18th-century print collectors. Such collections were therefore the fruit of chance more than the result of systematic printing, distributing, retailing or acquisition, as is further demonstrated by the fact that a good percentage of the engravings differ between the various bound compilations. As a result, the different order in which the various "books of proverbs," sub-sections and unnumbered plates appear in any particular volume can be understood as a demonstration of the compiler's notion of thematic coherence or collecting strategy rather than any original editorial intention on the part of Lagniet.

Very few engravings in the collections of *Illustres Proverbes* are signed, and variations in quality and execution in each bound volume suggest that there were a number of different engravers involved, even in the series of numbered prints. Certain names do appear occasionally: Jérôme David, Jaspar Isaac, a certain Leclerc and a Picart, whose names are followed by the word *delineavit* or *fecit*, indicating that they are the either the authors of the drawings or the engravers of the plates themselves. Lagniet himself signs in various versions of his name: "par Jacques Lagniet" (by Jacques Lagniet), J. Lagniet *fecit* and Lagniet *excudit*, which implies various forms of authorship at this time, ranging from the original drawing to the finished plate or the printed product.[21] The proverbs that feature on each of Lagniet's prints (sometimes at the bottom of the image, sometimes at the top, and often in the picture space) were current in 17th-century France and can be found in contemporary anthologies, such as the *Curosités françaises* by Antoine Oudin (1640) and the *Etymologie ou explication des proverbes français* by Fleury de Bellingen (1656).[22] Many of the engravings feature a variety of proverbs, which collectively provide a commentary on the action depicted.

A systematic comparison of all surviving compilations of Lagniet (and the other prints bound with the *Illustres Proverbes*) would permit the reconstruction of various series of prints, and doubtless bring to light images that have not yet been studied. For example, engravings on the theme of Lustucru (derived from the expression *l'eusse-tu cru* = "would you have believed it?") are more numerous in the Getty compilation, while fewer of these prints are to be found in the Paris volume.[23] Lustucru is a mythological blacksmith who appears in French satirical prints on marriage *mores* as of the 17th century: he "reforges" the heads of disobedient wives to make them more submissive to their husbands.[24] This visual treatment of a solution to instability in the gendered status-quo thrived in mid-17th-century Paris, at a moment in which both salon culture and the phenomenon of the *précieuses* were gathering momentum, soon to be mocked by Molière and his contemporaries.[25] Might Lustucru be seen as transmitting a certain grass-roots acknowledgement of the new roles being assumed by elite women, facetiously proposing a "solution" to any attempt at emulation on the part of ordinary wives? What is most striking in the many evocations of the "miraculous" forge and its clientele is the fact that women's *heads* are seen as being the source of trouble.[26] This *topos* belongs to a long tradition of satires on marriage: the marvelous mill (*moulin merveilleux*) that turns querulous old wives into docile young brides, the domestic dispute (*lutte des sexes*) where plates and cooking pots fly, and the fight for the hose (*lutte pour la culotte*) where women exchange their skirts for their husband's trousers, thereby appropriating both masculine authority and privilege.[27] The primary innovation of the Lustucru prints lies in the identification of the seat of problems between the sexes as being above all cerebral, and its topicality in terms of contemporary *salon* culture can hardly be denied.[28] Just as the series of "jealousy" plays by Molière—from *Sganarelle* (1660) to the *École des femmes* (1662)—proposed emerging new roles for women in juxtaposition to traditional ideas about their social identity, so too were printmakers engaged in the current debate on marriage and the relationship between the sexes.[29]

Amongst the many stock themes that appear in the *Illustres Proverbes* are, predictably, humorous evocations of the faults attributed to women, above all conjugal conflict and marital infidelity. An image in the second book of proverbs (featuring the number 14) is incongruously placed between a print (n°13) depicting a common man having his hair oiled, and another—signed by Lagnet [*sic*] and dated 1657—that makes fun of doctors (N°15). In the image bearing the number "14," female adultery is depicted as constituting a form of dishonesty equivalent to that practiced by an innkeeper who waters down wine in a barrel. While the innkeeper cheats his clients, his wife cheats on him with the baker boy (Fig. 10.2). The multiple inscriptions on the engraving refer to contemporary proverbs appropriate to the situation, such as "A pretty hostess is bad for the purse" and "[Drinking] Glasses and women are always in danger."[30] Female adultery is, however, hardly restricted to the humbler ranks of society. This *topos* again appears in a more elevated social circle in another plate (n°31), again curiously situated between an image of a foolish man who burns his house to keep warm (n°30) and a domestic scene with a henpecked husband (n°32). The plate that deals with adultery showcases another case of marital infidelity: an elderly and jealous husband has so persecuted his wife with his suspicions that he has brought about exactly that which he feared. Opening a chest in his wife's luxuriously appointed bedroom, the bearded old gentleman "looks for that which he does not want to find" (Fig. 10.3).[31] Discovering an elegant young gallant in hiding, he thus seals his own shame.

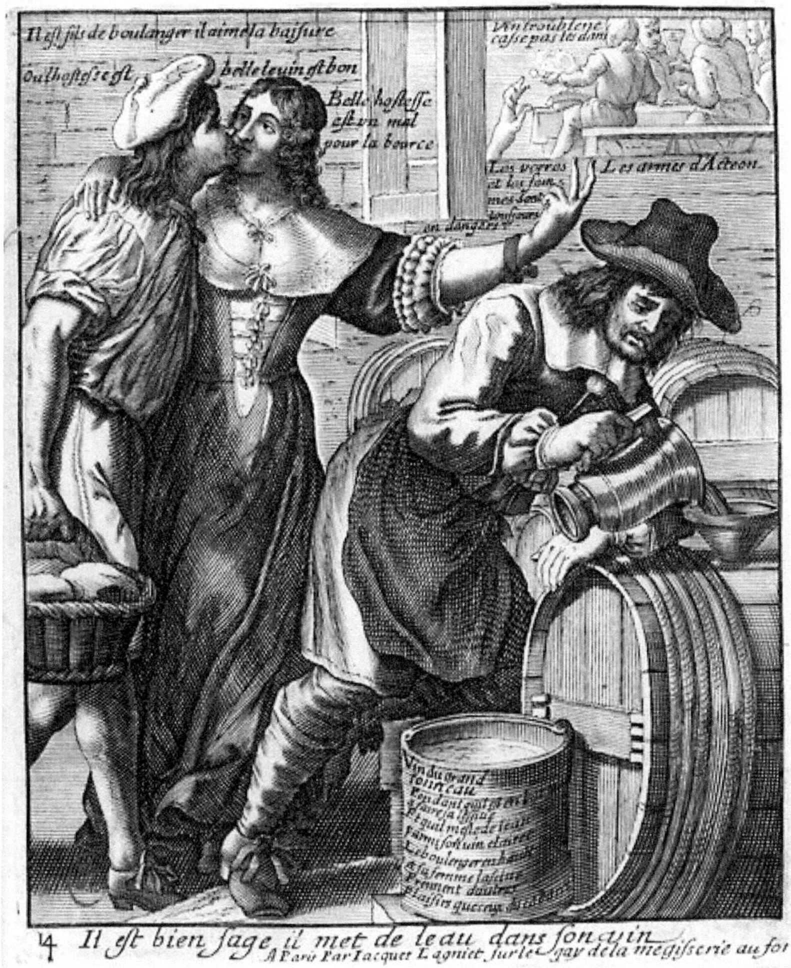
Il est fils de boulanger il aime la baisure
belle hostesse est un mal pour la bource
Les armes d'Acteon
14 Il est bien sage il met de leau dans son vin
A Paris Par Iacquet Lagniet sur le qay de la megisserie au for

10.2 Jacques Laignet, "He is very wise, he puts water in his wine," print n° 14 in *Le second livre ou est despaint les proverbes ioyeux*, Paris, c. 1660, engraving, Rés. Z-1746 in 8°, Bibliothèque Nationale de France, Paris

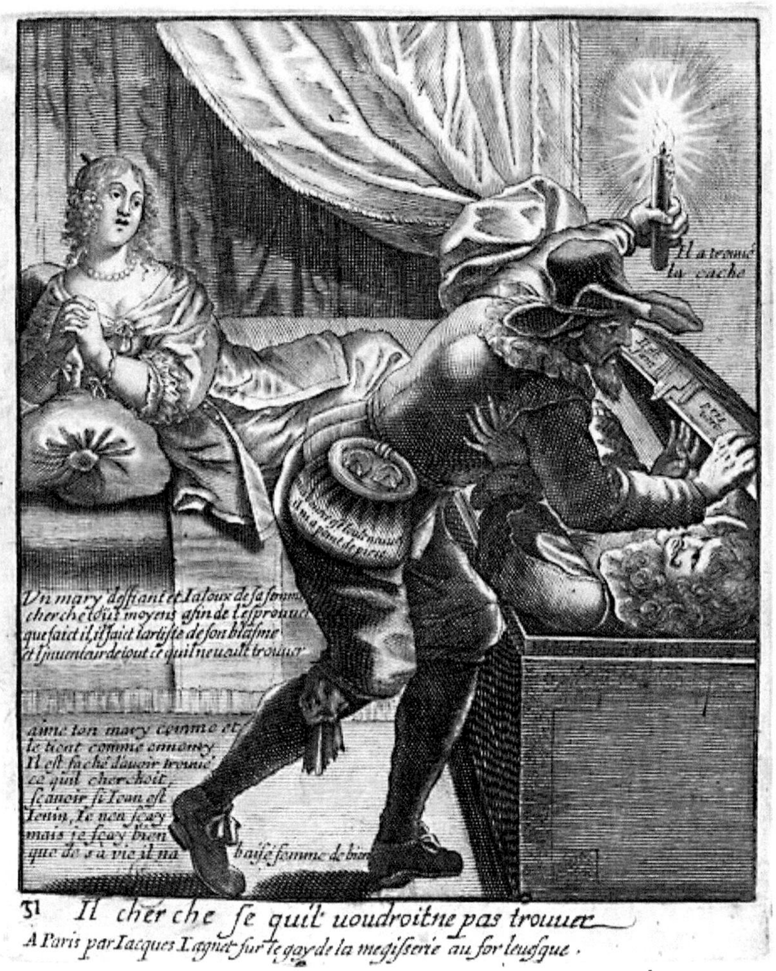
Il a trouué la cache
31 Il cherche se quil uoudroitne pas trouuer
A Paris par Iacques Lagniet sur le quay de la megisserie au for leuesque.

10.3 Jacques Lagniet, "He looks for that which he does not want to find," print n° 31 in *Le second livre ou est despaint les proverbes ioyeux*, Paris, c. 1660, engraving, Rés. Z-1746 in 8°, Bibliothèque Nationale de France, Paris

In these two examples, men of vastly different social classes are portrayed as being equally guilty of transgressing their familial and professional duty. The tavern keeper's dishonesty is reflected in that of his spouse, while the elderly gentleman's oppressive suspicion of his young and beautiful wife has ended up with her taking a young and handsome lover. Such images suggest that men who neglect either their professional ethos or a minimum of conjugal decorum cannot expect their wives to behave any better. While the first presents a moralizing equation whereby husbandly/professional dishonesty is compared to wifely/conjugal adultery, the second is close to contemporary farces. Playing in city squares as well as at the Hôtel de Bourgogne and Théâtre du Marais, popular farces had standard comic plots which featured jealous old husbands who were often impotent and predictably cuckolded, while flighty young wives sought solace in the arms of clandestine lovers.[32]

These two prints on adultery (and others like them) are part of a numbered series of illustrated proverbs whose purpose was undoubtedly to amuse, but they do not construct a more elaborate or continuous narrative with neighboring images. Not only is there a lack of a thematically coherent development or storyline between consecutively numbered engravings, but there is also a great variety in their presentation and execution. This diversity was probably due to a publishing ploy: the numbered images may have been issued one or more at a time as a "collectible" series, which suggests that novelty was more important than narrative in the retail commerce of the early modern print market.

Picart's *de facto* Series

While all the collated volumes bound under the name "Lagniet" feature a number of individual prints that specifically treat the subject of cuckoldry (there is even a series of six prints with the title: *La Cornologie*),[33] of specific interest in terms of the contemporary treatment of cuckoldry, impotence and adultery is a series of 12 engravings scattered throughout the Bibliothèque Nationale compliation. This series can be attributed to an engraver–printer–publisher called Pierre Picart, who belonged to a family of engraver–printer–retailers in mid-17th-century Paris.[34] The dates of these images are disputed, but it is generally agreed that they were printed between the later 1650s and the mid-1660s. Although some of the burin engravings from this series can be found in various print collections, the most complete set (12 in number) owes its survival to being bound in the Paris volume of Lagniet's *Illustres Proverbes*.[35] This *de facto* group was presumably issued as an open-ended series on the subject of domineering wives, cuckolded husbands and the consequences of female adultery, all stock themes in satirical prints and easy to sell. The prints all have a similar size (c. 20 × 13 cm), an identical layout and presentation, and all include an explanatory quatrain located in a separate space below the image, engraved directly on each plate by the same hand. Most, if not all, of the prints seem to be by the same engraver, and the uniform presentation suggests that this series can be safely attributed to the same workshop. One is signed "*Picart excudit*" (Fig. 10.4), and in two other prints (presumably meant to be successive), the location of a shop is spelled out on a continuous line at the bottom of the page: "*Soubz les charnie[rs] St Innocent a la maitreſſe porte qui donne dans la rue St. denis Avec privilege du Roy*" (Figs. 10.5 and 10.6).

Very little is known about the Picart family of engravers and print sellers. In his *Livre des peintres et graveurs*, the Abbé de Marolles mentions "two Picard" (spelled with a "d") who appear, like Lagniet, under the category of "mediocre engravers."[36] And again, as with Lagniet, the art critics and gazetteers of the time do not seem to have considered the work of this family of printer–engravers worthy of attention, although the family name (spelled with a "t" or a "d") appears repeatedly in records of marriages and baptisms amongst the community of Parisian booksellers, engravers and printers.[37] Various Picart also appear in a number of legal documents and guild regulations throughout the century, but as the address given on the engravings mentioned above was that of a property that originally belonged to the engraver–publisher Jacques Lagniet, and Lagniet's daughter married a certain Pierre Picart around 1670, the series in question was most probably a joint venture between father and (future) son-in-law.[38] The Picart engravings were certainly issued around the same period as Lagniet's *Illustres Proverbes* were being marketed, and were eventually collected and bound together due to their similar subject matter more than any other factor.[39]

Street Views

The first image that bears the words "*Picart excudit*" (Fig. 10.4) depicts a group of lower-class women assaulting a group of men—their husbands—who are interrupted in a game of ninepins they had been playing in the street. An explanatory text located in the image itself points out that "these are not women, these are devils" while the quatrain below elaborates upon the same theme, calling the women *diablesses* and listing the bodily injuries they inflict on their unresisting and pusillanimous husbands.[40] An inversion of gender roles is also implied by the aggressiveness of the women and the passivity of the men, most of whom have taken to their heels in fright. The time-tried misogyny of both text and image acts as a comic vehicle to amuse the viewer, while at the same time it reinforces the secondary content of the image: men who indulge in idle pastimes deserve such treatment because they are dissipating their time instead of earning an honest wage to support their family. Idle and irresponsible husbands have abdicated their role as the head of a household and thus deserve the bodily punishment they receive, just as an idle housewife might receive a physical reprimand on the part of her spouse.

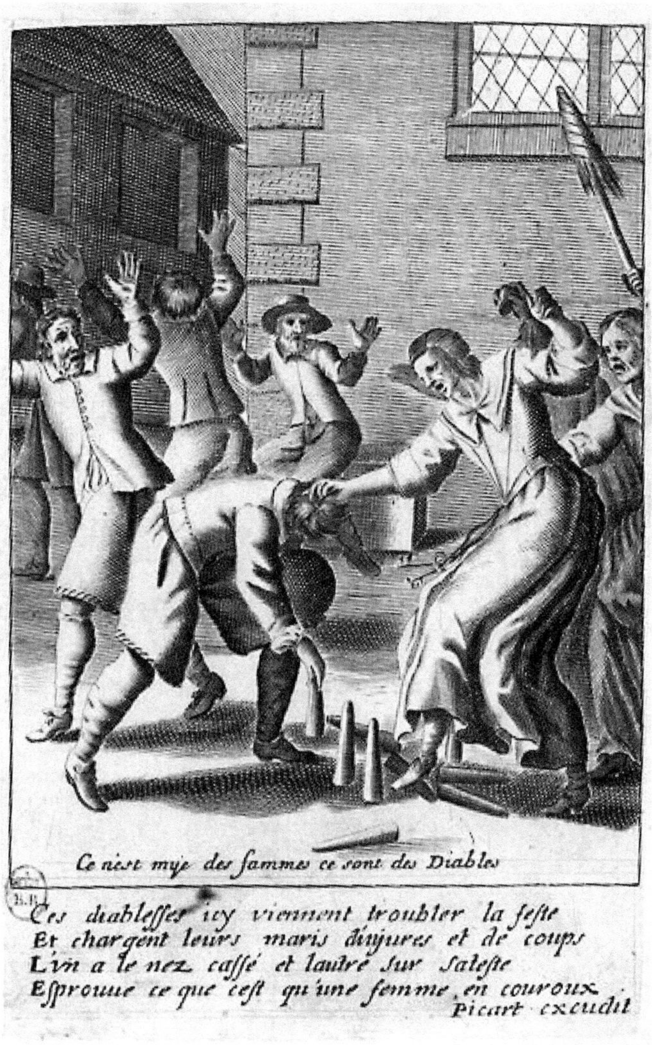

Ce n'est mye des fammes ce sont des Diables
Ces diablesses icy viennent troubler la feste
Et chargent leurs maris d'injures et de coups
L'vn a le nez cassé et l'autre sur sa teste
Esprouue ce que c'est qu'une femme en couroux
Picart excudit

10.4 Pierre (?) Picart, "These are not women, these are devils," bound in Jacques Lagniet, *Le second livre ou est despaint les proverbes ioyeux*, Paris, c. 1660, n.p., engraving, Rés. Z-1746 in 8°, Bibliothèque Nationale de France, Paris

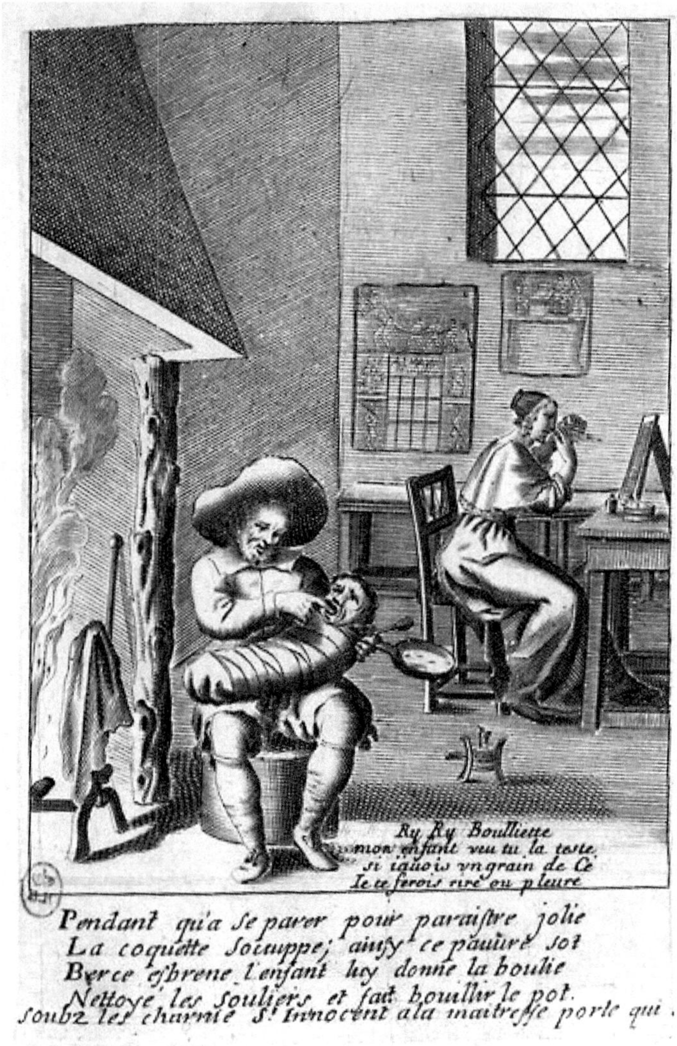

10.5 Pierre (?) Picart, "The topsy-turvy household," bound in Jacques Lagniet, *Le second livre ou est despaint les proverbes ioyeux*, Paris, c. 1660, n.p., engraving, Rés. Z-1746 in 8°, Bibliothèque Nationale de France, Paris

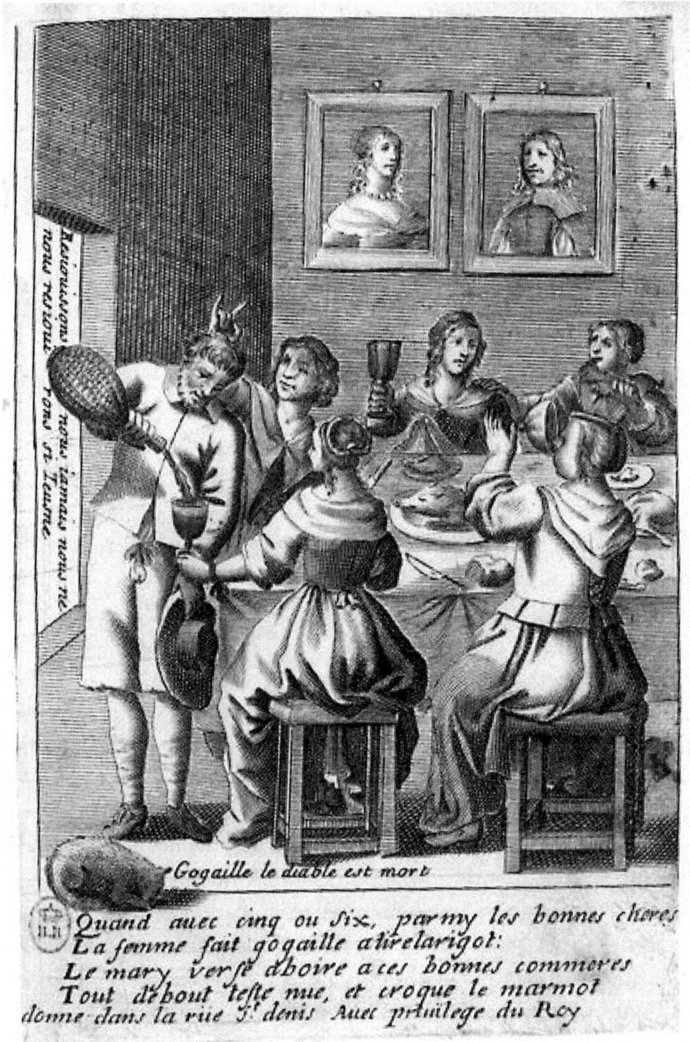
Resiouissons nous iamais nous ne
nous resiouirons si ieune
Gogaille le diable est mort
Quand auec cinq ou six, parmy les bonnes chores
La femme fait gogaille atirelarigot:
Le mary verse à boire a ces bonnes commeres
Tout debout teste nue, et croque le marmot
donne dans la rue S.t denis Auec priuilege du Roy

10.6 Pierre (?) Picart, "Eat hearty, the devil is dead!" (a husband waits on his wife and her friends), bound in Jacques Lagniet, *Le second livre ou est despaint les proverbes ioyeux*, Paris, c. 1660, n.p., engraving, Rés. Z-1746 in 8°, Bibliothèque Nationale de France, Paris

Ridicule with an intent to both denounce and correct is a recurring rhetorical strategy in social satire, as can be seen in a second print from this series, representing another scene in the public arena (Fig. 10.7). Here a group of women are spoiling their husband's meal at a tavern. The men cower and attempt to propitiate their wives' anger by making gestures of deference, hat in hand, but the harridans have no pity. Not only do they spoil their husbands' social life, but they also ruin their menfolk's sexual reputation: the tavern goers are defined as being cuckolds (*cocus*) in the text below the image.[41] According to early modern gender logic, dominant and scolding wives would inevitably cuckold their husbands, if they had not done so already: a subjugated husband had relinquished not just his authority as head of the household, but also the masculine privilege of promiscuity.[42] The primary moral message conveyed by the chaotic scene is that men should not be controlled by women; this type of social and conjugal disorder led to public humiliation. Of course the secondary—but equally important—message deals again with the distribution of household resources. Like street games, tavern dinners and drinking were a source of domestic contention insofar as such pastimes dissipated family funds, whence the conflict of interest between husband and wife.

This same theme appears in a contemporary print published by Jean Ganière (Paris, between 1640 and 1660) entitled "Dialogue of Dame Alison and Lubin, her husband, at the Tavern" (Fig. 10.8). This engraving is often cited by historians of print culture as a good example of the semi-public display of single sheet prints in this period: a confraternity image and other pictures (including graffiti) adorn the tavern wall.[43] As the dialogue featured at the top of the print points out, Alison must prostitute herself in order to feed her children (pictured in the foreground) because her good-for-nothing husband Lubin spends all the household funds at the tavern.[44] Fondled by the tavern-keeper, whose hand creeps close to her breast, she makes the sign of the horns in the direction of her drunken spouse. This print, like the Picart tavern scene, denounces the self-indulgence and irresponsibility of a husband whose sodden impassivity confirms his marital and sexual inadequacy. The child in the foreground who wastefully pours wine from a pitcher (visually echoing the man urinating in the back right corner) adds insult to injury, alluding to the waste of resources brought about by such a situation, but also the waste of his father's sexual emissions, no longer used in an appropriate way in the appropriate "vessel." Once again sexual disorder is the result of a husband not fulfilling his designated social role. Providing for a household automatically conferred authority on the *pater familias*, while failing to support a wife and children led to a series of social ills, not the least being prostitution on the part of the wife. Lubin ends the dialogue with the words: "Since you are so generous, you keep the bed and I'll keep the table, it's the way to be content."

The drunken husband in the Ganière print is portrayed as being a contented cuckold, but he is not a pimp. Men who prostituted their wives for their own gain were punished severely by the courts as being guilty of *maquerellage* (whore mongering), but a passive, complacent husband could

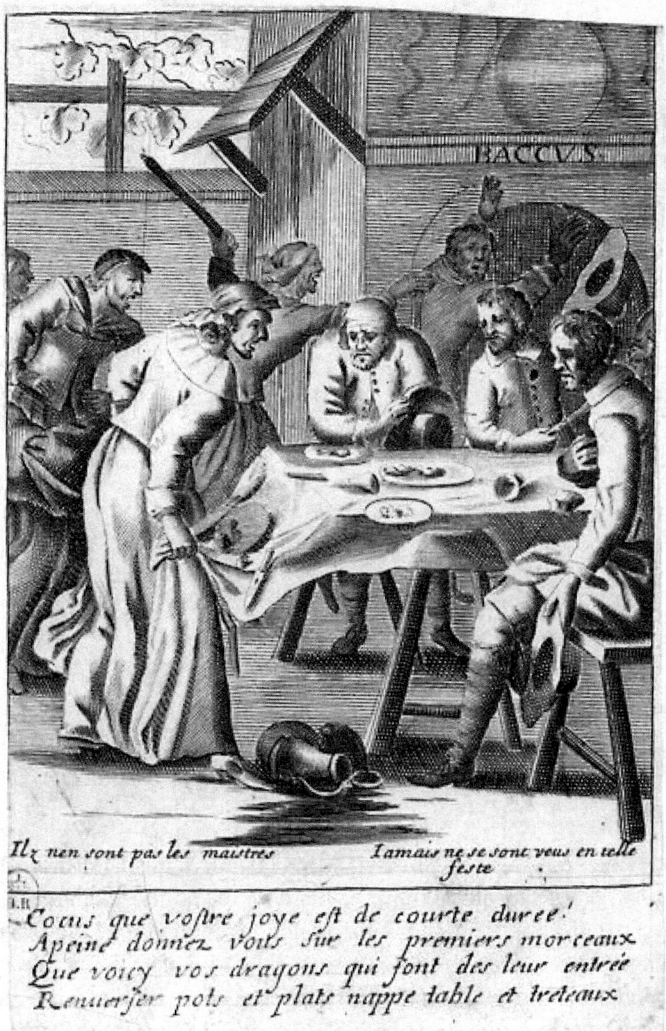
BACCVS
Ilz nen sont pas les maistres
Iamais ne se sont veus en telle feste
Cocus que vostre joye est de courte duree!
Apeine donnez vous sur les premiers morceaux
Que voicy vos dragons qui font des leur entrée
Renuerser pots et plats nappe table et treteaux

10.7 Pierre (?) Picart, "Women spoil their husbands' meal at the tavern," bound in Jacques Lagniet, *Le second livre ou est despaint les proverbes ioyeux*, Paris, c. 1660, n.p., engraving, Rés. Z-1746 in 8°, Bibliothèque Nationale de France, Paris

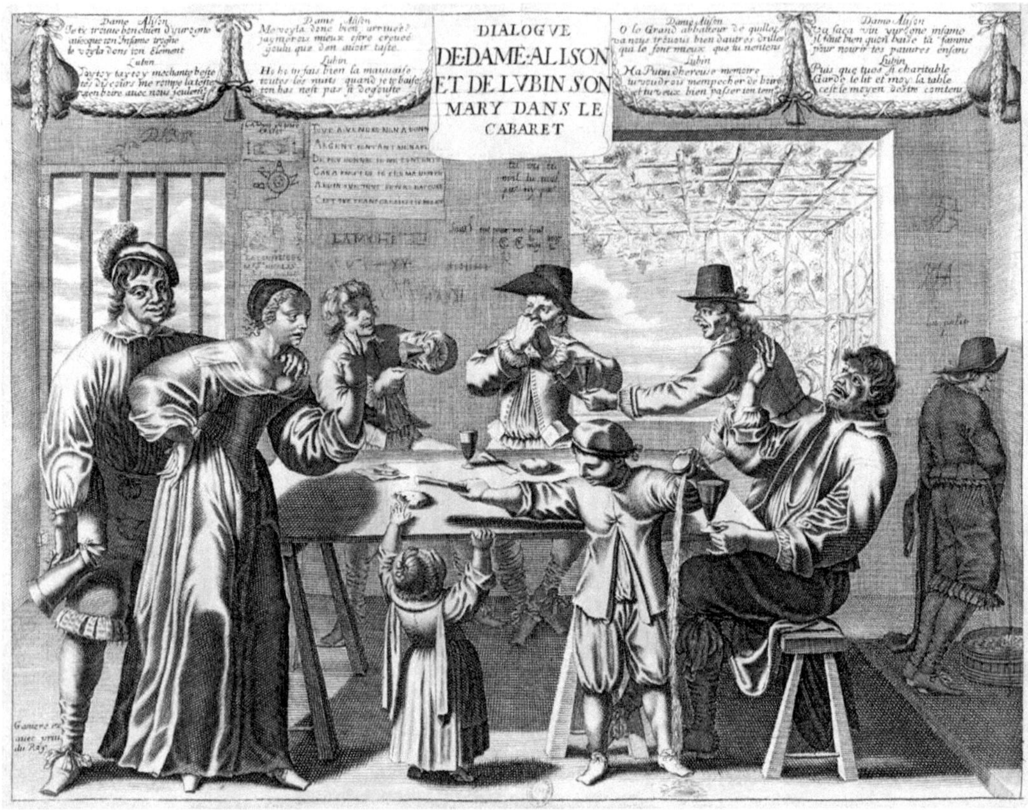

10.8 Jean Ganière, *Dialogue of Dame Alison and Lubin, her husband, at the Tavern*, Paris, 1640–1660, engraving, Tf2 Rés fol. p. 78, 29.5 × 39.6 cm, Bibliothèque Nationale de France, Paris

not be forced to correct his wife. In fact, only a husband (not a brother, father or son) could legally denounce his wife for adultery as he was the lawgiver in his household, with a power analogous to that of a king over his subjects.[45] The only exception to this rule was if the wife's infidelity became so publicly scandalous that the local magistrate was compelled to intervene in order to correct a clamorous case of social disorder. On the whole, however, legislators supported the principle that families should govern themselves, and if husbands were resigned or complicit, as long as the situation did not become a subject of public outrage (or a bad example for the rest of the community), then it was the husband's business and nobody else's.[46]

Another example of a henpecked husband in the Picart series—a shoemaker scolded by his wife in the street as he works—echoes both Ecclesiastes (7:26–9) and contemporary proverbs in the text at the top of the image which states that it is better to live under a ruined roof at the mercy of wind and rain than to have to live with a quarrelsome wife (Fig. 10.9).[47] The primary message of this satirical print is that the husband who does not control his scolding wife is, once again, guilty of abdicating his familial and social responsibility as the head of a household. Is this a "negative example" print, whereby the shrewish wife—arms akimbo—implies that this unfortunate state of affairs was all too

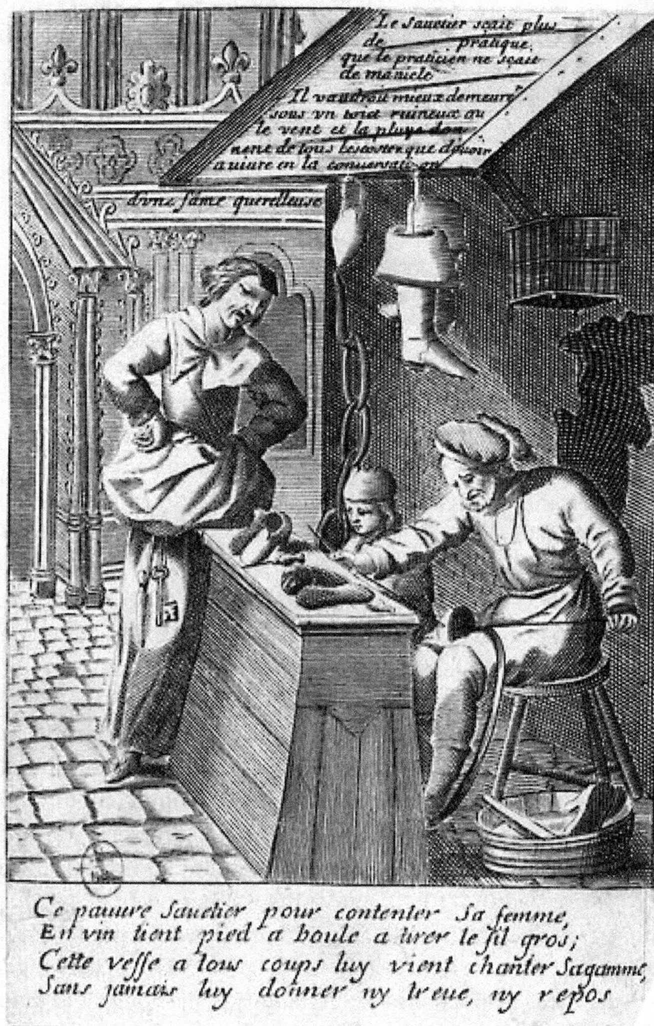
Le Sauetier scait plus
de pratique
d'vne fame querelleuse
Ce pauure Sauetier pour contenter Sa femme,
En vin tient pied a boule a tirer le fil gros;
Cette vesse a tous coups luy vient chanter Sagamme,
Sans jamais luy donner ny treue, ny repos

10.9 Pierre (?) Picart, "The poor shoemaker scolded by his wife," bound in Jacques Lagniet, *Le second livre ou est despaint les proverbes ioyeux*, Paris, c. 1660, n.p., engraving, Rés. Z-1746 in 8°, Bibliothèque Nationale de France, Paris

common? She also acts as a foil, evoking on a secondary level the opposite model: the current social ideal of chaste, silent and obedient womanhood.

The significant number of surviving prints dedicated to the *topos* of conjugal conflict, of which the Picart series is but one example among many, would seem to imply that the issue of domestic order—or rather, disorder—was a burning topic in 17th-century France.[48] To what extent might such obsessively recurring reminders of the joint responsibility of husband and wife imply problems of disorder on a larger scale, especially in the political arena? The analogy of the household as a microcosmic version of the state was, after all, widely recognized throughout Europe.[49] Until 1661, when Louis XIV assumed sole control of the kingdom, France had been effectively ruled by the young king's mother, the Queen-Regent Anne of Austria, in close collaboration with the Italian Cardinal Jules Mazarin (Giulio Raimondo Mazarino).[50] Excessive taxes and a heavy-handed style of government gave rise to a protest on the part of both the *petit peuple* and the bourgeoisie, encouraged and supported by magistrates and city parliaments in a widespread revolt known as the *Fronde* (1648–1653). Far from being a revolt against the crown or a contestation of the principle of monarchy, the uprising of the *Fronde* aspired to limit the absolutist powers of the sovereign and temper the burden of taxation.[51]

Engraver publishers such as Abraham Bosse and Jacques Lagniet belonged to a social and professional category that tended to sympathize with the *frondeurs*, which may have made both printmakers and their clientele inclined towards images with stock themes that could denounce social chaos while avoiding the censorship incurred by more explicit satirical prints.[52] By criticizing sexual and economic disorder in the contemporary household, printed pictures could still imply that the problem was more pervasive: like a negligent *pater familias*, the young king had not fulfilled his role as a *pater patriae*, letting "foreigners"—his mother and her purported lover/first minister—rule in his stead.[53] Parisian prints would thus seem to be echoing a widespread concern with regard to the chaotic state of the kingdom, implicitly accusing those responsible for the stability of the household-state of neglecting their designated roles. If Louis XIV had behaved as an irresponsible "head of household," it was no wonder that Paris and the rest of the kingdom had played the role of an errant and unfaithful wife.

Household Chaos

Moving off the street and into the private arena, the second of the signed prints in the Picart series features a topsy-turvy domestic scene (Fig. 10.5). Here a husband sits in front of the fire feeding a swaddled child while his wife preens in front of a mirror, seated at a table in the background. The quatrain points out that the wife is making herself look beautiful while the poor idiot (*pauvre sot*) of a husband takes care of household chores: he rocks and feeds the child, makes food, and even cleans shoes![54] The image plays on the notion that a man who takes on traditional female tasks is both stupid and ridiculous, for he has voluntarily abdicated the prerogatives of his sex. At the same time, the implication of the woman's care with her appearance is that she is prettying herself for someone other than her husband. Once again, a passive and feminized husband is seen as being the victim of his own folly; his wife is interested in another man and he—like a woman—is saddled with the baby.

A similar message is conveyed by another print from the same series depicting another type of domestic disorder: a woman brandishing a sword is chasing her husband out the door while their child cries on the floor (Fig. 10.10). Two lines of text at the bottom of the image specify that he who is not master in his house only gets what he deserves, and in fact what looks like either a stick or an empty scabbard (most probably the former as his apron identifies him as an artisan) lies on the floor next to his hat. He has not only lost his weapon and a primary symbol of his masculinity, but this metaphorical castration is emphasized by his being chased out hatless, a further insult to his social identity since hats (like sticks and swords) were manly attributes.[55] The quatrain refers to the time-tried metaphor of the crowing hen and the silent cock, a barnyard *topos* which not only implies the reversal of the natural order in the reversal of domestic roles, but also suggests that the husband's own bird—his virile member—was guilty of another kind of silence.[56] The implications with regard to male impotence could hardly be more explicit.[57]

Such a disorderly situation in a household leads to a variety of consequences that are depicted in other Picart prints from this series. Henpecked husbands are driven to join the *Confraternity of Cuckolds* (Fig. 10.11), where a man stands, hat in hand, in front of a tavern whose sign features the (cuckold's) horns. He has just put down a few coins in order to join the confraternity, signing himself up in a register of members which the quatrain below calls a "book of martyrs" (martyrs of marriage).[58] In the background hovers a crowd of men—identified by their dress as belonging to all social stations—who are waiting their turn to enroll. While real *confrairies des cocus* or *cornards* once reigned over periodic festivities, they had been subjected to systematic repression by both Church and State for more than a century by the time this print was engraved.[59] The confraternity pictured here is thus an entirely different type of organization, ironically seen as providing a group identity and tavern headquarters for hapless husbands to drown their sorrows in drink with others who are similarly afflicted.[60] Cuckoldry—like a kind of plague—is seen as making no distinction of class or situation: it strikes rich and poor, artisan and aristocrat alike.

Confraternities provided, amongst other things, a homo-social context for men of like interests, which is why the theme of the confraternity of martyred husbands was to enjoy a certain success in satirical prints, conferring an ironic afterlife to the joyous confraternities of *cocus* that had been so energetically suppressed in most of France. Another example is an anonymous *facétie* entitled *L'Origine des Cornes ou les Cornarts enregistrez,* where men of all

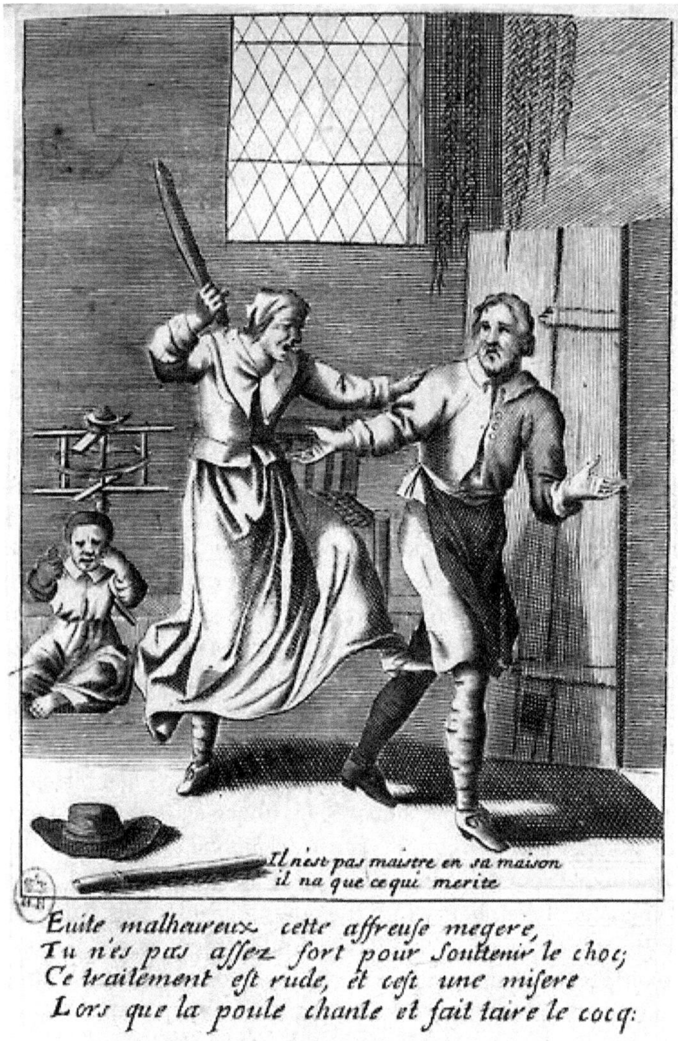
Il n'est pas maistre en sa maison
il na que ce qui merite
Euite malheureux cette affreuse megere,
Tu n'es pas assez fort pour Soustenir le choc;
Ce traitement est rude, et cest une misere
Lors que la poule chante et fait taire le cocq:

10.10 Pierre (?) Picart, "The henpecked husband is chased out of the house," bound in Jacques Lagniet, *Le second livre ou est despaint les proverbes ioyeux*, Paris, c. 1660, n.p., engraving, Rés. Z-1746 in 8°, Bibliothèque Nationale de France, Paris

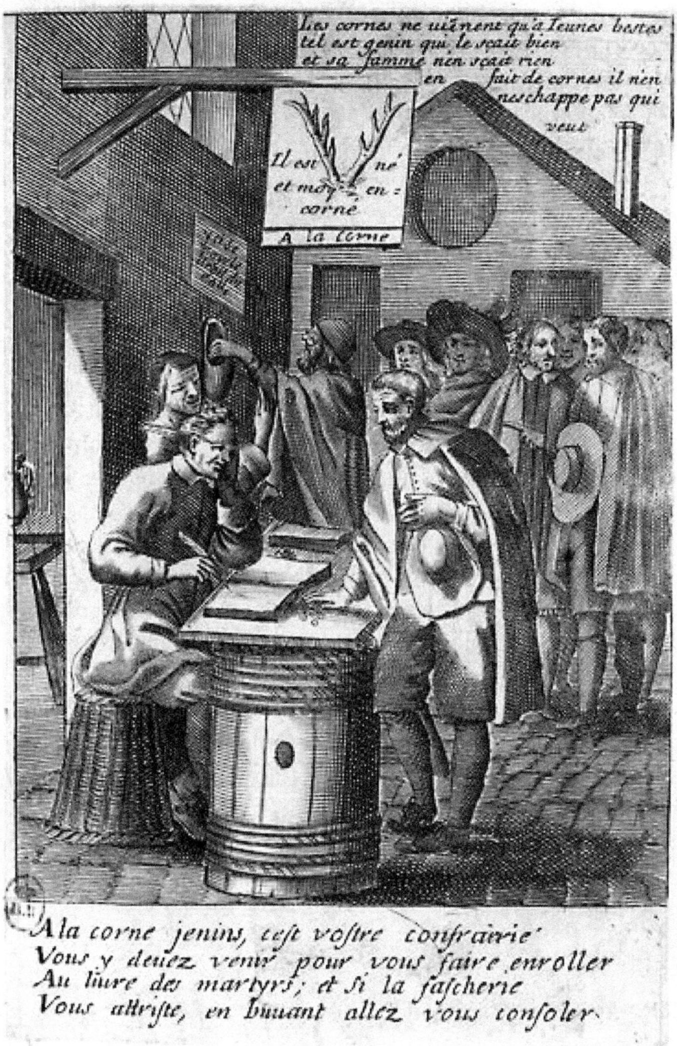
Les cornes ne uiēnent qu'a Ieunes bestes
tel est genin qui le sçait bien
et sa famme n'en sçait rien
en fait de cornes il n'en
n'eschappe pas qui
veut
Il est né
et moy en = corné
A la corne
A la corne jenins, c'est vostre confrairie
Vous y deuez venir pour vous faire enroller
Au liure des martyrs; et si la fascherie
Vous attriste, en buuant allez vous consoler.

10.11 Pierre (?) Picart, "The confraternity of cuckolds," bound in Jacques Lagniet, *Le second livre ou est despaint les proverbes ioyeux*, Paris, c. 1660, n.p., engraving, Rés. Z-1746 in 8°, Bibliothèque Nationale de France, Paris

ages, sporting horns of all sizes, sign up in a register.[61] Yet another print sold in Paris by Francois Guérard at the very end of the century proposes a confraternity for "martyred" husbands beaten by their wives and, by implication, also cuckolded,[62] while a somewhat later print shows women signing men up in a confraternity register and distributing the outward and visible sign of their common state: the cuckold's horns.[63] Finally, in the logic of 18th-century political satire, a post-revolutionary print from about 1790 refers to the time tried *topos* of cuckoldry as being an affliction that occurs at all levels of society, and thus a source of social equality.[64] Equally horned, Aristocrat and Bourgeois fraternally embrace in the great brotherhood of cuckoldry, while the text below states, somewhat redundantly: "Come on, no more social distinctions, this common misfortune makes us equals."[65] Although this latter example was printed much later than Picart's series, it serves as a reminder of the well-documented longevity of the theme of (con)fraternal cuckoldry, and brings home the fact that the 18th century was to see an overt use of the cuckold's horns in political prints and caricature.[66]

As a whole, the early modern print market seems to have been particularly fond of visual denunciations of domestic disorder, especially in regard to adulterous wives and subjugated husbands. The meek and passive acceptance attributed to cuckolds is depicted as a lamentably real and frequent social practice: a tendency to turn a blind eye towards wifely infidelity and a widespread resignation with regard to female philandering. In fact, given the social opprobrium to which cuckolds were subjected, the jokes at their expense and the shame and humiliation of criminal proceedings, many men may well have chosen to avoid public scandal. The theme of the confraternity of cuckolds thus implies that cuckolded husbands are many in number, a kind of silent majority at the base of the social fabric, a widespread—if hidden—household pathology.

Consequences of Cuckoldry

The remaining images in the Picart series deal specifically with the ills that result from conjugal infidelity. One plate features different actors but could be a direct sequel to the print where the husband is being chased—swordless and hatless—out of the house. The text reads: "Here she is finally free, she got rid of him / With hard blows and a kick in the ass (*pied dans le cu[l]*) / In order to entertain her lover / Who fills the cuckold's place" (Fig. 10.12).[67] An adulterous couple is portrayed sitting on a bed (the conjugal bed). The man puts coins into the woman's hand, while underneath the couple's feet two lines of text underscore the implications of the scene with a well-known saying of the time: "Women usually do not fall on their face but more often on their back."[68] Here the comparative elegance of the gentleman caller is a simple reflection on the fact that sexual promiscuity came easily to men of means, and in a cross-class encounter such as this one, each would gain by the transaction.

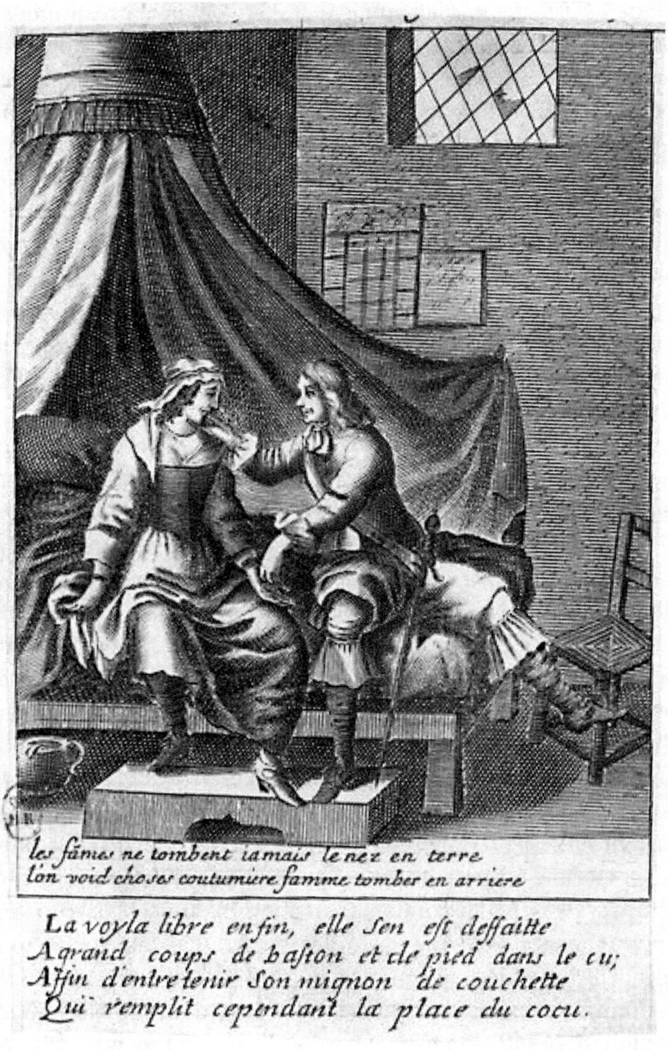
les fãmes ne tombent iamais le nez en terre
l'on void choses coutumiere famme tomber en arriere
La voyla libre enfin, elle Sen est deffaitte
A grand coups de baston et de pied dans le cu;
Affin d'entretenir Son mignon de couchette
Qui remplit cependant la place du cocu.

10.12 Pierre (?) Picart, "The adulterous wife and her lover," bound in Jacques Lagniet, *Le second livre ou est despaint les proverbes ioyeux*, Paris, c. 1660, n.p., engraving, Rés. Z-1746 in 8°, Bibliothèque Nationale de France, Paris

Nonetheless, the implication is that the woman is prostituting herself within her own household, while her husband is guilty of not fulfilling his role, neither in bed nor in society. As the quatrain below the image reiteratively points out, like the cuckoo bird, another man is about to lay his own egg in the cuckolds' nest.

The third print that bears the identification and address of the Picart as printer–retailers (Fig. 10.6) shows women economically exploiting a man under the domestic roof. Here a husband waits on his wife and a group of her friends who are seated around a table laden with choice meats (there is even the head of a suckling pig on a platter). One of the women (perhaps his wife?) makes the sign of the horns over his head as he pours wine into a goblet held by another woman. They are eating and dining at his expense, while at the bottom of the image, a cat sleeps next to the words of a contemporary toast: "Eat hearty, the devil is dead!"(*Gogaille, le diable est mort!*)[69] The quatrain develops the implications of the merry scene by pointing out that the husband is reduced to the level of a servant: he stands while they sit, he is hatless (a sign of subservience that has other implications, as has already been pointed out), and he must *croquer le marmot*—wait on their pleasure.[70] Historians of literary culture have pointed out a flurry of satirical pamphlets in mid-17th-century France that criticized female gatherings and women's talk. Humorous denigration of female gatherings and speech had long been standard *topoi* in both pictures and texts, but the proliferation of such time-honored topics at this point in time can probably be attributed to the phenomena of the *précieuses* and Parisian salons. Current events could always provide a new impetus for social satire, ranging from engravings denigrating the *Caquet des femmes* to the instant success of Molière's *Précieuses ridicules* (1659) and its imitators.[71]

One of the worst crimes that a woman could commit in conjunction with adultery was to abscond with money or household property. The Picart engraving on this theme is simpler in narrative details than most of the other prints in the series, and may be by another hand (Fig. 10.13). It nevertheless continues the narrative thread with regard to female infidelity, economic exploitation and domestic disorder. Here a woman of fairly humble social rank has just come out of a doorway, leaving the conjugal hearth with cooking implements and a big bundle. The quatrain points out that she is taking everything (including the cat) to furnish her lover's abode.[72] In addition to her theft of her husband's sexual and social honor, she has also robbed him of his household goods, goods that technically would not have belonged to her even if they had come into the house as part of her dowry. This kind of compound crime on the part of a married woman—adultery accompanied by theft—could even be punished by death; it constituted a criminal act considered to be the equivalent of murder, incest or sacrilege.[73]

In fact, the victim of adulterous amours was not seen as being limited to the cuckolded husband but included the whole family and, by extension, the entire community. Just as the cuckoo leaves its eggs in the nests of other birds, so does the adulterous woman present her family with an imposter. Or worse

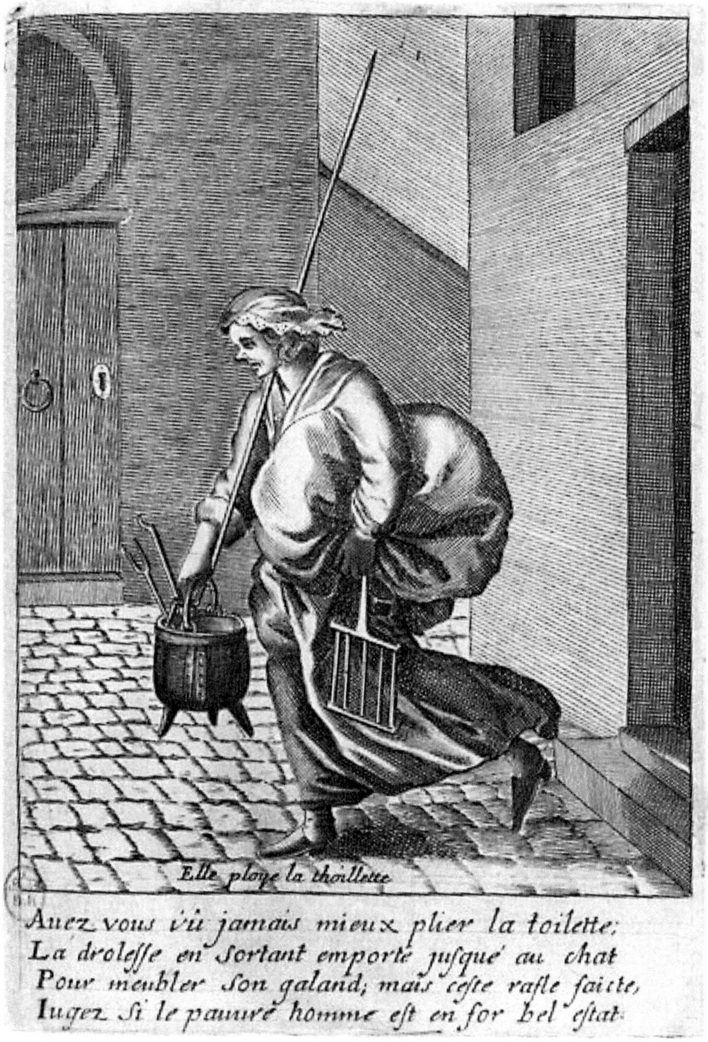
Elle ploye la thoillette
Auez vous vû jamais mieux plier la toilette;
La drolesse en sortant emporte jusque au chat
Pour meubler son galand; mais ceste rafle faicte,
Iugez si le pauure homme est en for bel estat.

10.13 Pierre (?) Picart, "The adulterous woman carries off household goods," bound in Jacques Lagniet, *Le second livre ou est despaint les proverbes ioyeux*, Paris, c. 1660, n.p., engraving, Rés. Z-1746 in 8°, Bibliothèque Nationale de France, Paris

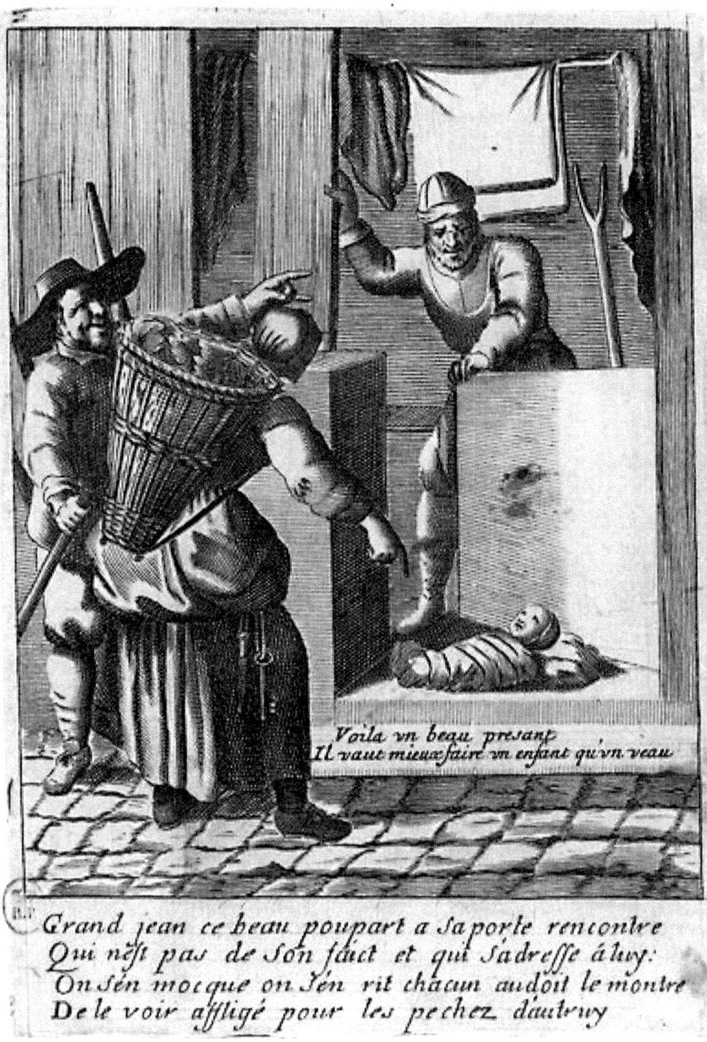
Voila vn beau presant
Il vaut mieux faire vn enfant qu'vn veau
Grand jean ce beau poupart a sa porte rencontre
Qui n'est pas de son faict et qui s'adresse á luy:
On s'en mocque on s'en rit chacun au doit le montre
De le voir affligé pour les pechez d'autruy

10.14 Pierre (?) Picart, "Grand Jean finds the abandoned infant," bound in Jacques Lagniet, *Le troisieme livre des proverbes contenan* [*sic*] *la vie des gueux*, Paris, c. 1660, n.p., engraving, Rés. Z-1746 in 8°, Bibliothèque Nationale de France, Paris

yet—as shown in another Picart print —a newly delivered mother can leave her offspring on a stranger's doorstep, and the man who discovers an abandoned infant on his threshold will suffer the mirth of passers-by (Fig. 10.14). Is this a case of 17th-century *shadenfreude* whereby "Grand Jean" (as the quatrain names him) finds himself the butt of neighborhood merriment, provoked both by this tangible result of someone else's sexual transgression and the dilemma of what to do with the child?[74] However the scenario might be read, the ostensible message is that the repercussions of female adultery are vast, and constitute a burden for all of society.

A Contemporary Debate

The marital mores denounced by Picart's group of images go beyond simple moral caveats with regard to topsy-turvy household relations; taken as a whole, they constitute a visual catalogue of social ills attendant upon domestic disorder. As has already been pointed out, prints deploring this state of affairs were hardly an isolated phenomenon and similar themes cropped up in all forms of social commentary in the course of the 17th century. Theatre, literary satire and scandal sheets also found inspiration and commercial success in treating such a consistently controversial topic, while the most successful dramatic theme on the Parisian stage was doubtless cuckoldry (or the suspicion thereof).[75] In Italian, Spanish and French farces playing in public squares, theatres and private palaces, jealous old husbands married to beautiful young wives provided a popular comic *topos* for all levels of the urban public.[76] When Molière first performed *Sganarelle ou le cocu imaginaire* at the Théâtre du Petit Bourbon on May 28, 1660, its immediate success had as much to do with the novel twist to its plot, as with its debt to traditional French face and suggestive language.[77] Totalling 131 performances during the lifetime of its author, between court (nine performances) and city (122 performances), the *Imaginary Cuckold* was by far the most often performed of Molière's plays, and gave rise—as did the earlier *Précieuses ridicules* (1659)—to a pirate publication of the play within a few months of its first showing.[78] Comedy, nonetheless, could also have a more serious moral agenda. Cuckoldry, domestic dynamics and fear of female philandering was seen as being an ongoing problem in contemporary society, one which playwrights sought to both expose and "cure" by means of ridicule.[79]

Like contemporary comic theatre, the moral agenda of satirical prints comprised a public shaming ritual, a kind of permanent *charivari* in visual culture.[80] While a mid-century surge of printed pictures "publicly" denounced bilateral conjugal transgressions as a negative example to be avoided, these same images also reinforced a "new" view of marriage based on a type of social contract rather than the more traditional and authoritarian model of household government. The participation of prints in the contemporary debate on gender relations faithfully echoes a period shift in the terms of discourse, moving away from the traditional invective aimed at women to a more considered evaluation of (shared) responsibility in the running of the domestic unit.[81] It does not seem entirely serendipitous that the multiplication of Parisian engravings on domestic disorder so closely parallels the basic premise of the *Fronde*: just as the Fronde challenged the abuse of royal power without contesting the political institution of kingship, so, too, were prints denouncing conjugal abuse without contesting the institution of marriage itself. In the years immediately before and after 1661, when Louis XIV personally took up the reins of his kingdom, satirical prints were harping on the inadequate exercise of patriarchy in the contemporary household. The social contract of the mid-17th-century domestic household was—like that of the kingdom itself—hardly being contested, but rather in need of the kind of strenuous reinforcement that the young king would bring to the next decades of his rule.

While comic theatre and humorous prints acted as light-hearted vehicles for more sober moral agendas, 17th-century legislation provided an institutional counterpoint to the representation of cuckoldry in entertainment media. In an historical study on the history of adultery in *Ancien Régime* France, the Belgian criminologist Régine Beauthier found that French magistrates paid particular attention to the issue of (female) adultery in the course of the 17th century.[82] Legislators took a serious approach to the troubling topic of wifely infidelity, describing it as being the source of a number of social ills, an insidious blight that attacked society and its institutions at the root. Contemporary treatises on civil and criminal law invariably reiterated the early modern *topos* according to which the *pater familias* was invested with the authority of Church and State, which meant that his role fulfilled both a religious and a civic function. Female adultery was therefore not just a private matter, but a public crime capable of undermining social, political and religious order. The jurist Claude Lebrun de la Rochette (1560–1630), whose volume *Le Procès civil et criminel* (first edition 1607) was published repeatedly throughout the 17th century, makes a list of the ills entailed by adultery: it was a form of larceny in that it passes off illegitimate children as heirs; it is a kind of homicide, in that the adulterous woman is responsible for murdering two souls, her own and her lover's; adultery is a kind of perjury before God and the Church, for marriage vows are broken; it is a sacrilege in that the woman's body, which should be a temple of the Holy Spirit, becomes a brothel for a whore. Finally, adultery is a form of idolatry in that the unfaithful woman worships her lover instead of her husband and the Holy Sacrament of marriage.[83] As far as the legal discourse was concerned, cuckoldry was a nefarious act with moral, economic and religious consequences; it was certainly no laughing matter.

Reconciliation?

With respect to the institutional approach to female adultery, wives accused of infidelity were subject to different treatment according to their husband's means and social status. The wives of the well-to-do could be consigned to convents, where their husbands had to pay for their room and board, while women from the less privileged classes (or Protestants) could be sent to an asylum or a hospital, along with public whores and other debauched women. The main difference between the convent and other options lay in the preventative detention that Catholic husbands could inflict on their wives, ordering them to repair to a religious community until their trial had been concluded. Other options for detainment—asylums, hospitals and prisons—did not require husbands to provide an allowance for their wives, but only accepted women after they had been sentenced by the courts. Preventative detention in a cloister thus remained a privilege of the wealthy. This of course did not stop men from trying to have their wives locked up in penal institutions with an accusation of adultery. As a result, in 1666, the *Parlements* of both Aix and Paris forbade husbands or any other men to bring women to such places of detention before the court had levied a sentence.[84]

Institutional incarceration was not the only solution with respect to feckless wives, as there also existed a number of strategies for conjugal reconciliation. While repeated denunciations of topsy-turvy households, cuckoldry and (implied) male impotence constitute the leitmotif of 10 out of the 12 prints in the Picart series, the last two images depart from this pattern with a particularly interesting variation. They both depict the upper classes and propose a solution to female adultery rarely (if ever) seen in visual media. Here the themes that animate the previous ten prints in the series—domestic disorder, male honor, sexual promiscuity and household finances—seem to have abruptly disappeared. One of these plates shows a scene of reconciliation: a man dressed as a lawyer with two heavy purses in hand takes his leave of a well-to-do couple in a domestic interior (Fig. 10.15). A line of text in the body of the image states: "She has come back, Denise," while the quatrain explains that the "coquette" of a wife, who has been abandoned by her lover, has sought out a learned lawyer to negotiate a *rapprochement* with her husband, obtaining both a pardon and a promise that he will treat her as well as before.[85] Reconciliation with an adulterous wife after a physical separation was not unknown in this period, but it was not quite as easy to bring about as this print implies.

Conjugal pardon and marital *rapprochement* were only considered feasible after a physical separation and legal mediation, or after an errant wife had learned her lesson during a period of incarceration. Two years was the minimum sentence for women convicted of adultery before a magistrate to be consigned to a convent, refuge or prison. While a husband might decide to avoid the publicity of the courts but nonetheless impose a separation—

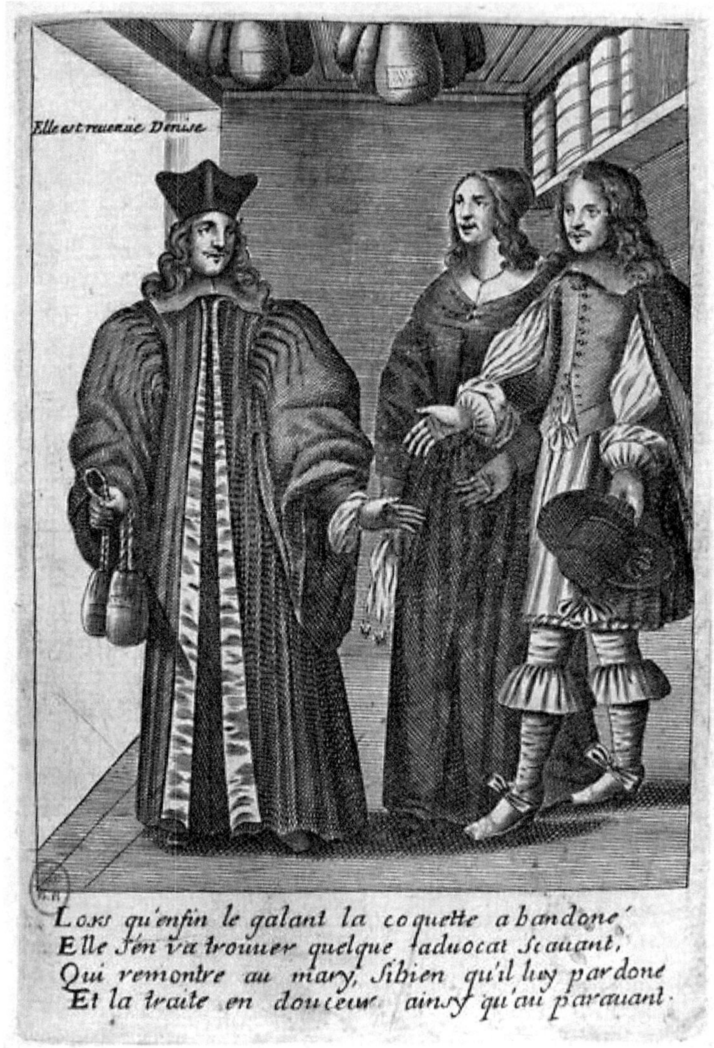
Elle est reuenue Denise
Lors qu'enfin le galant la coquette abandone
Elle s'en va trouuer quelque aduocat scauant,
Qui remontre au mary, s'ibien qu'il luy pardone
Et la traite en douceur ainsy qu'au parauant.

10.15 Pierre (?) Picart, "A scene of reconciliation," bound in Jacques Lagniet, *Le second livre ou est despaint les proverbes ioyeux*, Paris, c. 1660, n.p., engraving, Rés. Z-1746 in 8°, Bibliothèque Nationale de France, Paris

lodging his errant spouse with friends or in a convent—legal mediation was often instigated by the wife in order to shorten her period away from the conjugal residence. A somewhat later but nonetheless eloquent example dates from 1694, when Marie Gabrielle Perrault hired a lawyer to file a request for reconciliation. She declared that her husband, a *marchand espicier*, had visited her every day in the convent where he had placed her, giving her money and lots of little presents. On either side of the grille, they not only engaged in tender conversation, but also kissed through the bars. Despite these demonstrations of affection—witnessed by the nuns as well as by the convent prior—her husband seemed to be in no hurry to abbreviate the corrective lesson, declaring that she would remain in the convent until he was pleased to take her back.[86] A motivating factor in certain husbandly accusations of wifely adultery may have been the fact that the dowry of a woman convicted of conjugal infidelity was forfeit to her husband. Nevertheless, a wife was still of use, especially if she was still of childbearing age. Monthly fees paid out to a convent could mount up, and a repudiated wife did not give a man the option of remarrying to have legitimate heirs. The motivations for conciliation were thus many, and would always be easier to bring about if the wife's extra-conjugal *amours* had not created a public scandal, and the husband had not lost face.[87]

The last print in the Picart series shows an elegant couple strolling in a bucolic setting, arm in arm (Fig. 10.16). This is the only image of the series in which the satirical vein seems to fall flat, or maybe today's sensibilities prevent us from understanding its humor? With the exception of the sawed-off tree trunk behind the gentleman that may refer facetiously to his having been metaphorically "castrated" by his philandering wife, the whole is more difficult to decipher. The quatrain expresses mild surprise as to the tranquility of what had once been a "*mauvais ménage.*" As the verses point out somewhat incredulously: "He is far too good, and she now behaves herself, to the extent that everything is better than before."[88] The tumult of the artisan household where the husband was beaten, exploited, cuckolded and evicted is a far cry from this image of conjugal contentment. Is there perhaps a note of skepticism with respect to a solution that these two images suggest is reserved to the wealthy? Or might these prints also represent a grassroots attitude, a refractory attitude towards leniency in a period when magistrates were proposing reconciliation as an alternative to years of incarceration for errant wives?

Certainly the hypothesis according to which the metaphor of the disorderly household could be transposed onto the political arena might here be seen as a wry acknowledgement of the post-*Fronde* truce between the crown and the city, and might better explain the humorous implications of this last image for a contemporary audience. Like kings and priests, the power to pardon and forgive was the prerogative of the husband, but 17th-century legislation increasingly considered that the *onus* of feminine fault should be mitigated by husbandly misconduct. Spendthrift husbands, domestic violence and

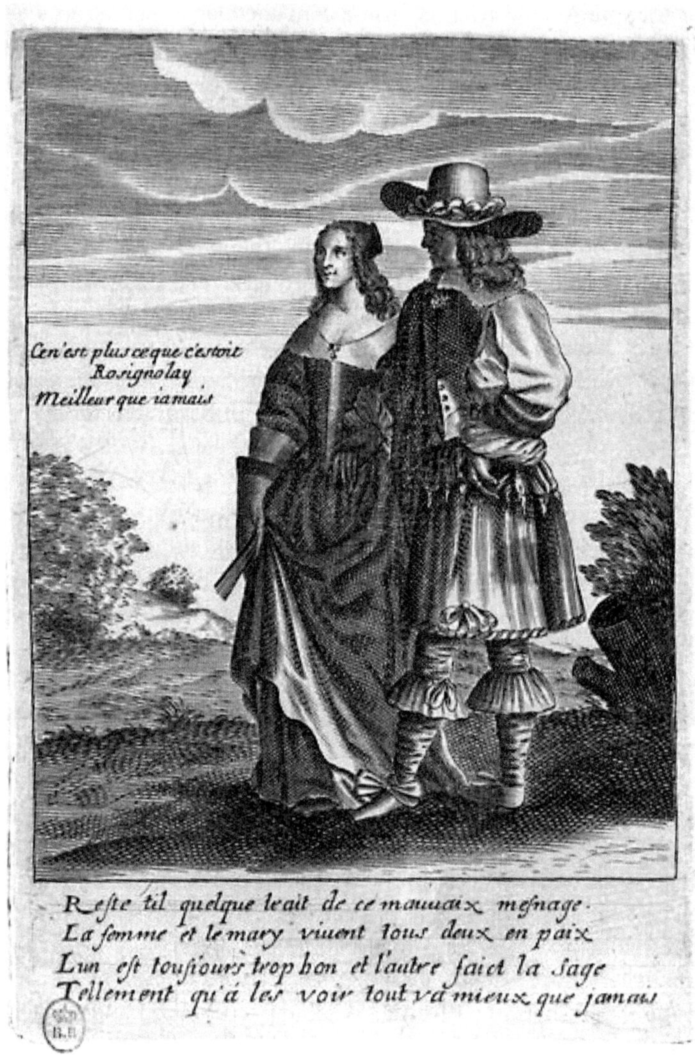
Ce n'est plus ce que c'estoit
Rosignolay
Meilleur que iamais
Reste til quelque leait de ce mauuaix mesnage.
La femme et le mary viuent tous deux en paix
Lun est tousiours trop bon et l'autre faict la Sage
Tellement qu'a les voir tout va mieux que jamais

10.16 Pierre (?) Picart, "Everything is better than before," bound in Jacques Lagniet, *Le troisieme livre des proverbes contenan* [*sic*] *la vie des gueux*, Paris, c. 1660, n.p., engraving, Rés. Z-1746 in 8°, Bibliothèque Nationale de France, Paris

flagrant commerce with whores were beginning to be treated as extenuating circumstances that could partly exonerate wifely infidelity.[89] Thus, to continue the *Fronde* analogy, the "misbehavior" of Paris and the provinces could also be read as a justifiable protest against an excessively authoritarian and financially abusive royal government. Like Picart's last print on the improbably reconciled couple, the royal pardon of Paris following the *Fronde* entailed an agreement regarding good behavior on both sides. As a result: "He [the King] is far too good, and she [the city] now behaves herself, to the extent that everything is better than before."

As the Picart series suggests, the Age of Absolutism provided an opportunity for print culture to express concern with the stability of the household/kingdom and the authority of the husband/sovereign, using as a vehicle a mid-level commercial product marketed to all levels of contemporary society. Should the increase in visual discourse on such topics be seen as a direct reaction to *salon* culture or a lingering echo of the *Fronde*? No matter what the original stimulus behind their creation, these images conveyed a collective reminder that the *pater patriae*, the city and individual households would do well to carry out their designated roles. At the grassroots level, these visual documents testify to the fact that printmakers certainly partook—opportunistically or serendipitously—in both political controversy and institutional strategies for social change.

Cultural products such as prints, plays and popular pamphlets may have exploited certain traditional themes that guaranteed commercial success, but their participation in contemporary social and political currents should not be underestimated. From a coded commentary on the *Fronde* revolt to an echo of shifts in marriage legislation, no one interpretation of the prints in this series can be asserted as being paramount. It is nonetheless certain that the mid-17th-century Parisian public, both high and low, was apt in the art of analogy, and particularly engaged by clever re-workings of contemporary issues, especially when entertainingly portrayed in popular prints.

Works Cited

Early Printed Sources (pre-1900)

Champfleury (Jules François Félix Husson), *Histoire de l'imagerie populaire*, Paris, Dentu, 1869.

Fournel, Victor, ed., *Les contemporains de Molière : recueil de comédies, rares ou peu connues jouées de 1650 à 1680 avec l'histoire de chaque théâtre*. Genève: Slatkine, 1863–1865.

Guyon de Sardière, Jean-Baptiste-Denis, *Catalogue des livres de la bibliothèque de feu M. J. B. Denis Guyon, chev. seigneur de Sardière, ancien capitaine au régiment du roi, & l'un des seigneurs du canal de Briare*. Paris, Barrois, Paris, Chez Barrois, Libraire, Quai des Augustins, 1759.

Herluison, Henri, *Actes d'état-civil d'artistes français : peintres, graveurs, architectes, etc. : Extraits des registres de l'Hôtel-de-ville de Paris, détruits dans l'incendie du 24 mai 1871.* Orléans: Herluison, 1873.

Lebrun de la Rochette, Claude, *Le Procez Civil et Criminel Contenant la methodique liaison du Droit et de la Practique Judiciaire civile et criminelle : Plus l'Eslection de la Jurisdiction des Eslerz sous un bref discours des Finances et Officiers d'icelles.* Rouen: Du Mesnil, 1640.

Marolles, Michel de, *Catalogue des Estampes et de figures en taille-douce avec un dénombrement des pièces qui y sont contenuës Fait à Paris en l'année 1666. Par M. De Marolles Abbé de Villeloin,* A Paris, Chex Frederic Leonard, ruë S. Jacques, à lEscu de Venise M.DC.LXVI.

Marolles, Michel de, *Le Livre des peintres et graveurs par Michel de Marolles, Abbé de Villeloin, revue et annoté par M. Georges Duplessis.* Paris: Plon, 1872.

Secondary Sources and Modern Editions

Adhémar, Jean and Dennery, Etienne, *Au Temps des Précieuses. Les Salons Littéraires au XVIIème siècle,* Exhibition Catalogue. Paris: Bibliothèque Nationale, 1968.

Amussen, Susan Dwyer, *An Ordered Society: Gender and Class in Early Modern England.* New York: Columbia University Press, 1994.

Avalon, Jean, "Lustucru, Opérateur Cephalique," *Les Nouvelles de l'Estampe,* 1968 (n°3), 98–124. Beam, Sara, "Les notables catholiques et la marginalisation de la culture populaire au XVIe siècle," *Histoire urbaine* 2:25 (2009): 105–25.

Beaumont-Maillet, Laure, *La guerre des sexes: XVe–XIXe siècles.* Paris : Bibliothèque Nationale, 1984.

Beauthier, Régine, *La Répression de l'adultère en France du XVIème au XVIIIème siècle: De quelques lectures de l'histoire.* Brussels: E. Story-Scientia, 1990.

Beik, William, *Louis XIV and Absolutism. A Brief Study with Documents.* London/New York: Palgrave Macmillan, 2000.

Bell, Rudolph, *How to Do It. Guides to Good Living for Renaissance Italians.* Chicago: University of Chicago Press, 1999.

Bourqui, Claude, *Les sources de Molière. Répertoire critique des sources littéraires et dramatiques.* Paris: SEDES, 1999.

Brizard, Mme. G., "La légende de Lustucru," *Revue de folklore français et de folklore colonial* 11:2 (1940): 37–44.

Burke, Peter, *The Fabrication of Louis XIV.* New Haven/London: Yale University Press, 1992.

Caldicott, C.E.J., *La Carrière de Molière entre protecteurs et éditeurs.* Amsterdam/Atlanta, GA: Rodopi, 1998.

Carrier, Hubert, *La presse de la Fronde (1648–1653): les Mazarinades,* Genève, Droz, 1989.

Carrier, Hubert, *Le labyrinthe de l'état: essai sur le débat politique en France au temps de la Fronde (1648–1653).* Paris: Honoré Champion, 2004.

DeJean,Joan, "Violent Women and Violence against Women: Representing the 'Strong' Woman in Early Modern France," *Signs* 29:1 (Autumn 2003): 117–47.

Duggan, Anne E., *Salonnières, Furies, and Fairies: The Politics of Gender and Cultural Change*. Newark: University of Delaware Press, 2005.

Esmonin, Edmond, "Un recueil de caricatures du XVIIe siècle. Les Illustres Proverbes de Lagniet," *Societé Dauphinoise d'ethnologie et dàrcheologie* (1958): 19–25.

Gaignebet, Claude, *À plus hault sens: l'ésotérisme spirituel et charnel de Rabelais*. Paris: Maisonneuve et Larose, 1986.

Gaignebet, Claude and Lajoux, Jean-Dominique, *Art profane et Religion populaire au Moyen Age*. Paris: Presses Universitaires de France, 1985.

Gérin, Pierre M., "Un genre littéraire bourgeois, le caquet," *Dalhousie French Studies* 14 (Spring–Summer 1988): 3–14.

Goldstein, Carl, *Print Culture in Early Modern France. Abraham Bosse and the Purposes of Print*. Cambridge: Cambridge University Press, 2012.

Grieco, Allen J., "From roosters to cocks: Italian Renaissance fowl and sexuality," in *Erotic Cultures of Renaissance Italy*, ed. Sara F. Matthews-Grieco. Farnham, UK/ Burlington, VT: Ashgate, 2010. 89–140.

Grimm, Jürgen, *Molière en son temps*. Paris/Seattle/Tübingen: Biblio17, *Papers on French Seventeenth Century Literature*, 1993.

Grivel, Marianne, *Le Commerce de l'estampe à Paris au XVIIe siècle*. Paris: Droz, 1986.

Guichemerre, Roger, *La comédie avant Molière 1640–1660*. Paris: Eurédit, 2009.

Hanley, Sarah, "Engendering the State: Family Formation and State Building in Early Modern France," *French Historical Studies* 16:1 (1989): 4–27.

Henderson, Katherine and McManus, Barbara F., *Half Humankind: Contexts and Texts of the Controversy about Women in England, 1540–1640*. Urbana: University of Illinois Press, 1984.

Howarth, William Driver, *Molière. A Playwright and His Audience*. Cambridge: Cambridge University Press, 1982.

Join-Lambert, Sophie and Préaud, Maxime, *Abraham Bosse, savant graveur. Tours, vers 1604–1676, Paris*. Paris/Tours: Bibliothèque nationale de France, Musée des Beaux-Arts de Tours, 2004.

Jones, Malcom, *The Print in Early Modern England: An Historical Oversight*. New Haven/London: Yale University Press, 2010.

Kinnaird, Joan K., "Mary Astell and the Conservative Contribution to English Feminism," *The Journal of British Studies* 19:1 (Autumn, 1979): 53–75.

Kramer, Michael (ed.), *La comédie de proverbes pièce comique, d'après l'édition princeps de 1633*. Geneva: Droz, 2003.

Kumin, Beat A. *Drinking Matters: Public Houses and Social Exchange in Early Modern Central Europe*. London/New York: Palgrave Macmillan, 2007.

Kumin, Beat A. and B. Ann Tlusty (eds.), *The World of the Tavern: Public Houses in Early Modern Europe*. Farnham, UK/Burlington, VT: Ashgate, 2002.

Kunzle, David, *The Early Comic Strip: Narrative Strips and Picture Stories in the European Broadsheet from c. 1450 to 1825* (*History of the Comic Strip*, Volume 1). Berkeley, CA: University of California Press, 1973.

Matthews-Grieco, Sara F., "Mary Astell, l'educatrice femminista," in *La storia al femminile, L'età barocca*, ed. Giulia Calvi. Roma/Bari: Laterza, 1992. 218–62.

Matthews-Grieco, Sara F., *Ange ou diablesse: La représentation de la femme au XVIe siècle*. Paris: Flammarion, 1992.

Michaut, Gustave, *Les Débuts de Molière à Paris*. Geneva: Slatkine Reprints, 1986 (from first edition. Paris: Hachette, 1922–1925), 3 vols.

Mongrédien, Georges, *La vie quotidienne des comédiens au temps de Molière*. Paris: Hachette, 1966.

Moxey, Keith, *Peasants, Warriors, and Wives: Popular Imagery in the Reformation*. Chicago: University of Chicago Press, 1989.

Muchembled, Robert, *Culture populaire et culture des élites dans la France moderne (XVe-XVIIe siècle)*. Paris: Flammarion, 1978.

Nicholson, Eric A., "Dry Mocks and Wet Smocks: Displacements of Sex Scandals on the English Comic Stage, 1595–1625," in *Place and Displacement in The Renaissance*, ed. Alvin Vos, vol. 132. Binghampton, NY: Medieval and Renaissance Texts and Studies, 1995. 25–50.

Park, Katharine, *Secrets of Women. Order, Generation, and the Origins of Human Dissection*. New York: Zone Books, 2006.

Perry, Ruth, "Mary Astell and the Feminist Critique of Possesive Individualism," *Eighteenth-Century Studies* 23:4, Special Issue: *The Politics of Difference* (Summer, 1990): 444–57.

Perry, Ruth, *The Celebrated Mary Astell: An early English feminist*. Chicago: University of Chicago Press, 1986.

Pitsch, Marguerite, "Un médecin imaginaire au XVIIe siècle: Lustucru Opérateur céphalique," *Aesculape* (Juillet, 1957): 41–50.

Préaud, Maxime with Casselle, Pierre, Grivel Marianne and Le Bitouzé, Corinne *Dictionnaire des éditeurs d'estampes à Paris sous l'Ancien Régime*. Paris: Promodis, 1987. 20–22.

Ruggiero, Guido, *Machiavelli in Love: Sex, Self, and Society in the Italian Renaissance*. Baltimore: Johns Hopkins University Press, 2006.

Scott, Virginia, *Molière. A Theatrical Life*. Cambridge: Cambridge University Press, 2000.

Scribner, Robert W., *For the Sake of Simple Folk: Popular Propaganda for the German Reformation*. Oxford: Clarendon Press, 1994.

Simons, Patricia, *The Sex of Men in Premodern Europe: A Cultural History*. Cambridge: Cambridge University Press, 2011.

Trexler, Richard, "La prostitution florentine, au XVIeme siècle," *Annales: Economies, Sociétés Civilisations* 36 (1981): 9834–1015.

Turner, David, *Fashioning Adultery. Gender, Sex and Civility in England, 1660–1740*. Cambridge: Cambridge University Press, 2002.

Weigert, Roger-Armand, *Inventaire du fonds français, graveurs du XVIIe siècle. Bibliothèque nationale, Cabinet des estampes*. Tome IV. Paris: Bibliothèque nationale, 1961.

Wilbur, Richard, "Introduction" to "The Imaginary Cuckold or Sganarelle" in *School For Husbands and Sganarelle, or The Imaginary Cuckold, by Moliere*. Boston: Mariner Books, 1994. 85–9.

Zika, Charles, *The Appearance of Witchcraft: Print and Visual Culture in Sixteenth-Century Europe*. London/New York: Routledge, 2007.

Notes

1 I have a deep debt of gratitude to Maxime Préaud, Conservateur Général of the Département des Estampes of the Bibliothèque Nationale de France in Paris, whose generous comments, publications and unpublished research have been of inestimable value for this essay. Equal recognition goes to the Herzog August Bibliothek in Wolfenbüttel, which provided a haven for concentrated research in the summer of 2013. Heartfelt thanks are also due to the friends and colleagues who contributed to this essay: Eric Nicholson, for his generous suggestions regarding 17th-century French theatre; Molly Bourne and Matteo Duni, fellow contributors to this volume, for their patient comments and close readings; Alexandra Korey and Allen J. Grieco, for generously assuming the role of target readers for this essay in its final stages.

2 For a selection of some of the satirical works against women and the institution of marriage that appeared in print between the closing decades of the 16th century and the 1630s, see the website of the University of Victoria (Canada), which also provides transcriptions: http://mariage.uvic.ca/toc.htm?docFilter=satire.

3 On the survival rates of single sheet prints at the low and middling level of the 17th-century print market as opposed to finer engravings, such as those of Abraham Bosse, see: Carl Goldstein *Print Culture in Early Modern France. Abraham Bosse and the Purposes of Print* (Cambridge: Cambridge University Press, 2012), 1.

4 On the collection of the Abbé de Marolles, see the introduction to *Le Livre des peintres et graveurs par Michel de Marolles, Abbé de Villeloin, revue et annoté par M. Georges Duplessis*, Paris, Plon, 1872, 8–9. "Popular" engravings are those produced at the middle to low levels of the print market which can even be quite finely or very coarsely executed and—while made primarily for a middle-range audience of shopkeepers, artisans and merchants —had an appeal that bridged all social strata of society, Cf. Marianne Grivel, *Le Commerce de l'estampe à Paris au XVIIe siècle* (Paris: Droz, 1986), 198–203. In 1660 Marolles defined the range of his print collection of over 100,000 pieces as being worth between 10 *sols* and 10 *louis d'or* (Grivel, 230).

5 This quantitative, if approximate, conclusion is due to an examination of the impressive British Library online collection of "popular" prints between c. 1580 and 1680, and to 20 years of work on Italian prints which seem to have suffered even more under the Counter Reformation than did the English print under Cromwell. On "popular" prints representing, amongst other subjects, wittols and cuckolds, see Malcom Jones, *The Print in Early Modern England: An Historical Oversight* (New Haven/London: Yale University Press, 2010). It is also significant that David Turner's book entitled *Fashioning Adultery. Gender, Sex and Civility in England, 1660–1740* (Cambridge: Cambridge University Press, 2002) commences with the Restoration.

6 On the audience of middle-range print publishers and contemporary comic theatre see: Goldstein, 9, 80–82, 163–4; Georges Mongrédien, *La vie quotidienne des comédiens au temps de Molière* (Paris, Hachette, 1966), 161, 178–9; Jürgen Grimm, *Molière en son temps* (Paris/Seattle/Tübingen: Biblio17), *Papers on French Seventeenth Century Literature*, 1993, 43–5.

7 On print makers as commercial opportunists see Sophie Join-Lambert and Maxime Préaud, *Abraham Bosse, savant graveur. Tours, vers 1604–1676, Paris* (Paris/Tours: Bibliothèque nationale de France, Musée des Beaux-Arts de Tours, 2004); Grivel, *passim*; Goldstein, 9–10. Of course this was hardly a characteristic limited to the 17th-century print market, but characterized the printed picture from the beginning of commercial print making.

8 On Bosse's sympathies with the Fronde see Goldstein, 116 (Fig. 45), 153–4. In 1651, Bosse, Lagniet and one of the Picart family signed a document in defense of the Parisian print trade against foreign competition. This document is transcribed in Maxime Préaud, Pierre Casselle, Marianne Grivel, Corinne Le Bitouzé, *Dictionnaire des éditeurs d'estampes à Paris sous l'Ancien Régime* (Paris: Promodis, 1987), 20–22.

9 Goldstein, chapter 3, 56–84.

10 Goldstein, 52 (Fig. 17); William Driver Howarth, *Molière. A Playwright and His Audience* (Cambridge: Cambridge University Press, 1982) (Plate IIb); Virginia Scott, *Molière. A Theatrical Life* (Cambridge: Cambridge University Press, 2000), 117 (Fig. 5).

11 Robert W. Scribner was one of the first historians to explore effectively the role of printed pictures in social and religious change: *For the Sake of Simple Folk: Popular Propaganda for the German Reformation* (Oxford: Clarendon Press, 1994). See also the author's *Ange ou diablesse: La représentation de la femme au XVIe siècle* (Paris: Flammarion, 1992). For other attempts at using prints as a primary source that attempt to trace the strategic relationships between visual discourse and social history see: Keith Moxey, *Peasants, Warriors, and Wives: Popular Imagery in the Reformation* (Chicago: University of Chicago Press, 1989), and Charles Zika, *The Appearance of Witchcraft: Print and Visual Culture in 16th-Century Europe* (London: Routledge, 2007).

12 It would seem that Lagniet can be credited with inventing the series of single-sheet illustrated proverbs, although Italian multi-vignette broadsheets with illustrated proverbs were already circulating in the second half of the 16th century (eg. Nicoló Nelli, *Proverbii,* 1564) and ended up in Parisian collections of entertaining engravings (BNF Cab.Est. Tf1&Tf2 Rés). In his *Catalogue des Estampes et de figures en taille-douce avec un dénombrement des pièces qui y sont contenuës. Fait à Paris en l'année 1666. Par M. De Marolles Abbé de Villeloin* (A Paris, Chex Frederic Leonard, ruë S. Jacques, à lEscu de Venise M.DC.LXVI), Michel de Marolles lists a "book" by Jacques Lagniet: "Grotesques au sujet de divers Proverbes recueillies dans un livre par Jacques Lagniet, où il y a 209 pièces" (p. 156, entry CDXX).

13 Entry LXXIII bears the title: "Médiocres graveurs" and lists under this qualification "Humbelot et Ganière, Lagnect [Lagniet], Vanloch , Jolain, Roussel, d'Auroux, Guérin" as well as "Picard, Piquet, Isac, Blandin, Michel Pelais, l'Huilier, François de la Roussière." *Le Livre des peintres et graveurs par Michel de Marolles, Abbé de Villeloin* 29. On Lagniet see also Grivel, 154–7.

14 It is in fact thanks to Michel de Marolles that some of the more "popular" and thus rarer engravings of French, Italian, German and Dutch print culture came to be conserved in the Print Cabinet of the Bibliothèque Royal (now Bibliothèque de France).

15 Département des Imprimés, Réserve, Livres Rares, Z1746. I would like to thank Jean-Marc Chatelain, Conservateur à la Réserve des livres rares, Bibliothèque nationale de France, for having provided information on the collector, Jean-Baptiste-Denis Guyon de Sardière (1674–1759), whose catalogue of books—listing the volume in question—was printed in the middle of the 18th century: *Catalogue des livres de la bibliothèque de feu M. J. B. Denis Guyon, chev. seigneur de Sardière, ancien capitaine au régiment du roi, & l'un des seigneurs du canal de Briare*. Paris, Barrois, Paris, Chez Barrois, Libraire, Quai des Augustins, 1759, 120, entry 1135.

16 According to Edmond Esmonin, the *Bibliothèque de Méon* had a volume comprising 504 pieces which is believed to have ended up in England in the 19th century (Edmond Esmonin, "Un recueil de caricatures du XVIIe siècle. Les Illustres Proverbes de Lagniet," *Societé Dauphinoise d'ethnologie et d'archeologie* (Grenoble, 1958), 19. The Getty volume, which was bound at some point in the 18th century, can be accessed online at: http://archive.org/details/recueildesplusil00lagn. The Bibliothèque Nationale de France volume (Rés. Z-1746) is now also consultable online at: http://gallica.bnf.fr/ark:/12148/btv1b86267983.r=lagniet+proverbes.langEN. Other compiled volumes can be found at the Bibliothèque de l'Arsenal, the Cabinet des Estampes (BNF) in Paris, the Princeton Library, the Huntington Library, the University of Amsterdam, the Albertina, the British Library, and doubtless in many other collections.

17 Maxime Préaud, Conservateur Général of the Département des Estampes in Paris (who is perhaps the greatest living expert on French 17th-century prints) has suggested to the author that the motivation behind the collecting of Lagniet prints may have been a fascination with "street language" and popular French culture in addition to the amusement provided by the visual *topoi.*

18 The characters appearing in the third book on beggars are evidently inspired by Jacques Callot's *Les Gueux* (c. 1621).

19 Humor related to bodily functions was widespread in Europe from the Middle Ages though the early modern period. For France, the work of the historian anthropologist Claude Gaignebet is perhaps the most useful. See for example: *À plus hault sens: l'ésotérisme spirituel et charnel de Rabelais,* Paris, Maisonneuve et Larose, 1986 and, with Jean-Dominique Lajoux, *Art profane et Religion populaire au Moyen Age* (Paris: Presses Universitaires de France, 1985).

20 Till Eulenspiegle was a trans-European comic character, whose adventures and pranks forms appear in some of the earliest narrative print series, ancestors of the comic strip; see David Kunzle, *The Early Comic Strip: Narrative Strips and Picture Stories in the European Broadsheet from c. 1450 to 1825* (History of the Comic Strip, Volume 1), (Berkeley: University of California Press, 1973).

21 Also spelled: Lagnet, Lagner. Lagnier, L'Agnet. etc.: See Esmonin, 20.

22 Ibid., 20.

23 The Getty volume has a *de facto* sub-series of images dealing with *Lustucru* and the *Moulin Merveilleux* that is scattered through the volume where wives (and sometimes husbands) are "re-forged" or "ground" in order to make them more agreeable, younger, more beautiful, and so on. Some of those bound in the Paris volume can be found on the University of Victoria (Canada) website "Le Mariage sous l'Ancien Régime": http://mariage.uvic.ca/.

24 On Lustucru see Joan DeJean, "Violent Women and Violence against Women: Representing the 'Strong' Woman in Early Modern France," *Signs* 29:1 (Autumn, 2003): 117–47; Jean Avalon, "Lustucru, Opérateur Cephalique," *Les Nouvelles de l'Estampe* 3 (1968): 98–124; Marguerite Pitsch, "Un médecin imaginaire au XVIIe siècle : Lustucru Opérateur céphalique," Aesculape, Juillet, 1957, 41–50; M. and G. Brizard, "La légende de Lustucru," *Revue de folklore français et de folklore colonial* 11:2 (1940): 37–44; Champfleury, *Histoire de l'imagerie populaire* (Paris: Dentu, 1869), 226 and *passim.*

25 On salon culture (which developed exponentially as of the 1620s) and the extension of its agenda into contemporary theater see Howarth, 51–6.

26 In a logical variant, women attack Lustucru's forge en masse to take their revenge and, in one example, husbands of all ages and stations in life are taken to a "brain operator" (opérateur céphalique) so that they will be kinder to their wives. See chapter 3 on *Lustucru, opérateur céphalique* in Laure Beaumont Maillet, *La guerre des sexes: XVe–XIXe siècles* (Paris: Bibliothèque Nationale, 1984), 24–39.

27 For an overview of prints representing these themes in 16th- and 17th-century French prints see Beaumont-Maillet's useful compilation (*supra*, note 26).

28 The bibliography on salon culture is vast. On its influence on contemporary society, see Anne E. Duggan, *Salonnières, Furies, and Fairies: The Politics of Gender and Cultural Change* (Newark, Delaware, University of Delaware Press, 2005) as well as the exhibition catalogue: *Au Temps des Précieuses. Les Salons Littéraires au XVIIème siècle* (Paris: Bibliothèque Nationale, 1968).

29 Scott, 118–9; Goldstein, 9.

30 " *Belle hostesse est un mal pour la bource* [*sic*] " and " *Les verres et les femmes sont toujours en dangers* [sic]. " Another inscription identifies the tavern as being at the sign of the "Arms of Acteon."

31 " Il cherche ce qu'il voudroit ne pas trouver."

32 Roger Guichemerre, *La comédie avant Molière 1640–1660* (Paris: Eurédit, 2009). See also Victor Fournel (ed.), *Les contemporains de Molière: recueil de comédies, rares ou peu connues jouées de 1650 à 1680 avec l'histoire de chaque théâtre* (Genève: Slatkine, 1863–1865). The "trickster tricked" topos, where both men and women achieve a type of justice through equal transgressions, is a plot with a long pedigree. It is to be found in medieval fabliaux, Italian *novelle*, French *nouvelles*, and in satires of marriage such as the 15th-century Les quinze joyes de marriage.

33 A subset of six prints featuring a title page with the words *La Cornologie* is also most complete in the (non-paginated) Paris volume (pages 284, 293, 295 out of 311 in the digital version available at: http://gallica.bnf.fr/ark:/12148/btv1b86267983/f1.image.r=Lagniet.langFR).

34 On the overlapping and often undistinguishable roles played by the artisans working in the 17th century print market, see: Goldstein, Grivel, Préaud et al., 1987.

35 The pages are not numbered, but the Picart engravings in question can be found at pages 205–14, 280–81 (of 311) of the digital version.

36 Entry LXXIII suggests that there were two "Picard" printmakers active in the same period. The entry bears the title: "Médiocres graveurs" and lists under this qualification (my italics) "Humbelot et Ganière, Lagnect [Lagniet], Vanloch , Jolain, Roussel, d'Auroux, Guérin, *L'un et l'autre Picard,* Piquet, Isa[a]c, Blandin, Michel Pelais, l'Huilier, François de la Roussière." *Le Livre des peintres et graveurs par Michel de Marolles, Abbé de Villeloin,* 28. Two other Piccard/Picart were documented by Henri Herluison, *Actes d'état-civil d'artistes français: peintres, graveurs, architectes, etc.: Extraits des registres de l'Hôtel-de-ville de Paris, détruits dans l'incendie du 24 mai 1871,* Orléans, Herluison, 1873; "Jean Piccard, graveur en taille douce à Paris," 1637, 344; "Pierre Picart, marchand graveur en taille douce et bourgeois de Paris," 1681, 346.

37 Various Picart/Picard appear in legal documents and guild regulations throughout the century. Préaud et al., 1987, *passim.*

38 Pierre Picart married Françoise Perronne Lagniet, daughter and sole heir of Jacques Lagniet (10 April 1675) (Archives nationales, Minutier central, XXXVIII-6-26 Nov. 1675). The house at Fort l'Evêque, on the Quai de la Mégisserie, is in fact a former address of Lagniet. My thanks to Maxime Préaud for this information.

39 There were, in fact, two engravers (cousins?) known by the name Pierre Picart who were active in Paris in the mid-17th century. The one responsible for this series of engravings is located just off rue St. Denis in 1668. Might this be this same Pierre Picart who moves to Lagniet's workshop when he marries Françoise Péronne Lagnet [*sic*] (probably around 1670 as Françoise was baptized in 1650, and their first child was baptized in 1672). In 1675, at the death of Lagniet, Pierre Picart takes over his father-in-law's printing paraphernalia. Grivel, 364–5.

40 "Ces diablesses icy viennent troubler la feste / Et chargent leurs maris d'injures et de coups / L'un a le nez cassé e l'autre sur sateste / Esprouve ce que cest qu'une femme en courroux."

41 "Cocus que vostre joye est de courte durée / Apeine donnez vous sure les premiers morceaux / Que voicy vos dragons qui fond des leur entrée / Renverser pots et plats nappe table et treteaux."

42 As the other essays in this volume amply demonstrate, this is a widely accepted premise that appears in literature, drama, medicine, canon law, and of course visual culture. The premise is based on current medical theory, according to which women were naturally lustful, and for reasons of health needed to have frequent carnal concourse. A lack of attention from a husband could therefore motivate a wife to seek solace elsewhere, and should her adultery be discovered, her husband's lack of manliness would become public knowledge. On medical theory and women's health needs see: Patricia Simons, *The Sex of Men in Premodern Europe: A Cultural History* (Cambridge: Cambridge University Press, 2011); Katharine Park, *Secrets of Women. Order, Generation, and the Origins of Human Dissection* (New York: Zone Books, 2006); Rudolph Bell, *How to Do It. Guides to Good Living for Renaissance Italians* (Chicago: University of Chicago Press, 1999).

43 Roger-Armand Weigert, *Inventaire du fonds français, graveurs du XVIIe siècle. Bibliothèque nationale, Cabinet des estampes*. Tome IV (Paris: Bibliothèque nationale, 1961), 314–15; Préaud et al., 1987, 130–32, 319; Grivel, 202, 303. Jean Ganière also published a number of caricatures against Spain and Spaniards, perhaps an indirect criticism of the Queen Regent Anne of Austria who was, after all, a Spaniard (Grivel, 155).

44 Dialogue, top left: Dame Alison / Je t'y trouve bon chien d'yurogne / avecque ton Infame trogne / te voyla dans ton Element Lubin / Tay toy tay toy mechante beſte / tes discours me rompe la teſte. / vien boire avec nous seulemt Dame Alison / Me voyla donc bien arriuée? / jaymerois mieux estre creueé / goulu que den avoir taſte. Lubin / Ho ho tu fais bien la mauuaiſe / toutes les nuits quand je te baiſe / ton bas neſt pas si degouſte Dialogue, top right : Dame Alison / O le Grand abbatteur de quilles / va nous trõuous bien dautres drilles /qui le font mieux que tu nentens Lubin / Ha Putin dhereuse memoire / tu voudrois mempecher de boire / et tu veux bien paſser ton tems Dame Alison / Va ſ Va vin yurogne infame / il faut bien quon baise ta famme / pour nourir tes pauures enfans Lubin /Puis que tu es ſP charitable / Garde le lit et moy la table / cest le moyen destre comtens.

45 Sarah Hanley, "Engendering the State: Family Formation and State Building in Early Modern France," *French Historical Studies* 16:1 (1989): 4–27; Susan Dwyer Amussen, *An Ordered Society: Gender and Class in Early Modern England* (New York: Columbia University Press, 1994).

46 Perhaps the most useful book on adultery legislation in early modern France is that of Régine Beauthier, *La Répression de l'adultère en France du XVIème au XVIIIème siècle : De quelques lectures de l'histoire*, Brussels, E. Story-Scientia, 1990. According to an *Arrêt du Parlement de Paris* (1er juillet 1606), either the Procurer du Roi or the Procureur Fiscal could take a husband to court, even if "le mari ne se plaigne point de la conduit de sa femme et qu'il n'ait connivé à ce désordre." The reasoning behind this was not only the bad example set for the rest of the community, but a complacent husband was seen as also encouraging debauchery. However, when a husband pimped his wife the Procureur "peut accuser le mari de macquerellage et la femme d'adultère." See Beauthier, 60–66, 80–82. Nevertheless, Lebrun de la Rochette's treatise on criminal law points out that a woman cannot be considered guilty of adultery "… quand le mary ou par sa negligence, ou par occasion par luy recherchées, ou par autres moyens, a occasionné l'adultère de sa femme: ou si luy mesme en a été le macquereau … Ou quand le mary sçachant la vie desbordée de la femme, la dissimule et passé sous silence, cinq ans entiers (qui est la vraye prescription de ce crime)." There are in all seven conditions listed by Lebrun de la Rochette where the husband shares responsibility for the wife's adultery (*Le Procez Civil et Criminel Contenant la methodique liaison du Droit et de la Practique Judiciaire civile et criminelle: Plus l'Eslection de la Jurisdiction des Eslerz sous un bref discours des Finances et Officiers d'icelles* [Rouen: Du Mesnil, 1640], 14–16).

47 A few lines of text inteserted into the picture space (on the roof) state: "Il vaudroit mieux demeruer sous un toit ruineux qu le vent et la pluye donnent de tous les costez que davoir a vivre en la conversation d'une fame querelleuse." The quatrain states: "Ce pauvre Savetier pour contenter Sa femme, / En vin tien pied a boule a tirer le fil gros; / Cette vesse a tous coups lui vient changer sa gamme / Sans jamais lui donner ny treve, ny repos."

48 For an overview of prints representing these themes in 16th- and 17th-century French prints see Beaumont-Maillet's useful compilation (*supra*, note 26).

49 See *supra* note 45.

50 For a brief biography of Louis XIV in terms of his public image see: Peter Burke, *The Fabrication of Louis XIV* (New Haven/London: Yale University Press, 1992). Most critical prints and pamphlets were not criticizing the King so much as his entourage, discrediting the Queen and Mazarin and suggesting the role a good ruler should play. See for example "A Mazarinade against the Queen and the Cardinal" in William Beik, *Louis XIV and Absolutism. A Brief Study with Documents* (London/New York: Palgrave MacMillan, 2000), 29–35.

51 Hubert Carrier, *Le labyrinthe de l'État: essai sur le débat politique en France au temps de la Fronde (1648–1653)* (Paris: Honoré Champion, 2004).

52 Akin to the kind of "gentle fun" that could criticize in order to correct: Burke, 135–6.

53 Prints and pamphlets from the period of the *Fronde* (generally designated as *Mazarinades* given their lively critique of the Cardinal), repeatedly accused Mazarin of being the lover of Anne of Austria, although there is no proof of this type of relationship between the Spanish Queen and her Italian advisor. Hubert Carrier, *La presse de la Fronde (1648–1653): les Mazarinades* (Genève: Droz, 1989).

54 "Pendant qu'à se parer pour paraistre jolie / La coquette soccupe; ainsy ce pauvre sot / Berce esbrenne l'enfant lui donne la boulie / Nettoye les souliers et fait bouillir le pot." Shoes are often used in 17th-century prints as a sign of subjugation, especially when men kneel to put a shoe on a woman's foot. See for example Pierre Brebiette, "Le pauvre badin," Paris, 1630–1640, reproduced in Beaumont-Maillet, 55, Fig. 44. Most of the Picart engravings (wrongly identified as "Laignet") and number of the prints mentioned in this essay may be found at: http://mariage.uvic.ca/.

55 Hats were an object of symbolic contention in early modern Europe. On hat snatching in Renaissance Florence, see: Richard Trexler, "La prostitution florentine, au XVIeme siècle," *Annales: Economies, Sociétés Civilisations* 36 (1981): 9834–1015. In 17th-century England, women's fashion adopted men's hat styles, which gave rise to satirical pamphlets and prints, see: Katherine Henderson and Barbara F McManus *Half Humankind: Contexts and Texts of the Controversy about Women in England, 1540–1640* (Urbana: University of Illinois Press, 1984).

56 "Evite malheureux cette affreuse megere / Tu n'es pas assez fort pour soutenir le choc; / Ce traitement est rude, et cest une misère / Lors que la poule chante et fait taire le coq."

57 On bird analogies for male sexuality see: Allen J. Grieco, "From roosters to cocks: Italian Renaissance fowl and sexuality," in *Erotic Cultures of Renaissance Italy*, ed. Sara F. Matthews-Grieco (Farnham, UK/Burlington, VT, Ashgate, 2010), 89–140; Guido Ruggiero, *Machiavelli in Love: Sex, Self, and Society in the Italian Renaissance* (Baltimore: Johns Hopkins University Press, 2006), 98–103.

58 "A la corne jenins, cest vostre confrairie / Vous y devez venir pour vous faire enroller / Au livre des martyrs; et si la fascherie / Vous attriste, en buvant allez vous consoler."

59 On the repression of such confraternities in early modern France see, for example, Sara Beam, "Les notables catholiques et la marginalisation de la culture populaire au XVIe siècle," *Histoire urbaine* 2:25 (2009): 105–25; Robert Muchembled, *Culture populaire et culture des élites dans la France moderne (XVe–xviie siècle)* (Paris: Flammarion, 1978).

60 On taverns see: Beat A. Kumin and B. Ann Tlusty, eds., *The World of the Tavern: Public Houses in Early Modern Europe* (Farnham, UK/Burlington, VT: Ashgate, 2002); Beat A. Kumin, *Drinking Matters: Public Houses and Social Exchange in Early Modern Central Europe* (London/New York: Palgrave Macmillan, 2007).

61 *L'Origine des Cornes ou les Cornarts enregistrez*, Collection Michel Hennin. Estampes relatives à l'Histoire de France. Tome 57, Pièces 5016–5084, période: 1680, Q155960.

62 This print is reproduced in Beaumont-Maillet, 94, Fig. 90 and can also be found at http://mariage.uvic.ca/.

63 *A la Grande confrérie*, A Paris chez Daumont rue de la Feronnerie à l'Aigle d'or, RESERVE FOL-QB-201 (93). Collection Michel Hennin. *Estampes relatives à l'Histoire de France*. Tome 93, Pièces 8093–170, période: 1730–1731.

64 Bibliothèque nationale de France, département Estampes et photographie, RESERVE FOL-QB-201 (120). Digital reproduction at: http://gallica.bnf.fr/ark:/12148/btv1b8410983q.r=Allons+plus+de+Distinction+.langEN.

65 "Allons plus de Distinction ce malheur commun nous rend égaux." Bibliothèque nationale de France, département Estampes et photographie, Collection Michel Hennin. Estampes relatives à l'Histoire de France. Tome 120, Pièces 10490–613, période: 1789, RESERVE FOL-QB-201 (120). Available online at: http://gallica.bnf.fr/ark:/12148/btv1b8410983q.r=.langEN. In a period when satirical prints have widely adopted the horns of the cuckold to imply the political incompetence of kings and political leaders, this print implies that social equality extends to men—or at least to the aristocracy and the bourgeoisie—in the domestic context as well as the political arena.

66 As was the early 19th century, see for example the print on Napoleon's return from Elba entitled *Le cocu authentique*, RESERVE QB-370 (71)-FT 4, Recueil. Collection de Vinck, 1770–1870. vol. 71 (pièces 9302–76).

67 The quatrain states: "La voyla libre enfin sen est deffaite / Agrand coups de baston et de pied dans le cu; / Affin dentretenir son mignon de couchette / Qui remplit cependant la place du cocu."

68 "Les fẽmes ne tombent iamais le nez en terre / l'on void choses coutumiere fame tomber en arrière."

69 "Gogaille, le diable est mort!" Michael Kramer, ed. *La comédie de proverbes pièce comique, d'après l'édition princeps de 1633*, Droz, 2003. This play had quite an editorial success in the course of the 17th century (17 known editions by 1715) moving into the Bibliothèque Bleue in the 18th century, 12–13. *Dictionnaire Historique Littré*, http://www.littre.org/definition/gogaille gogaille (go-ghâ-ll', ll mouillées, et non gogâ-ye) s.f. Terme populaire .1 Repas joyeux. Faire gogaille. Être en gogaille. Enfin on danse, on fait gogaille [Scarron, Virg. VI]. The two couple portraits on the back wall suggest a comfortable household, while the family cat (often associated with women in domestic scenes) is contentedly curled up on the bottom margin of the image, thereby underscoring the contentedness of the female company.

70 "Quand avec cinq ou six parmy les bonnes cheres / La femme fail gogaille a tirelarigot: / Le mary verse aboire a ces bonnes commeres / Tout debout teste nue, et croque le marmot."

71 Goldstein, 72–3. On the *caquet des femmes* see: Pierre M. Gérin, "Un genre littéraire bourgeois, le caquet," Dalhousie French Studies 14 (Spring–Summer, 1988): 3–14. On the success of the *Précieuses ridicules* and its imitators see also Gustave Michaut, *Les Débuts de Molière à Paris* (Genève: Slatkine Reprints, 1986) (from first edition [Paris, Hachette, 1922–1925], 3 vols.).

72 "Avez-vous vû jamais mieux plier la toilette: / La drolesse en sortant emporte jusqu'au chat / Pour meubler son galand; mais ceste rafle faicte / Iujez Si le pauvre hommeest en for bel estat."

73 Beauthier, 146–7, Arrêt Parelment d'Aix, November 18, 1656. See also case 1637, 148.

74 "Grand jean ce poupart a sa porte rencontre / Qui nest pas de son faict et quji s'addresse áluy: / On s'en mocque on s'en rit chacun audoit le montre / De le voir affligé pour les pechez d'autruy."

75 Scott, 109–10.

76 On farces pre-Molière see : Guichemerre, passim and Claude Bourqui, *Les sources de Molière. Répertoire critique des sources littéraires et dramatiques* (Paris: SEDES, 1999).

77 Although "imaginary" cuckolds had already appeared in a couple of Italian farces, this variant was still a relative novelty. Bourqui, 43–50; Richard Wilbur, Introduction to "The Imaginary Cuckold or Sganarelle" in *School For Husbands and Sganarelle, or The Imaginary Cuckold, by Moliere.* (Boston: Mariner Books, 1994), 85–9.

78 Molière died in 1670. C. E. J. Caldicott, *La Carrière de Molière entre protecteurs et éditeurs* (Amsterdam/Atlanta: Rodopi, 1998), 175.

79 Grimm, "Sociologie du comique chez Molière," 159–62.

80 On the *charivari*, see the essay by M. A. Katritzky in this volume. This kind of literary displacement is nothing new. See for example Eric A. Nicholson, "Dry Mocks and Wet Smocks: Displacements of Sex Scandals on the English Comic Stage, 1595–1625," in *Place and Displacement in The Renaissance*, ed. Alvin Vos, vol. 132 (Binghampton, NY: Medieval and Renaissance Texts and Studies, 1995), 25–50.

81 Mary Astell was one of the first "feminist" writers to make the connection between political theory and gender politics in marriage. See for example Joan K. Kinnaird, "Mary Astell and the Conservative Contribution to English Feminism," *The Journal of British Studies* 19:1 (Autumn, 1979): 53–75; Ruth Perry, *The celebrated Mary Astell: An early English feminist* (Chicago: University of Chicago Press, 1986); Ruth Perry, "Mary Astell and the Feminist Critique of Possesive Individualism," *Eighteenth-Century Studies* 23:4, Special Issue: The Politics of Difference (Summer, 1990), 444–57; Sara F. Matthews-Grieco, "Mary Astell, l'educatrice femminista," in *La storia al femminile, L'età barocca*, ed. Giulia Calvi (Roma & Bari: Laterza, 1992), 218–62.

82 Beauthier examines above all "recueils d'arrets," compilations (usually by legislators) of judgments of interesting cases. By the 17th century, adultery cases were tried only in secular courts. Until 1670, when Louis XIV imposed uniform legislation on all of France, precedent continued to play a particularly important role in court cases.

83 Lebrun de la Rochette had editorial success throughout the century. So far I have found editions of this treatise dated 1607, 1611, 1615, 1616, 1619, 1622, 1623, 1624, 1626, 1640, 1661, 1665 and later. There are doubtless more.

84 Beauthier, 82–3.

85 "Lors qu'enfin le gallant la coquette abandoné / Elle s'en va trouver quelque advocat scavant / Qui remontre au mary, Sibien qu'il luy pardone / Et la traite en douceur ainsy qu'au paravant."

86 Beauthier, 114–15, and a case from 1671, 117–18.

87 On reconciliation: Beauthier, 110–29.

88 "Reste til quelque trait de ce mauvais mesnage / La femme et le mary vivent tous deux en paix / Lun est toujours trop bon et l'autre fait la sage / Tellement qu'a les voir tout va mieux que jamais."

89 On more tolerant treatment for errant wives and the weighing of mitigating circumstances see Beauthier, 51–2, 142–4, 257–8.

Index

Platter, Thomas 61, 64, 67

For Product Safety Concerns and Information please contact our EU representative GPSR@taylorandfrancis.com Taylor & Francis Verlag GmbH, Kaufingerstraße 24, 80331 München, Germany

Batch number: 10726322

Printed by Printforce, the Netherlands